Diminished Ovarian Reserve and Assisted Reproductive Technologies

Orhan Bukulmez

Editor

Diminished Ovarian Reserve and Assisted Reproductive Technologies

Current Research and Clinical Management

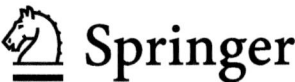 Springer

Editor
Orhan Bukulmez
Division of Reproductive Endocrinology and Infertility
Department of Obstetrics and Gynecology
The University of Texas Southwestern Medical Center
Dallas, TX
USA

ISBN 978-3-030-23234-4   ISBN 978-3-030-23235-1   (eBook)
https://doi.org/10.1007/978-3-030-23235-1

This Springer imprint is published by the registered company Springer Nature Switzerland AG
The registered company address is: Gewerbestrasse 11, 6330 Cham, Switzerland

To our patients trusting us for their care and to my wife, Lark, and my daughter, Stella, for enduring countless days and hours of my absence in their lives, I dedicate this book with deepest appreciation.

Foreword I

Receiving word of Professor Bukulmez's manuscript brings to mind the natural convergence of the streams of translational research. As social and economic issues have changed our reproductive habits, along comes in vitro fertilization (IVF) and the imperative to comprehend, diagnose, and contend with ovarian aging. The success of cancer therapy further sharpens the lens of planning for the survivor's reproductive future. These massive shifts in female reproduction have driven both the basic and clinical sciences to contend with this new world. Progress in the clinical approaches to decreasing ovarian reserve has gone from just tinkering with the protocols to being evidence-based, leading-edge issues.

Dr. Bukulmez and his collaborators have been working in this area for years. Fortunately, their success can be made available by this book. Many couples and individuals will benefit from what is here. It dovetails and enhances the laboratory findings that also are in the moment of discovery and searching for clinical application. Many hints are here in this book and it should be read as more than a manual. The astute observer of this movement will find clues here for the coming decade.

This book gives me special gifts, including the fulfillment of the mentor's responsibilities. I have worked with its editor for decades and seen him conquer the everyday problems of the aspiring scientist and the heavy weight of clinical responsibility, without losing his compass or giving in to the deteriorating environment for the clinician-scientist. The release of this book documents his success; but even more, it shows Dr. Bukulmez and his work to be at the right moment to take our increasing knowledge of ovarian aging/reserve at the flow and to bring others along. Read it and use it to build onto the future when "all will be explained."

New Haven, CT, USA   Frederick Naftolin, MD, PhD
New York, NY, USA

Foreword II

The history of in vitro fertilization (IVF) procedures at The University of Texas Southwestern (UT Southwestern) Medical Center began in the early 1980s. One of the young faculty (Dr. Guzick) initiated the IVF Program and was successful in providing care for a couple in the first IVF pregnancy at UT Southwestern. However, the success rates were low at that time. Patients received human menopausal gonadotropins and human chorionic gonadotropin for stimulating follicle growth and triggering ovulation, respectively. The follicles were monitored primarily by serum estradiol measured by radioimmunoassay (RIA) which was a cumbersome system and occasionally by abdominal/pelvic ultrasound. The eggs were retrieved by laparoscopy and needle aspiration of follicles. At that time, we did not have micro cameras and video monitors, so visualization of the follicles was by direct observation via the laparoscope.

In 1986, I became the division director and the fellowship director of Reproductive Endocrinology and Infertility (REI) at UT Southwestern. In 1987, I hired a former fellow, Dr. Odum, to become director of our IVF Program. Dr. Guzick had left to join the program at the University of Pittsburgh. My first plan was to send Dr. Odum to Norfolk, Virginia, to learn the new technique of retrieving eggs via a transvaginal ultrasound with an attached needle. This technique allowed for easier and improved egg retrieval and higher success rates. Dr. Odum left for Texas Tech University in 1989. For the next 20 years, a number of former fellows served as IVF Program directors, i.e., Dr. Bradshaw, Dr. Kutteh, Dr. Chantilis, and Dr. Attia. The standard treatment included various forms of gonadotropins plus gonadotropin-releasing hormone agonists and antagonists. We also developed a donor egg program in the mid-1990s.

In 2010, our department recruited my former fellow, Dr. Orhan Bukulmez, to become the REI division director and IVF Program practice and medical director. Dr. Bukulmez focused on improving IVF outcomes of couples failed elsewhere and especially those women with expected poor ovarian response, diminished ovarian reserve, and/or advanced reproductive age. As a novel approach in UT Southwestern IVF Program, now called as Fertility and Advanced Reproductive Medicine, he instituted the minimal and mild stimulation protocols for IVF in women with diminished ovarian reserve and/or advanced reproductive age. Currently both of these issues clearly are very common associated factors of infertility, mostly due to delayed childbearing of women. Today, majority of our fertility patient population at our Fertility and Advanced Reproductive Medicine at UT Southwestern consists of women with advanced reproductive age and/or diminished ovarian reserve, and most are those who did not have successful IVF cycles elsewhere. Being successful in terms of achieving live birth in such patients resulted in increasing reputation of the IVF Program at UT Southwestern.

In addition, Dr. Bukulmez developed a fertility preservation program primarily for cancer patients and women who are delaying childbirth and updated third-party reproduction programs. Our program is now renowned for its personalized, patient-centered, and cost-effective IVF approaches, which require profound understanding and applications of reproductive endocrinology. This is in my opinion leading to more advanced training of our REI fellows who will be more capable of helping so-called poor prognosis patients for IVF, hopefully resulting in more research in this field.

Two of our fellows were instrumental in starting to analyze the minimal and mild stimulation protocols' impact. Following a review paper on diminished ovarian reserve and advanced reproductive and assisted reproduction, Dr. Beverly Reed published a paper entitled "Use of Clomiphene Citrate in Minimal Stimulation in In Vitro Fertilization Negatively Impacts Endometrial Thickness" supporting frozen embryo accumulation over multiple cycle rather than considering fresh embryo transfer. Dr. John Wu has recently submitted his thesis entitled "Differential Effect of Ovarian Stimulation Protocols on Endometrial Histomorphology and Gene Expression" showing endometrial impact of conventional and minimal stimulation protocols. Now, our fellow, Dr. David Prokai, has been working on a large dataset for in-depth analysis of minimal and mild stimulation IVF cycles and their frozen embryo transfer outcomes.

In summary, the use of personalized and customized IVF approaches and their rationale for women with diminished ovarian reserve including minimal and mild stimulation protocols implemented by Dr. Bukulmez along with the related patho-physiology and upcoming technologies will be discussed in detail in the following chapters. Dr. Bukulmez is supported by an esteemed team of authors.

I am proud of what our IVF team has achieved with the management of women with diminished ovarian reserve, and I am already looking forward to seeing the successive editions of this book.

Dallas, TX, USA   Bruce R. Carr, MD

Preface

When I started my career as a fertility physician in the mid-1990s, I realized that some women would not respond to controlled ovarian stimulation (COS) while requiring higher doses of gonadotropins than other age-matched women. Because high-dose gonadotropins per se did not result in satisfactory outcomes, various COS and adjuvant treatment regimens were considered for such women. Most of these patients were in their early or late 30s again reflecting the age-related decline in ovarian response, echoing the fact that natural conception rates drop with female aging. However, some younger women in their 20s and early 30s were also responding to assisted reproductive technology (ART) treatment with low oocyte and embryo yield. In the early 1990s as a trainee, we did not have an adequate understanding of what is now known as antral follicle count (AFC), and we were frequently checking basal FSH and estradiol (E2) levels. Upon seeing normal FSH and E2 values, we were frequently perplexed why this particular patient's COS response was low. We usually proceeded with clomiphene citrate (CC) challenge test which was somewhat cumbersome for patients, but again we believed this test would be better than basal FSH and E2 levels to assess the ovarian oocyte reserve problems leading to low inhibin secretion, which was biologically detected as increased FSH level after using CC. Then, we had more profound understanding of AFC, which was complemented by then "new" ovarian reserve marker called anti-Mullerian hormone (AMH), after going through some other tests for ovarian reserve assessment. Eventually, we could somewhat predict why poor response occurred, or we could figure out who the poor responder might be if the patient did not have any prior ART cycles. Shortly, the term "diminished ovarian reserve" (DOR) met with widespread acceptance. In the 1990s, the age of the females pursuing our services were mostly between 20s and mid-30s.

Especially by the turn of the twenty-first century, the demographics of women presenting to fertility clinics began to show profound changes. Many women were postponing marriage or childbearing. Women started to consider having babies in their early or late 30s or even later. Many such women, already anxious about their reproductive aging, turned to ART to fulfill their dreams to have babies. However, poor ovarian response (POR) with this demographic shift became a more frequent problem. The definition of advanced reproductive age (ARA) was considered when the female age was at or above 35 years. Ovarian reserve assessment with both ultrasound and serum tests turned into one of the checklist items before COS for ART. The patients with predicted DOR were subjected to many different COS protocols mostly with high daily doses of gonadotropins which increased the cost of ART. In my earlier years as an ART physician, our community was also favoring fresh embryo transfers since frozen embryo transfers were resulting in much lower live birth outcomes. In addition, the transfer of multiple embryos was exercised frequently, hoping to improve success in women with POR or DOR. These approaches actually resulted in inferior results in terms of clinical pregnancy and take-home baby rates, some of which was due to unintended consequences of transferring multiple embryos. Many women failing with fresh embryo transfers were undergoing multiple high-dose COS cycles to have more fresh transfers with multiple embryos.

First in vitro fertilization (IVF) in the UK was performed via natural cycle. Then, the first American IVF baby was made possible with gonadotropins albeit at low doses. Since ovarian stimulation with gonadotropins increased the efficiency of IVF process through the recruitment of numerous follicles and retrieval of multiple oocytes, this approach quickly became the norm in all IVF cycles. The doses of daily gonadotropins were usually kept high. In the 1990s, a movement advocated decreasing the amount of gonadotropins used in ART cycles. As a new fertility physician at that time, I noticed that there was a group in the UK promoting minimal stimulation for IVF. However, my initial perception was the pregnancy rates per cycle with fresh transfers after such minimal stimulation seemed to be low. When I was practicing at Hacettepe University in Turkey, we were included in a multicenter double-blind randomized clinical trial in Europe on a recombinant (rec-) FSH preparation. The objective of this study was to assess whether increased doses of rec-FSH, with advancing female age between the ages of 30 and 39, could improve the number of oocytes collected during ART treatment. The study showed that higher doses of rec-FSH did not improve age-related decline in oocyte yield. In fact, post hoc analysis suggested that lower ovarian stimulation doses were associated with improved outcomes especially in women older than 33 years of age. This study was eye-opening for me and shaped my future approach to the care of women with DOR and/or ARA or those with expected POR. Shortly after this study was published, I left my faculty position in Turkey to complete the obstetrics and gynecology (OBGYN) residency training in the USA. Since I aspired to continue my career in ART in the USA as well, I applied to reproductive endocrinology and infertility (REI) fellowship-training programs. I was accepted to my current institution for REI training, The University of Texas Southwestern (UT Southwestern) Medical Center in Dallas, Texas. Professor Frederick Naftolin, as the chairman of the Department of OBGYN at Yale University, supported my residency, fellowship, and faculty applications in the USA and mentored me along the way. Professor Bruce Carr recruited me to his fellowship program and then welcomed me back to UT Southwestern as the division director of REI, from The University of Florida where I took a faculty position right after my fellowship. My focus at UT Southwestern was to develop the ART program.

While practicing at UT Southwestern, I noticed that the majority of the patients were presenting to pursue their fertility care after experiencing POR and/or poor embryo quality resulting in no pregnancy elsewhere. I was then very well aware of the mild stimulation approaches for IVF from the pioneers in Western Europe and Asia, especially in Japan. There was already a busy ART center focusing on mild and minimal stimulation approaches in New York City in the USA. Inspired by these practices, I started our minimal/mild stimulation program for DOR and/or ARA patients or those with history of POR with conventional high-dose COS protocols. I had strong support from Drs. Huai Liang Feng, Jianming Li, and Zexu Jiao as our ART laboratory directors. Our REI fellows were very instrumental in implementation and close monitoring of these protocols. As I can agree with another US pioneer on minimal stimulation from St. Louis, Missouri, these protocols seem to be easy for the patient but intense for the ART team. Taking advantage of the era of profoundly successful outcomes with frozen embryo transfers, we started a multiple-cycle approach for minimal/mild stimulation for frozen embryo accumulation and planned elective transfer of thawed embryos while minimizing multiple pregnancy rates. Therefore, it was not easy for patients as well since it was a long process. Without the trust and perseverance of our patients, we would not have been able to witness the successful live birth outcomes from women who were primarily recommended donor oocytes to conceive through ART. Cost savings from cycle charges and low-dose injectable medications also helped with this multiple-cycle paradigm. We learned a lot along the way, and we were looking forward to having a venue to present our experiences. I appreciated the synchronicity of timing when Springer approached me to create a book on DOR and ART.

The distinguished authors of this book include seasoned ART physicians and academicians from the USA and abroad. Dr. Wei Shang, chief of IVF at PLA Navy General Hospital, contributed from Beijing, China. Dr. Gurkan Bozdag was my resident when I was a faculty member in Hacettepe University and now is a renowned professor at the same institution. Dr. Hakan Duran and I both attended the same medical school and then the same residency program at Hacettepe University. Then, we both repeated the residency and the fellowship programs in the USA. Dr. Duran has profound ART experience, having his REI training at an institution where the first IVF baby was born in the USA. Dr. Erkan Buyuk was also a graduate of the medical school at Hacettepe University and completed his training in the USA, currently directing an REI fellowship program, with an academic interest in ovarian aging and fertility preservation. Dr. Bala Bhagavath and I are the same year graduates of REI fellowship program at UT Southwestern. He is a clinically busy academician in ART and in minimally invasive surgery. Dr. Kotaro Sasaki and I met when we were trying to recruit him for our reproductive research program since we were very impressed with his work on artificial ovary development. Currently an investigator at the University of Pennsylvania, he graciously wrote a chapter on the same topic. Dr. Zexu Jiao is our current ART laboratory director relentlessly working on optimizing lab protocols for DOR and/or ARA patients. Dr. Karla Saner is our andrology, reproductive endocrinology laboratory supervisor, closely involved in our clinical operations. I could not put the ART program together focusing on women with DOR and/or ARA without the strong support and genuine enthusiasm of our REI fellows trained at UT Southwestern. Among my fellows, Drs. Beverly Reed, John Wu, and David Prokai worked closely with me as the authors, witnessing the outcomes of our ART approaches while also focusing on important research projects. Our most recent fellow, Dr. Jennifer Shannon, was involved with the project as well. I am thankful to all the authors and coauthors for their contribution, especially at a time when all of us are having continuously increasing daily demands and responsibilities.

I hope this book is comprehensive enough to be a starting point of reading for clinicians, researchers, trainees, and perhaps for anyone who is interested in knowing more about diminished ovarian reserve and ART. I believe the readers can assure some foundation about ART treatment in general while reviewing various ART approaches and adjuvant treatment modalities. This book may seem to be somewhat heavy on minimal and mild stimulation protocols. However, this was not intended to be another literature review on such protocols, but rather we focused on providing some recipes and their scientific rationale for practitioners who are willing to offer these protocols to their patients with DOR and/or ARA. In addition, future prospects section reviews some emerging technologies and research, which may be applicable for fertility patients with DOR.

Lastly, I look forward to having a second edition of this book with more international collaboration, leading to more editors and authors in the near future. I hope the information presented can help to shape the current and future practice of ART through personalizing the treatment considering the ever-changing demographics and the needs of our patients.

Dallas, TX, USA   Orhan Bukulmez

Contents

Contributors

Karla Saner Amigh, PhD, HCLD Fertility & Advanced Reproductive Medicine Clinic at University of Texas Southwestern Medical Center, Dallas, TX, USA

Bala Bhagavath, MBBS University of Rochester Medical Center, Rochester, NY, USA

Melis Bozan, MD Hacettepe University School of Medicine, Ankara, Turkey

Gurkan Bozdag, MD Department of Obstetrics and Gynecology, Hacettepe University School of Medicine, Ankara, Turkey

Orhan Bukulmez, MD Division of Reproductive Endocrinology and Infertility, Fertility and Advanced Reproductive Medicine Assisted Reproductive Technologies Program, Department of Obstetrics and Gynecology, University of Texas Southwestern Medical Center, Dallas, TX, USA

Erkan Buyuk, MD Montefiore's Institute for Reproductive Medicine and Health, Department of Obstetrics and Gynecology & Women's Health, Albert Einstein College of Medicine, Montefiore Medical Center, Bronx, NY, USA

Hakan E. Duran, MD Department of Obstetrics and Gynecology, Division of Reproductive Endocrinology and Infertility, University of Iowa, Iowa City, IA, USA

Zexu Jiao, MD, PhD, HCLD Division of Reproductive Endocrinology and Infertility, Fertility and Advanced Reproductive Medicine Assisted Reproductive Technologies Program, Department of Obstetrics and Gynecology, University of Texas Southwestern Medical Center, Dallas, TX, USA

Alexander Kucherov, MD Montefiore's Institute for Reproductive Medicine and Health, Department of Obstetrics and Gynecology & Women's Health, Albert Einstein College of Medicine, Montefiore Medical Center, Bronx, NY, USA

David Prokai, MD Division of Reproductive Endocrinology and Infertility, Fertility and Advanced Reproductive Medicine Assisted Reproductive Technologies Program, Department of Obstetrics and Gynecology, University of Texas Southwestern Medical Center, Dallas, TX, USA

Beverly G. Reed, MD IVFMD, Irving, TX, USA

Kotaro Sasaki, MD, PhD Department of Biomedical Sciences, University of Pennsylvania School of Veterinary Medicine, Philadelphia, PA, USA

Trisha Shah, MD Montefiore's Institute for Reproductive Medicine and Health, Department of Obstetrics and Gynecology & Women's Health, Albert Einstein College of Medicine, Montefiore Medical Center, Bronx, NY, USA

Wei Shang, MD Reproductive Medicine Center, Department of Obstetrics and Gynecology, Sixth Medical Center, Chinese PLA General Hospital, Beijing, China

Jennifer Shannon, MD Division of Reproductive Endocrinology & Infertility, Department of Obstetrics and Gynecology, University of Texas Southwestern Medical Center, Dallas, TX, USA

Volkan Turan, MD Department of Obstetrics and Gynecology, Yeni Yuzyil University School of Medicine, GOP Hospital, Istanbul, Turkey

Rachel M. Whynott, MD Department of Obstetrics and Gynecology, REI Division, University of Iowa, Iowa City, IA, USA

John Wu, MD Division of Reproductive Endocrinology and Infertility, Fertility and Advanced Reproductive Medicine Assisted Reproductive Technologies Program, Department of Obstetrics and Gynecology, University of Texas Southwestern Medical Center, Dallas, TX, USA

Part I
The Paradigm of Diminished Ovarian Reserve, Conventional & Adjuvant Treatment Approaches for Assisted Reproductive Technologies

Chapter 1
Introduction: The Scope of the Problem with Diminished Ovarian Reserve

Orhan Bukulmez

1.1 Definitions: Fertility, Fecundability, and Fecundity

Per the American Society for Reproductive Medicine (ASRM), fertility is defined as the capacity to produce a child [1]. Fecundability is defined as the probability of pregnancy per month. Strict definition of fecundability is the probability of conceiving in a given ovulatory menstrual cycle. Fecundity, on the other hand, is the probability to have a live birth within a single menstrual cycle. Monthly fecundability is highest during the first 3 months of trying, and about 80% of the couples achieve pregnancy within the first 6 months of trying. Again, per ASRM, infertility is defined as the failure to achieve a successful pregnancy after 12 months or more of regular unprotected intercourse or sperm exposure. However an earlier evaluation for possible treatment after 6 months without conception for women over age 35 years is recommended [2]. This recommendation is because fertility declines with female aging. Monthly fecundability rates decline by close to 50% between the ages of 35 and 39 years as compared to the same rates noted between the ages of 19 and 26 years [1].

1.2 Female Age

The classic data on the rate of natural pregnancy per female age graph shows that the natural conception rates decline from early to mid-30s and steeper decline is expected after 40 years of age (Fig. 1.1). Not surprisingly, in the United States, the

O. Bukulmez (✉)
Division of Reproductive Endocrinology and Infertility, Fertility and Advanced Reproductive Medicine Assisted Reproductive Technologies Program, Department of Obstetrics and Gynecology, University of Texas Southwestern Medical Center, Dallas, TX, USA
e-mail: Orhan.Bukulmez@UTSouthwestern.edu

© Springer Nature Switzerland AG 2020
O. Bukulmez (ed.), *Diminished Ovarian Reserve and Assisted Reproductive Technologies*, https://doi.org/10.1007/978-3-030-23235-1_1

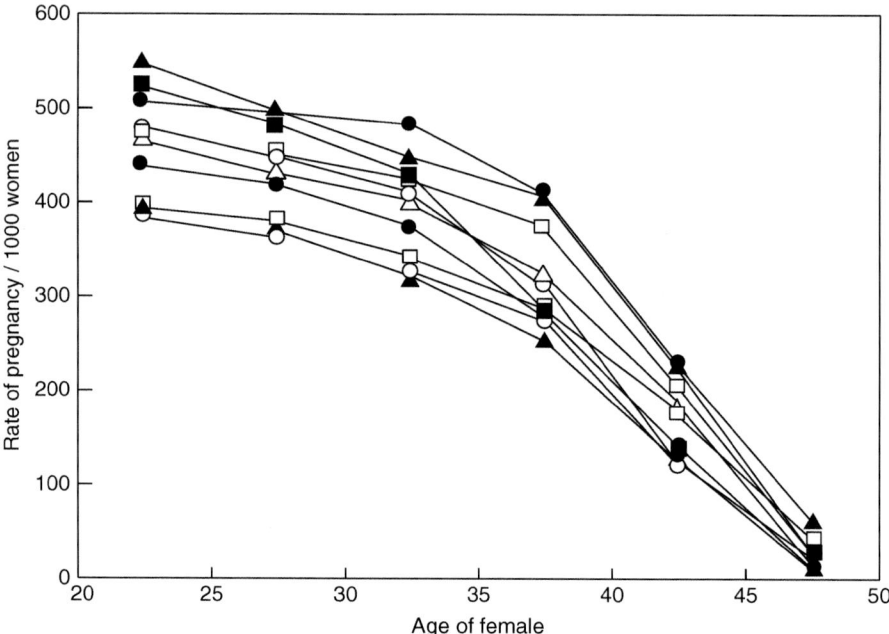

Fig. 1.1 Pregnancy rate per 1000 women in different populations from 1700 to 1950, with permission [1]

Society for Assisted Reproductive Technology's (SART) annual assisted reproductive technology treatment outcome report clearly shows that pregnancy and live birth rates decline with advancing female age (Fig. 1.2) https://www.cdc.gov/art/pdf/2015-national-summary-slides/ART_2015_graphs_and_charts.pdf. Female age is in fact the most important determinant of live birth with in vitro fertilization (IVF) treatment. This data also suggests that decline in live birth rates with treatment starts in the early 30s; then this decline becomes more pronounced after the mid-30s; and steeper decline is seen at and after age of 40.

The fertility trends at least in OECD (Organisation for Economic Co-operation and Development) countries suggest that the age of first birth in women is increasing around the globe. The average mean age of women at first birth has risen by almost 3 years in the last two decades in OECD countries (Fig. 1.3). In the United States, while birth rate decline is observed in teenage girls and in women between 20–29 and 30–34 years of age, birth rate increase is noted within the age groups of 35–39 and 40–44 years old. Therefore, females are postponing their pregnancies until later years of the reproductive period.

OECD (2016), "The average mean age of women at first birth has risen by almost three years in the last two decades: Mean age of women at first birth, 1995 and 2014 (or nearest year)," in *General context indicators*, OECD Publishing, Paris, https://doi.org/10.1787/soc_glance-2016-graph37-en.

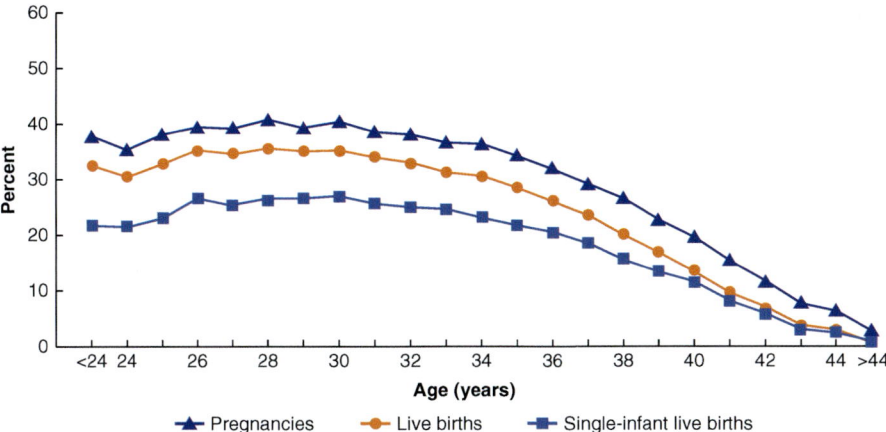

Fig. 1.2 SART 2015 Assisted Reproductive Technology (ART) summary report: percentage of pregnancies, live births, and single-infant live births by age of woman as a result of ART treatment (https://www.cdc.gov/art/pdf/2015-national-summary-slides/ART_2015_graphs_and_charts.pdf)

The most important reflection of delayed child-bearing in females is fertility decline as expected by advancing age. This fertility decline is associated with diminished ovarian reserve and diminished oocyte/embryo quality with aging. Diminished ovarian reserve itself may also be noted at any age when the women present with infertility. Although female fertility decreases with aging, the pace of reproductive decline can be different in each woman [3].

1.3 Paradigm of Diminished Ovarian Reserve as a Clinical Reflection of Poor Ovarian Response in Assisted Reproductive Technology

Diminished ovarian reserve (DOR) is one of the recent challenges clinicians and patients alike face in fertility treatment. Since the controlled ovarian stimulations became a norm in assisted reproductive technology (ART) cycles, it has been realized that some women just do not respond well to ovarian stimulation, while others suffer from ovarian hyperstimulation syndrome (OHSS). Therefore, the terms "poor responder" and "high responder" have been used, respectively.

There are various definitions of these terms but we can first review various definitions of DOR. National ART Surveillance System guideline defines DOR as "reduced fecundity related to diminished ovarian function; includes high FSH or high estradiol measured in the early follicular phase or during a clomiphene citrate challenge test; reduced ovarian volume related to congenital, medical, surgical or other causes; or advanced maternal age (>40)" [4].

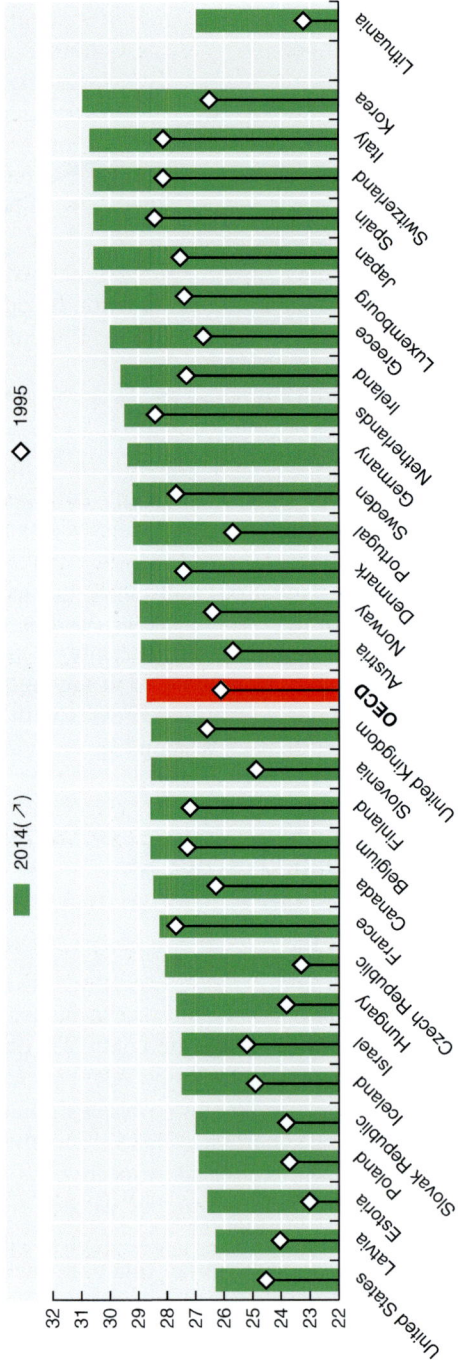

Fig. 1.3 The mean age of women at first birth has risen by almost 3 years in the last two decades

Definition of assisted reproductive technology per Office of the Federal Register (USA) is as follows: "*Assisted reproductive technology (ART)*—All treatments or procedures that include the handling of human oocytes or embryos for the purpose of establishing a pregnancy. This includes, but is not limited to in vitro fertilization and transcervical embryo transfer, gamete intrafallopian transfer, zygote intrafallopian transfer, tubal embryo transfer, oocyte or embryo cryopreservation, oocyte or embryo donation, and gestational surrogacy. ART does not include assisted insemination using sperm from either a woman's partner or sperm donor." [5]

In the same federal registry document, DOR was defined as a condition of reduced fecundity related to diminished ovarian function based on clinical assessment; often indicated by FSH $\geq$ 10 mIU/ mL or AMH < 1 ng/mL (https://www.gpo.gov/fdsys/pkg/FR-2015-08-26/pdf/2015-21108.pdf).

In the National ART Registry of the United States, in 2005 the DOR diagnosis is present in an average of 8.2% of ART cycles, while 39.9% of ART cycles were performed in women younger than 35 years of age. In 2015, the same registry shows that 31% of the ART cycles has the DOR diagnosis, while 38.1% of the ART cycles were from women <35 years of age. DOR diagnosis can be as high as 69% [6]. Therefore, DOR diagnosis is much more frequently made, while the proportion of women at or $\geq$35 years of age undergoing ART has increased by close to 2%. This discrepancy may be due to the more widespread use of ovarian reserve assessment before ART. In addition, more couples may be visiting fertility centers for infertility associated with DOR, and DOR may be becoming a more frequent indication for ART.

1.3.1 Poor Ovarian Response per European Society of Human Reproduction and Embryology

The European Society of Human Reproduction and Embryology (ESHRE) came up with a consensus definition for poor ovarian response (POR) for in vitro fertilization [7]. The Bologna criteria for POR is shown in Table 1.1. Many studies on POR used differing criteria and reported variable conclusions whether

Table 1.1 The "Bologna criteria" for poor ovarian response (POR): two out of three should be present[a]

1. Advanced maternal age $\geq$ 40 years or any other risk factor for POR
2. A previous POR defined as $\leq$3 oocytes with conventional ovarian stimulation
3. An abnormal ovarian reserve test: AFC < 5–7 or AMH < 0.5–1.1 ng/mL

AFC antral follicle count, AMH anti-Mullerian hormone
[a]Two previous cycles with POR after maximal stimulation are sufficient to define POR in the absence of advanced maternal age and abnormal ovarian reserve test

any particular IVF stimulation protocol results in better IVF outcomes [8]. The rationale was if there is a unified definition for POR, future research could be performed on such patient populations to come up with a unified global IVF treatment protocol for such patients. Shortly after its implementation, the criticisms followed since once again, one unified paradigm did not fit all. Although the majority of the POR may be due to DOR, some POR cases just cannot be explained with Bologna criteria. In addition, POR definition heavily relies on conventional IVF stimulation protocols, which mostly focus on retrieving as much oocytes as possible after a treatment cycle, since in such protocols it is believed that the number of oocytes retrieved is the most important treatment outcome parameter to predict clinical pregnancy and live birth. The Bologna criteria actually indirectly supports high-dose IVF stimulation protocols as the legitimate treatment approaches for such patients by mentioning about poorly defined "maximal stimulation" (Table 1.1).

Various endocrine and ultrasound markers and even some dynamic tests have been utilized to predict POR. Accordingly, POR has been defined by various criteria until the Bologna criteria for POR was recommended through consensus so that such patients could be defined in a unified manner so that the treatments can also be unified in such patients [7].

However, recently these criteria have been the focus of criticism since some patients showing poor response simply do not meet the Bologna criteria. This is in spite of the complaints that there was no accepted definition of POR, and therefore it will always be difficult to compare the results in published studies. In addition, POR may be due to systemic inflammatory diseases, nutritional disorders, advanced stage cancers without presence of the DOR per the age, AMH, and AFC criteria. Then Bologna consensus may not meet the needs. The criteria used for all such definitions relies on the female age equal or above 40 years, the serum markers like anti-Mullerian hormone (AMH) and ultrasound markers like antral follicle count (AFC), the number of oocytes collected in prior treatment cycles, highest estradiol levels achieved, and history of gonadotoxic treatments or ovarian surgery. Still the threshold levels for AFC and AMH vary in the latest Bologna criteria, while measurement of these two parameters is open to subjective and methodological biases, respectively [4, 9].

The AFC assessment of ≥ 2 mm antral follicles by transvaginal ultrasound as a marker of ovarian aging was first reported in 1996 by a study performed in volunteers aged between 22 and 42 years [10]. The authors noted that antral follicle counts decreased by aging. This measurement later evaluated to be one of the best predictors of ovarian response [11, 12]. Over the years, there were debates about the upper limit of antral follicle size or diameters measured by ultrasound. Diameters between 2 and 10 mm were included in some guidelines like Rotterdam criteria defining polycystic ovary morphology [13]. However, to better assess the controlled ovarian stimulation outcome, different upper thresholds less than 10 mm were proposed. One study reported that the number of antra follicles 2–6 mm decreased by age, but those between 7 and 10 mm stayed constant [14]. It was demonstrated that AMH expression is strongly observed in secondary, preantral, and small antral follicles up to the diameter of 4–6 mm. The AMH expression then decreases with further follicle growth and disappears in follicles measuring >8 mm in diameters. As expected, AMH expression is not observed in primordial follicles, and it is only weakly expressed in some primary follicles [15]. It was reported that the antral follicles measuring between 2 and 6 mm could be the best predictor for the number of mature oocytes retrieved at oocyte retrieval and was strongly associated with serum AMH levels [9]. Therefore, it is reasonable to focus on antral follicles between 2 and 6 mm while performing AFC.

1.3.2 Poor Ovarian Response Criteria per Prognostic Factors

There is another recent classification of patients with expected POR. The Patient-Oriented Strategies Encompassing IndividualizeD Oocyte Number (POSEIDON) group proposed a classification of POR patients into four groups per age; the presentation of unexpected POR, if previously stimulated, predicted poor prognosis, AFC, and AMH levels [16]. The main reasons for this new stratification effort for POR was due to the fact that Bologna criteria is disregarding female age effects on pregnancy outcomes regardless of the number of oocytes retrieved. The authors intended to change the paradigm from POR to low prognosis concept. Therefore, clinically more relevant criteria were suggested. They brought two new groups for defining low-prognosis patients according to how they responded to a conventional ovarian stimulation for IVF. First one is "suboptimal response" defined as the retrieval of four to nine oocytes, which is associated, at any given age, with a significantly lower live birth rate compared with normal responders defined those with 10–15 oocytes, in which authors supported this definition by quoting a retrospective study [17]. Second one is "hyporesponse" for those needing higher dose of gonadotropins and prolonged stimulation to retrieve more than three oocytes which may be due to genetic issues as authors quoted another study to support this definition [18]. Then the age threshold of 35 years in relevance to expected embryo aneuploidy rate, and AMH and AFC, as the ovarian reserve markers are also included to define groups. This is also a more dynamic assessment since it includes before, during, and after stimulation observations. POSEIDON classification of low-prognosis patients is summarized in Table 1.2.

The authors believe that the low prognosis concept will better help to personalize ART treatment protocols. It may also lead to define those patients with genetic polymorphism related to gonadotropins and their receptors [16].

Table 1.2 POSEIDON group for low prognosis for assisted reproductive technology treatment

Group	Subgroup	Description
1		Age < 35 years with acceptable pre-stimulation ovarian reserve (AFC ≥5, AMH ≥1.2 ng/mL) and with an unexpected poor or suboptimal ovarian response
	1a	Fewer than four oocytes
	1b	Four to nine oocytes after standard ovarian stimulation, who, at any age, have a lower live birth rate than age-matched normal responders
2		Age ≥ 35 years with acceptable pre-stimulation ovarian reserve (AFC ≥5, AMH ≥1.2 ng/mL) and with an unexpected poor or suboptimal ovarian response
	2a	Fewer than four oocytes
	2b	Four to nine oocytes after standard ovarian stimulation, who, at any age, have a lower live birth rate than age-matched normal responders.
3		Age < 35 years with poor ovarian reserve pre-stimulation parameters (AFC <5, AMH <1.2 ng/mL)
4		Age ≥ 35 years with poor ovarian reserve pre-stimulation parameters (AFC <5, AMH <1.2 ng/mL)

Modified from [16]

1.4 Conclusion

Women are postponing their pregnancies due to various reasons as also discussed in ovarian and hypothalamic aging section. The fertility decline is noted in women starting from late 20s to early 30s. This is mostly related to decrease in ovarian reserve, which we define as the quantity decline and decrease in oocyte quality, which we consider as quality decline. Poor ovarian response criteria per ESHRE has been heavily based on quantity decline, while the age criteria which mostly reflects quality, as will be discussed in Chap. 2, is included when the female age is ≥40 years. Although Bologna criteria was proposed to achieve more unified definitions for research, it introduced its own inherent problems due its assumptions, which may not reflect the prognosis. Recently, attempts are made to have more individualized criteria for POR focusing on expected low prognosis by POSEIDON group. Regardless, the diagnoses of DOR in ART cycles are increasing, while most of the women with POR are those with DOR. These women are a heterogeneous group who may require personalized approaches for ART treatments.

References

1. Practice Committee of the American Society for Reproductive Medicine in collaboration with the Society for Reproductive Endocrinoogy, Infertility. Electronic address, ASRM@asrm.org, Practice Committee of the American Society for Reproductive Medicine in collaboration with the Society for Reproductive Endocrinology, Infertility. Optimizing natural fertility: a committee opinion. Fertil Steril. 2017;107(1):52–8.

2. Practice Committee of American Society for Reproductive Medicine. Definitions of infertility and recurrent pregnancy loss: a committee opinion. Fertil Steril. 2013;99(1):63.
3. Practice Committee of the American Society for Reproductive Medicine. Testing and interpreting measures of ovarian reserve: a committee opinion. Fertil Steril. 2015;103(3):e9–e17.
4. Pastore LM, Christianson MS, Stelling J, Kearns WG, Segars JH. Reproductive ovarian testing and the alphabet soup of diagnoses: DOR, POI, POF, POR, and FOR. J Assist Reprod Genet. 2018;35(1):17–23.
5. Centers for Disease Control and Prevention (CDC), Department of Health and Human Services (DHHS). Reporting of pregnancy success rates from Assisted Reproductive Technology (ART) programs. Federal Register Notices. 2015;8(165):51811–9. https://www.gpo.gov/fdsys/pkg/FR-2015-08-26/pdf/2015-21108.pdf.
6. Center for Disease Control and Prevention. Archived ART Reports and Spreadsheets. 2015 and 2005.
7. Ferraretti AP, La Marca A, Fauser BC, Tarlatzis B, Nargund G, Gianaroli L, et al. ESHRE consensus on the definition of 'poor response' to ovarian stimulation for in vitro fertilization: the Bologna criteria. Hum Reprod. 2011;26(7):1616–24.
8. Polyzos NP, Devroey P. A systematic review of randomized trials for the treatment of poor ovarian responders: is there any light at the end of the tunnel? Fertil Steril. 2011;96(5):1058–61.e7.
9. Jayaprakasan K, Deb S, Batcha M, Hopkisson J, Johnson I, Campbell B, et al. The cohort of antral follicles measuring 2-6 mm reflects the quantitative status of ovarian reserve as assessed by serum levels of anti-Mullerian hormone and response to controlled ovarian stimulation. Fertil Steril. 2010;94(5):1775–81.
10. Ruess ML, Kline J, Santos R, Levin B, Timor-Tritsch I. Age and the ovarian follicle pool assessed with transvaginal ultrasonography. Am J Obstet Gynecol. 1996;174(2):624–7.
11. Bancsi LF, Broekmans FJ, Eijkemans MJ, de Jong FH, Habbema JD, te Velde ER. Predictors of poor ovarian response in in vitro fertilization: a prospective study comparing basal markers of ovarian reserve. Fertil Steril. 2002;77(2):328–36.
12. Eldar-Geva T, Ben-Chetrit A, Spitz IM, Rabinowitz R, Markowitz E, Mimoni T, et al. Dynamic assays of inhibin B, anti-Mullerian hormone and estradiol following FSH stimulation and ovarian ultrasonography as predictors of IVF outcome. Hum Reprod. 2005;20(11):3178–83.
13. Rotterdam, Eshre Asrm-Sponsored Pcos Consensus Workshop Group. Revised 2003 consensus on diagnostic criteria and long-term health risks related to polycystic ovary syndrome. Fertil Steril. 2004;81(1):19–25.
14. Haadsma ML, Bukman A, Groen H, Roeloffzen EM, Groenewoud ER, Heineman MJ, et al. The number of small antral follicles (2-6 mm) determines the outcome of endocrine ovarian reserve tests in a subfertile population. Hum Reprod. 2007;22(7):1925–31.
15. Weenen C, Laven JS, Von Bergh AR, Cranfield M, Groome NP, Visser JA, et al. Anti-Mullerian hormone expression pattern in the human ovary: potential implications for initial and cyclic follicle recruitment. Mol Hum Reprod. 2004;10(2):77–83.
16. Poseidon Group, Alviggi C, Andersen CY, Buehler K, Conforti A, De Placido G, et al. A new more detailed stratification of low responders to ovarian stimulation: from a poor ovarian response to a low prognosis concept. Fertil Steril. 2016;105(6):1452–3.
17. Drakopoulos P, Blockeel C, Stoop D, Camus M, de Vos M, Tournaye H, et al. Conventional ovarian stimulation and single embryo transfer for IVF/ICSI. How many oocytes do we need to maximize cumulative live birth rates after utilization of all fresh and frozen embryos? Hum Reprod. 2016;31(2):370–6.
18. Alviggi C, Pettersson K, Longobardi S, Andersen CY, Conforti A, De Rosa P, et al. A common polymorphic allele of the LH beta-subunit gene is associated with higher exogenous FSH consumption during controlled ovarian stimulation for assisted reproductive technology. Reprod Biol Endocrinol. 2013;11:51.

Chapter 2
Ovarian and Hypothalamic Aging

Alexander Kucherov and Erkan Buyuk

2.1 Female Reproductive Aging

While life expectancy for women increased significantly over the last century from 48.3 years in 1900 to 81.3 years in 2014 [1], the age at menopause stayed relatively stable at 49–52 years [2, 3]. Female reproduction depends on complex and coordinated interactions among the hypothalamus, the pituitary, and the ovaries, and these interactions are independent of the life span of a woman. For many years, female reproductive aging was viewed as simply the end product of oocyte depletion and ovarian failure. However, several recent studies challenge these observations [4]. Although menopause is ultimately defined by ovarian failure, convergent lines of evidence now suggest that hypothalamic-pituitary axis (HPA) dysfunction may also play a role in reproductive senescence [5]. It is possible that aberrant responsiveness to estrogen feedback and abnormal gonadotropin release patterns may contribute to accelerated consumptive exhaustion of the remaining ovarian follicles.

Over the past several decades, women have increasingly delayed childbearing [6], mainly due to professional/educational goals, financial barriers, and lack of a partner [7–9]. As a testimony to these trends, from 2005 to 2014, there has been an approximate 64% increase in in vitro fertilization (IVF) cycles reported to the Center for Disease Control, alongside an increase in the diagnosis of diminished ovarian reserve as an etiology for IVF from 8% to 32% [10]. As a result, understanding the physiological and cellular mechanisms of female reproductive aging has become an area of intense scientific interest because opportunities may exist to extend fertility, retard multisystem disease progress, and improve the overall

A. Kucherov · E. Buyuk (✉)
Montefiore's Institute for Reproductive Medicine and Health, Department of Obstetrics and Gynecology & Women's Health, Albert Einstein College of Medicine, Montefiore Medical Center, Bronx, NY, USA
e-mail: ebuyuk@montefiore.org

© Springer Nature Switzerland AG 2020
O. Bukulmez (ed.), *Diminished Ovarian Reserve and Assisted Reproductive Technologies*, https://doi.org/10.1007/978-3-030-23235-1_2

quality of life for aging women. This chapter reviews our current understanding of the independent contributions of the ovary and HPA axis to female reproductive aging.

2.2   Female Reproductive Aging and the Ovary

The ovaries are probably the only organs whose peak potential is reached long before first use! The maximum number of oocytes in humans is reached by the fifth month of in utero life, at which time they are surrounded by a single layer of flat squamous granulosa cells, forming the primordial follicle. Ovarian reserve is defined as the quantity and the quality of the oocytes remaining in the ovaries [11] and is reflected by this primordial follicle pool. After reaching the maximum number, the oocyte numbers continuously decline thereafter, until near depletion at the time of menopause. The original dogma was that female vertebrates acquire their complete complement of primordial follicles before birth [12–14]. However, this conceptual view of female gametogenesis was challenged, at least in mice, by studies suggesting that the gamete pool in the ovary is not finite but instead continuously replenished with gonadal stem cells derived from the bone marrow [15–19]. In addition, there is a growing body of evidence that stem cells may exist on the surface epithelium of the adult human ovary [20, 21], some of which appear to spontaneously differentiate into oocyte-like structures in vitro [20, 22]. In either case, the menopause generally occurs in the sixth decade of life and is defined by the loss of ovarian function. Although women start their reproductive lives with as many as 500,000 oocytes, by the time of the last menstrual period, the ovaries contain <1000 oocytes [23]. Ovarian follicular depletion and aging is a continuous process that begins after women attain maximum fertility, between 20 and 29 years of age, at which time a relatively steady state of follicular attrition is maintained until age 35–37. Around this age, despite normal gonadotropin production and eugonadism, most women begin to experience an accelerated depletion of primordial follicles available for recruitment, ovulation, and potential fertilization [24]. However, more recent studies suggest that this follicular attrition is not as steep as originally thought, and a smoother decline in oocyte numbers, rather than biphasic attrition rates, was proposed (Fig. 2.1) [25].

Of note, this altered ovarian physiology commences long before the appearance of overt clinical signs and/or symptoms suggestive of the menopausal transition (i.e., menstrual irregularity and vasomotor symptoms). As women continue to age, oocyte depletion accelerates dramatically, and clear signs of diminished ovarian reserve are manifest such as elevated follicle-stimulating hormone (FSH), erratic ovarian steroid production, and menstrual irregularities. Of importance is the observation that the reduction in the number of primordial pool parallels the steep reductions in fertility observed in the latter half of the fourth decade [26].

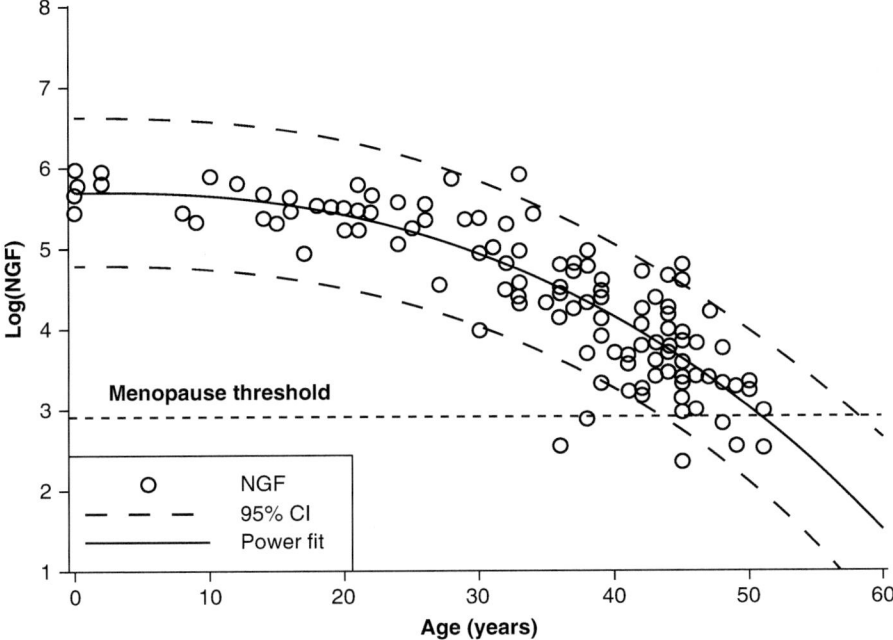

Fig. 2.1 Ovarian follicular attrition

2.2.1 *Markers of Ovarian Aging*

A distinctive feature of ovarian aging is the accelerated depletion of primordial follicles associated with reduced numbers of antral follicles. Ovarian reserve is a major predictor of the age at which natural menopause occurs, and monotropic rise of FSH is a recognized harbinger of impending ovarian failure [27]. Although FSH is traditionally used to predict the response to controlled ovarian hyperstimulation in the infertile population, and elevated FSH levels often coexist in women with clinical evidence of diminished ovarian reserve, serum FSH is neither the best predictor of reduced fertility nor prognostic of timing of onset of menopause [28]. Consequently, there have been great efforts made to identify the best markers for ovarian aging [29].

AMH and inhibin-B [30] have emerged as useful biomarkers for assessing ovarian reserve in infertility populations. Both markers are glycoproteins belonging to transforming growth factor β superfamily and produced by granulosa cells of preantral and early antral follicles. Hence, their serum levels correlate with antral follicle density. Inhibin B restrains early follicular FSH rises [31], and AMH affects folliculogenesis by altering the sensitivity of primordial follicles destined for recruitment, keeping the primordial follicle pool in abeyance [32]. Notably, serum inhibin B and AMH levels decrease with age [29, 33, 34]. Compared with FSH, inhibin B and AMH are better early serum predictors of diminished ovarian reserve, mainly due to cycle-to-cycle fluctuations in serum FSH levels [33, 35]. However, low serum AMH levels are not necessarily associated with a reduced rate of conception among those without a diagnosis of infertility [36]. On the other hand, AMH is one of the best predictors of the number of oocytes retrieved during an assisted reproductive technology (ART) cycle [37–40]. Moreover, its levels remain relatively stable during the menstrual cycle and, hence, can be measured anytime during the cycle [41]. As a result, it is commonly used in clinical practice to guide the therapy during controlled ovarian hyperstimulation (COH) cycles. Human and rodent studies suggest that reduced serum AMH levels may be the most sensitive indicator of diminished ovarian reserve and impending ovarian failure. Although reductions in AMH and inhibin B predate obvious ovarian failure, the mechanisms precipitating these changes remain unclear, and routine testing as a device just to predict menopause is, at present, unwarranted.

As stated previously, ovarian aging is invariably associated with decreased numbers of primordial and early antral follicles. Thus it is not surprising that a decrease in basal antral follicle count (AFC), as determined by ultrasound, is associated with diminished ovarian reserve [42]. Like AMH, AFC is another strong predictor of the number of oocytes retrieved during an ART cycle. This basic tenet has resulted in the use of the AFC by infertility specialists to predict ovarian responses to ovarian stimulation with exogenous gonadotropins and to assist clinicians as they counsel patients about the likelihood of treatment success [43].

2.2.2   Mechanisms of Ovarian Aging

Whether ovarian failure begins prematurely or during the "normal" perimenopause, the outcome is the same: primordial follicular pool depletion, subfertility, ovarian insufficiency, and hypergonadotropic hypogonadism. The time that it takes women to deplete their primordial follicle pool varies with environmental factors and personal genetic background. As discussed briefly above, controversy regarding whether follicular depletion is a biexponential versus a monophasic process persists [24–26]. The biexponential model for ovarian aging argues that when follicular reserve reaches a critical threshold of 25,000 in the mid to late 30s, follicular depletion accelerates. In contrast, the monophasic model proposes a constant rate of accelerated follicular depletion. Nonetheless, each model is consistent in their interpretation that overall follicular depletion increases with age. It should be noted that more than 99% of developing follicles undergo atresia prior to ovulation. Since women have approximately 500,000 oocytes at the time of menarche and this number decreases to roughly <1000 at the time of final menstrual period, roughly 1000 oocytes are lost each month throughout reproductive life span via mechanisms thought to involve apoptosis (programmed cell death) of the granulosa cells [44, 45], although the link between follicle depletion and granulosa cell apoptosis is controversial. For example, data among patients undergoing in vitro fertilization (IVF) demonstrated an increased rate of granulosa cell apoptosis in the preovulatory portion of the menstrual cycle in younger women (ages 23–30), with a greater antral follicle count, compared with older women (ages 35–45) [46]. However, within this older age group, these differences primarily existed among women who also had a reduced number of antral follicles. This suggests that decreased rates of granulosa cell apoptosis only exist within the setting of a reduced number of follicles. Moreover, dysregulation of receptors in older women, mainly receptors for bone morphogenetic protein (BMPR1B), FSH, and LH, may suppress the mitogenic growth rate in healthy follicles as demonstrated by reduced granulosa cell apoptosis [46]. Whereas the hormonal changes associated with impending ovarian failure are well-characterized [47], the mechanisms responsible for increased rates of follicular depletion and granulosa cell apoptosis are not well-defined.

A wide array of mechanisms and pathways are implicated in ovarian aging (Table 2.1). These include, among others, genetic and metabolic influences, environmental and metabolic factors, mitochondrial dysfunction, oxidative stress, role of stem cells and telomerases, and others. The following sections explain the association between these factors and ovarian aging.

Table 2.1 Factors implicated in ovarian aging

Genetic and epigenetic factors
Breast cancer 1 (*BRCA1*)
Meiotic recombination 11 homolog 1 (*MRE11*)
RAD51 Recombinase (*RAD51*)
Ataxia telangiectasia mutated (*ATM*)
Histone modifications
Mitochondrial factors
Mitochondria size and number
Sirtuin 1 (*SIRT1*)
Coenzyme Q
Decaprenyl diphosphate synthase subunit 2 (*PDSS2*)
Caseinolytic peptidase P (*CLPP*)
Mammalian target of rapamycin (*mTOR*)
Oxidative stress
Reactive oxygen species
Superoxide
Hydrogen peroxide
Hypochlorous oxide
Germline stem cells
Hippo signaling pathway
Mammalian sterile 20-like protein kinase 1 (*MST1*)
Large tumor suppressor homolog 1 (*LATS1*)
Telomeres
Telomerases
Sirtuin 1 (*SIRT1*)
Cohesin stromal antigens 1 and 2 (*SA1* and *SA2*)

Table 2.1 (continued)

Metabolic factors
Cumulus granulosa cells/pentose phosphate pathway
Sirtuins (*SIRT1, SIRT 3* and *SIRT6*)
Sphingosine 1 phosphate
Ceramide
Environmental factors
Cigarette smoking
Caffeine intake
Radiation exposure
Chemotherapy
Low socioeconomic status
Extensive pelvic surgery
Chronic psychologic stress
Toxins
Vinylcyclohexene diepoxide (VCD)
Caloric restriction
Peroxisome proliferator-activated receptor gamma coactivator 1-alpha (*PGC-1α*)
Forkhead box O1 (*FOXO1*)
Lipids
Others
Micro RNAs
TATA-box binding protein-associated factor 4B (*TAF4B*)
Mov10 like RISC complex RNA helicase (*MOV10L1*)

2.2.2.1   Genetic and Epigenetic Factors

Ovarian aging appears coincident with a decrease in expression of genes which produce double-stranded DNA repair proteins [48]. For instance, expression of the genes *BRCA1, MRE11, Rad51,* and *ATM,* but not *BRCA2,* decreases with oocyte aging [48]. Gene mutations may also play a direct role in ovarian reserve. Patients with germline *BRCA1* mutations are noted to have decreased AMH levels [48, 49], primordial follicle count [50], and increased oocyte DNA damage with double-stranded DNA breaks [50] compared to age-matched controls. Cumulus cells from older patients are also noted to have increased expression of angiogenic genes; this finding is hypothesized to be a countermeasure to increased age-related hypoxia encountered by oocytes [51]. The oocytes of older women are noted to contain greater numbers of "clusters" of de novo gene mutations compared to younger women; these appear to be sites which are associated with double-stranded DNA breaks [52]. This is hypothesized to be due to deregulated DNA recombination, particularly at chromosomes 8, 9, and 16 [52], although it is not clear if this leads to increased risk of aneuploidy during meiosis.

Epigenetic factors are also associated with ovarian aging. Histone modification, the modification of the terminal amino acid of histones, plays a role in normal cell cycle regulation and chromosome segregation during meiosis. Recent mouse studies have demonstrated that older mice were noted to have decreased levels of methylation of lysine residues on oocyte histones, compared to younger mice. Such a decrease in histone modification is one plausible explanation for the increase in meiotic errors associated with chromosome segregation noted in older females. DNA methylation, leading to either expression or suppression of gene activity, also plays a role in appropriate gene expression during gametogenesis. The effect of ovarian aging on DNA methylation is less clear; one study found decreased amount of direct DNA methylation in the oocytes of older females compared to young mice [53, 54].

2.2.2.2 Role of Mitochondria and Mitochondrial Dysfunction

Low levels of mitochondrial DNA have been demonstrated in patients with premature ovarian insufficiency (POI) as well as patients who demonstrate a poor response to ovarian hyperstimulation during fertility treatments [55]. These findings have also been discovered in older mice when compared to younger mice [56]. Conversely, elevated mitochondrial DNA levels in embryos are associated with decreased implantation rates during IVF, decreased embryo viability, and increased risk of aneuploidy [57, 58]. The pathophysiology for these differences have not been completely elucidated but it is suggested that higher mitochondrial DNA copy number is reflective of increased oocyte and embryonic stress [58], a finding supported by the determination that reactive oxygen species (ROS) levels are greater in older mouse oocytes exposed to hydrogen peroxide, when compared to younger mice [56]. The mitochondria of oocytes from primary follicles also tend to be smaller in older mice when compared to younger mice. However, no such association was found in oocytes from other types of follicles [56].

Oocyte aging is associated with mitochondrial dysfunction [59], with a coincident decrease in oxidative phosphorylation and ATP levels [60]. This finding may be affected by maternal age. A bovine model demonstrated that oocytes subjected to decreased ATP levels and increased ROS levels appeared to have decreased oocyte competence (as measured by their blastulation rate after fertilization) in older but not younger cows. This may be mediated by SIRT1, an upstream regulator of mitochondrial biogenesis, the expression of which was noted to be elevated in younger cows after exposure to agents leading to mitochondrial dysfunction. These findings suggest that younger oocytes may have better regulatory mechanisms and improved mitochondrial resilience when compared to older oocytes [61].

Coenzyme Q (CoQ) is a complex of multiple proteins required to maintain mitochondrial stability; disruptions in this pathway may increase mitochondrial instability [60]. Aging appears to lead to decreased expression of enzymes responsible for

CoQ production, like decaprenyl diphosphate synthase subunit 2 (*PDSS2*) [60, 62]. Conditional disruption of *Pdss2* in mouse oocytes leads to premature ovarian insufficiency phenotype that can be prevented by the addition of CoQ to the maternal diet [60]. In addition, CoQ supplementation to the diet of older mice led to an increased number of ovulated eggs after stimulation, lower mitochondrial copy numbers, and an increased litter size when compared to young controls [62].

Activity of mitochondrial caseinolytic peptidase P (*CLPP*), which cleaves misfolded proteins and is critical for normal mitochondrial function, has also been implicated in oocyte mitochondrial function, oocyte and embryo development. *Clpp* gene knockout mice demonstrate accelerated depletion of ovarian reserve and impaired oocyte and embryo development, likely through activation of the mTOR pathway. Upregulation of the mTOR pathway leads to decreased oocyte count, possibly by increased follicular atresia and depletion [58].

2.2.2.3 Oxidative Stress

Reactive oxygen species (ROS) are hypothesized to cause cellular aging, and elevated ROS levels have been implicated in decreased rates of oocyte maturation, fertilization, embryo development, and pregnancy rates [63]. Specifically, superoxide, hydrogen peroxide, and hypochlorous oxide contribute to oocyte aging and have been demonstrated to increase zona pellucida dissolution time, alter ooplasm microtubule dynamics, and increase cortical granule loss; these findings were most pronounced in older oocytes [64]. Antioxidants have been investigated in an attempt to slow this process. Mouse models treated with N-acetyl-L-cysteine (NAC), a potent antioxidant, have increased litter sizes and improved oocyte quality when compared to age-matched controls [63]. Melatonin, a free radical scavenger, has similarly been shown to decrease ROS levels, decrease rates of oocyte apoptosis, slow the decline in mitochondrial membrane potential, and increase the likelihood of embryo development from porcine oocytes [65].

One method of detecting evidence of oxidative stress of oocytes has been through the use of Raman spectroscopy. This method utilizes principal component analysis, and significant differences have been detected in the lipid and protein components of young mouse oocytes when compared to oocytes with damage induced by ROS and to oocytes from older mice. Interestingly, the oocytes with ROS-induced damage appeared to exhibit levels of oxidative stress similar to older oocytes which have not been exposed to exogenous ROS damage [66]. This method may prove useful in the future in evaluating oxidative damage to the oocytes in a noninvasive manner to predict oocyte quality.

2.2.2.4 Stem Cells

There is emerging evidence that germline stem cells (GSCs) play a role in continued oocyte production after birth, contrary to the standard model that mammals are born with all of the oocytes they will have in their lifetime and that these oocytes do not replenish themselves [12, 13, 67–69]. A trial investigating this theory has demonstrated that grafting aged ovarian tissue from germ cell-specific transgenic mice into the ovary of a young wild-type host resulted in the production of immature follicles and the co-expression of markers of primordial oocytes [67]. Other trials suggest that menopause may be a result of defects in replenishing the oocytes, rather than resulting solely from their depletion [69]. FSH plays a critical role in ovarian signaling, and FSH receptor defects in ovarian surface stem cells and the ovarian surface epithelium (OSE) may play a role in the development of POI [68]. The Hippo signaling pathway, which regulates oocyte polarity and egg chamber structure, as well as cancer stem cells, is also involved in changes which occur surrounding normal and pathologic ovarian aging in mice. More specifically, the mRNA and protein expression of the upstream kinase; mammalian sterile 20-like protein kinase 1, *MST1*; and large tumor suppressor homolog 1 (LATS1) is decreased in the ovarian cortex of old mice when compared to young mice [70].

Stem cells have been used to recover function in setting of premature ovarian aging (POA), such as after exposure to ovotoxic chemotherapy. However, at the present time, there is no cure for premature ovarian aging or POI. Recently, human amniotic epithelial cells (hAECs) and human amniotic mesenchymal stem cells (hAMSCs) were investigated in a mouse model to determine their efficacy for this purpose. hAMSCs have been shown to increase the proliferation rate of ovarian granular cells from POI. This supports the proposition that stem cells may be used in cases of POI in the future [71].

2.2.2.5   Telomeres

Telomeres are genomic structures located at the ends of linear chromosomes and are composed of TTAGGG repeat tracks in vertebrates including humans [72]. They help differentiate the ends of the chromosomes from exposed or damaged DNA and prevent their recognition by the DNA repair mechanisms as breaks in the DNA. Hence, they play a role in the protecting chromosomal DNA from degradation, recombination, loss, and fusion. The telomeric repeats of DNA sequences are shortened highly variably with each cell division. Telomere shortening occurs as a result of damage from ROS, and this process is implicated in the cellular aging. NAC, as discussed above, has been demonstrated to "rescue" oocytes and embryos with ROS-induced telomere shortening and apoptosis [63]. Estrogen also appears to play a role in preventing telomere shortening. Estrogen deficiency, via disruption of the aromatase gene, leads to shortening of telomeres and reduced granulosa cell proliferation in a mouse model. In this same model, exogenous replacement of estrogen, bypassing its production by aromatase, reverses these effects; increased telomere activity and length, as well as normal ovarian granulosa cell growth, was noted [73]. SIRT1, previously mentioned as an upstream regulator of mitochondrial biogenesis and which acts as a deacetylase, promotes repair of double-stranded DNA breaks. Cohesins SA1 and SA2 mediate sister chromatid cohesions at telomere sites. Together, SIRT1 and cohesins are noted to have increased expression in the cumulus cells of women who have robust response to ovarian hyperstimulation, and SIRT1 elevations were positively correlated with telomere length. Finally, SIRT1 mRNA levels in older women (age > 38) were noted to be twice as high as younger women (age < 34). Taken together, these findings suggest that SIRT1 and cohesins SA1 and SA2 play a role in telomere homeostasis [74].

2.2.2.6 Metabolic Factors

Many different metabolic factors have been investigated regarding their effect on ovarian aging. The mechanism by which oocytes are prevented from premature aging (both pre- and post-ovulatory) is not clear. Current research suggests that cumulus cells play a critical role in this process. Specifically, oocytes can utilize pyruvate or lactate to prevent premature aging but that glucose itself requires cumulus cells to facilitate this process; in addition, it appears that activation of the pentose phosphate pathway, rather than glycolysis, is the mechanism by which this occurs [75].

Sirtuins are NAD-dependent deacetylases and are known to play a role in regulating metabolism, cell proliferation, and genome stability. As previously mentioned, SIRT1 is one of these factors; however, other sirtuins, such as SIRT3 and SIRT6, are hypothesized to play a similar role. In several different murine ovarian aging models, all three of these sirtuins were demonstrated to be positively correlated with ovarian reserve, and decreased levels were associated with ovarian aging, decreased number of primordial follicles, and increased number of atretic follicles [76]. SIRT1 has also been demonstrated to protect against porcine oocyte aging in vitro [77]. Sphingosine-1-phosphate (SIP) and ceramide are two sphingolipids found in oocytes, and the balance of the two is what determines whether or not a cell undergoes apoptosis in many human tissues. Increasing intracellular SIP via the addition of an oral SIP analog in a rat model led to an increase in the ratio of non-apoptotic primordial follicles, as well as higher levels of mean AMH, when compared with controls [78].

2.2.2.7 Environmental Influence

Exogenous influences affect the rate of ovarian follicular depletion and ovarian reserve. Cigarette smoking [79], radiation exposure [80], low socioeconomic status [81], chemotherapy [82, 83], extensive pelvic scarring from pelvic surgery, and chronic psychological stress [84] have all been identified as ovotoxic and associated with ovarian senescence.

Environmental toxins can adversely affect ovarian aging. The toxin 4-vinylcyclohexane diepoxide (VCD), an industrial chemical found in insecticides, flame retardants, rubber tires, and plasticizers, has been shown to selectively destroy primordial and antral follicles. Mice treated with VCD experience accelerated follicular atresia/apoptosis, hypergonadotropic hypogonadism, and premature ovarian failure within 120 days of exposure to the toxin. Similarly, Siberian hamsters treated with VCD were noted to have a reduced number of primordial follicles and produced fewer offspring than untreated animals [85]. VCD is thought to mediate its ovotoxic properties through inhibition of the kit signaling pathway that will be discussed below, which is responsible for cell survival mechanisms. This leads to activation of apoptotic pathways [84, 86, 87].

Whereas many environmental factors negatively influence ovarian aging, rodent studies of the role of caloric restriction in longevity also reported delayed ovarian senescence and reduced follicle atresia in calorie-restricted rodents (50% of body weight compared with control) [88, 89]. Caloric restriction is hypothesized to alter the transcription of peroxisome proliferator-activated receptor gamma coactivator 1-alpha (*PGC-1α*) and the forkhead family of transcription factors (*FOXO*), which may decrease granulosa cell apoptosis and oocyte atresia [90]. Although a modest restriction of caloric intake is associated with an extended reproductive life, data for humans in this regard are nonexistent and remain uninvestigated.

Lipid metabolism may play a role in ovarian aging. One study demonstrated that follicular fluid extracted from oocytes in older women (age > 35) undergoing IVF had greater abundance of 11 different lipids, such as sphingomyelin, diacylglycerol, and triacylglycerol, whereas younger women (age ≤ 35) had a greater abundance of 4 other lipids, such as phosphatidylcholine, phosphatidylethanolamine, and phosphatidylinositol phosphate. This suggests that differential lipid metabolism and pathways may play a role in oocyte aging, perhaps by influencing downstream cascade of metabolic products [91].

There is emerging evidence that caffeine may improve reproductive outcomes in vitro for patients undergoing assisted reproductive technologies. For instance, studies have demonstrated that the addition of caffeine to oocyte culture media appears to inhibit oocyte fragmentation and spindle degradation in aged porcine oocytes [92]. A separate study demonstrated that aging porcine oocytes incubated with caffeine for 24 hours demonstrated an increase in the expression of proteins related to stress response and cell adhesion among others [93]. Caffeine appears to decrease separation of cumulus cells, maintain spindle morphology, and increase the fertilization rate, but not inhibit zona pellucida hardening [94] in mouse oocytes. Human studies on this topic are lacking and require investigation prior to making definitive determinations about efficacy in humans. The role of caffeine in human fertility has been debated since at least the 1980s. Several retrospective studies initially demonstrated possible increased risk of infertility; however, these studies were limited by small sample size and lack of controlling for confounders [95, 96]. More recent studies, larger and appropriately controlled, suggest that caffeine does not play a major role in human infertility [97, 98]; several Danish cohort studies demonstrated that there is no association between primary infertility and caffeine intake [97, 99], and current consensus does not support the theory that moderate caffeine intake leads to infertility [100]. In addition, recent retrospective human studies have demonstrated no difference in the outcomes of fertility treatments with regard to caffeine intake. For instance, one study demonstrated no difference in the number of high-quality oocytes retrieved, implantation rate, clinical pregnancy rate, or live birth rate, based on caffeine consumption [101]. There is a paucity of data regarding evaluation of ovarian reserve and caffeine intake in infertile women, although the lack of a difference between the number of oocytes retrieved suggests that there may not be a link overall. Earlier studies on caffeine also suggested its role in DNA repair inhibition [102]. In addition, a recent prospective cohort study investigating maternal dietary intakes in early pregnancy suggested that maternal caffeine intake was associated with low birth weight, lower birth length, smaller head circumference, and shorter gestational age [103].Therefore, further research is needed to fully elucidate the relationship, or lack thereof, between caffeine and ovarian reserve.

A mouse model has been used to investigate a potential role for diosgenin, a naturally occurring steroidal saponin found in yam. Diosgenin is known to have anti-inflammatory and antiproliferative activities and were given to mice orally for 3 months. Aging mice fed with diosgenin were noted to have increased AMH levels compared to age-matched controls; however, no statistically significant increase in number of primary follicles, oocytes retrieved, or fertilization rate with IVF was noted [104]. Further study is needed prior to making recommendations regarding the use of this compound.

2.2.2.8 Other Mechanisms That Affect Ovarian Aging

MicroRNAs (miRNA) are short-sequence RNA molecules which are involved in posttranscriptional cleavage of mRNA, leading to a targeted reduction in protein expression [105]. Ovarian miRNA expression has recently been investigated with regard to its expression in the ovaries of Ames dwarf mutant mice (df/df), which have extended life spans. Of the 46 miRNAs which were detected in which expression levels changed with age of the mice, only 3 were commonly regulated between the 2 phenotypes, and the most commonly expressed miRNAs were involved in cell regulation and apoptosis. In addition, between the 2 groups, 23 miRNAs were exclusively regulated in young mice, 12 exclusively in old mice, and 12 in both age groups. This indicates that ovarian age has a differential impact on gene expression depending on age and genotype [105]. Some miRNAs in MII oocytes play a role in controlling pluripotency, chromatin remodeling, and early embryo development; altered regulation of these miRNA may be related to ovarian aging [106]. Another method of posttranscriptional modification comes via the *TAF4B* gene. *TAF4B* codes for a protein of the same name, which is a component of a large ovarian protein complex required for fertility in mice. The deficiency of the gene that produces TAF4B leads to a rapid decline in oocyte quantity and POI. This appears to occur by reducing transcription of mov10 like RISC complex RNA helicase (*MOV10L1*), an RNA helicase; this demonstrates that TAF4B plays a role in posttranscriptional control of gene regulation in the ovary [107].

When a critical level of oocyte depletion is reached, menopause occurs. Mouse models have been developed to aid in this study and in order to attempt to mimic the physiologic changes of menopause. In mice, the kit receptor is part of a critical signaling apparatus in primordial germ cells, which start in the primordial streak and migrate to the genital ridges [108]. A mouse model with c-kit knockout mice leads to a substantial reduction in the number of germ cells as birth, to less than 5% of normal mice. These mice also experience altered cholesterol, gonadotropin, and steroid hormone levels, in addition to decreased bone density and cardiac function. As these changes mimic human menopause, this mouse model has the potential to become a valuable tool for future study [108].

2.2.3 Animal Models for Accelerated Folliculogenesis in Ovarian Aging

Insulin-like growth factor (IGF)-1 and FSH provide the primary survival signal to granulosa cells and suppress their apoptosis [109]. With aging, both IGF-1 production [110, 111] and the ability of estradiol to increase IGF-1 are reduced [112]. Knockout of mouse IGF-1 results in arrested folliculogenesis [113], suggesting that IGF-1 plays a role in ovarian aging. FSH, on the other hand, is the main hormone orchestrating folliculogenesis in the ovaries [114]. Knocking out FSH receptors in mouse models (FORKO) leads to infertility mediated by severely impaired folliculogenesis [115].

The FOXO proteins are transcription factors that regulate granulosa cell survival. They participate in cell cycle arrest and apoptosis [116]. FOXO1 interacts with the activin pathway to promote IGF transcription and cell survival. Conversely, it interacts with the bone morphogenic protein-2 (BMP2) pathway to promote apoptosis. The balance of these interactions is critical for normal follicle development [117]. FOXO3A, on the other hand, regulates folliculogenesis by suppressing follicular growth [118]. *FOXO3A*-null mice exhibit accelerated primordial follicular depletion and experience early ovarian aging [119]. Interestingly, mice which are both *FOXO1*-null and *FOXO3*-null experience abnormal follicle development, reduced granulosa cell apoptosis, and reduced response to gonadotropins [117].

2.3 Female Reproductive Aging and the Hypothalamic-Pituitary Axis

The hallmark of female reproductive aging is the declining ovarian reserve. Final menstrual period is marked by the almost complete exhaustion of the ovarian follicular pool. However, changes in the hypothalamic pituitary axis have been documented long before any acyclicity becomes apparent, especially in rodent models. Ovaries from aged rats resume ovulation when transplanted to young oophorectomized rats [120];similarly, acyclic rats may start ovulating in response to external stimuli [121]. These findings suggest that hypothalamic/pituitary signals may actually start reproductive senescence. However, it should be kept in mind that there is a major difference between species in reproductive senescence. Rodents undergo acyclicity well before complete depletion of their oocytes, whereas primates stop menstruating following complete depletion. This section focuses on how the HPA affects female reproductive aging.

2.3.1 Neuroendocrine Changes

Earliest stages of reproductive aging in women are characterized by a decrease in inhibin B and AMH secretion from the ovaries. These changes are associated with loss of negative feedback on FSH that increases before any cycle irregularity ensues [122]. Although both serum and follicular fluid activin A levels increase with aging [122–124], these changes are not universal [125]. Increase in serum activin A does not necessarily correlate with FSH [126]. The fact that the effect of activins is offset readily by follistatin [124], due to almost irreversible binding kinetics of follistatin to activin, suggests that activin acts in a more autocrine/paracrine rather than endocrine fashion. The increase in serum FSH levels is not due to decrease in serum estradiol levels. Rather, estradiol increases during the mid- and late follicular phase of the menstrual cycle in the late reproductive stages [127] together with urinary estrogen metabolites [128]. These findings suggest that the secretory capacity of follicular unit is maintained in older women [129], possibly due to increased aromatase activity stimulated by a rise in FSH [130].

2.3.1.1 Rodents

During transition from cyclicity to acyclicity, LH release is temporally delayed and diminished in middle-aged rats [131]. This attenuation is temporally correlated to decrease in the GnRH gene expression during the proestrus [132]. Decrease in GnRH secretion is neither related to decreased number of GnRH neurons [131, 133] nor to a defective GnRH secretory process [134–136]. In fact, GnRH neuronal activation is reduced during this transition, in such a way that only half of the GnRH neurons express c-fos, marker of GnRH neuronal expression, in middle-aged rats compared to young rats [136]. Reduced sensitivity to vasoactive intestinal peptide (VIP), which carries the time of day information to GnRH neurons, may also be responsible for reduced activation of GnRH neurons [137]. IGF-1 receptor signaling may be necessary for GnRH activation under estrogen-positive feedback conditions. Hence, reduced IGF-1 signaling in middle-aged rats may also contribute to decreased GnRH activation [112]. Aging in rats is also associated with decreased glutamatergic input to GnRH neurons [138, 139], glutamatergic-mediated GnRH release [134], and glutamate receptor subunits expressed on GnRH neurons [140], all of which may contribute to attenuated GnRH neuronal activation. Gamma-aminobutyric acid (GABA) is the main inhibitory neurotransmitter in the central nervous system. GABAergic signaling is increased in middle-aged rats, possibly due to elevated levels of the enzyme GAD67 that synthesize GABA [141]. Moreover, the ratio of glutamatergic to GABAergic cells that regulate the GnRH neurons is increased in middle-aged rats [142], further contributing to inhibition of GnRH signaling. Noradrenaline (NE) concentrations increase in the preoptic area just before ovulation [143, 144]. Cells from this area project directly to GnRH neurons. Decrease in NE concentrations and increased NE turnover may also be responsible for decreased GnRH activation that leads to impaired LH release in middle-aged rats [145]. Brain estrogen receptor (ER) gene expression is also altered in aging rodents. Estrogens can feedback to GnRH neurons directly via ERβ (estrogen receptor beta) or indirectly via ERα/ERβ through glial interactions [146]. *ERα* gene expression is reduced in periventricular preoptic nucleus of old rats, whereas *ERβ* expression is reduced in the cortex and supraoptic nucleus of middle-aged irregularly cycling and old rats compared to young rats [147]. Kisspeptin is a neuropeptide important in the regulation of ovulation and follicular development through control of pulsatile release of GnRH [148]. When compared to young rats, kisspeptin-expressing cells are significantly reduced in aged rats in the arcuate nucleus, suggesting lowered kisspeptin expression with aging [149]. Moreover, the sensitivity of anteroventral periventricular kisspeptin neurons to estrogen-positive feedback may also be responsible for reduced kisspeptin secretion leading to delayed or absent LH release in middle-aged rats [150]. Unlike kisspeptin, RFamide-related peptide 3 (RFRP3) is found in the dorsal medial hypothalamus and acts to inhibit GnRH release [151–153]. *RFRP3* gene expression increases with aging in rats, which may lead to decrease in GnRH release [154].

Contrary to decrease in LH levels, FSH levels are elevated during this transition [155]. This increase can be attributed to decreasing inhibin levels, as well as alterations in GnRH secretion and pulsatility, similar to menopausal transition in humans. These studies suggest that the neuroendocrine control of GnRH secretion during middle age in female rats occurs through multiple transmitters at various levels, which culminate in decreased secretion in GnRH that leads to delayed and insufficient LH secretion resulting in acyclicity.

2.3.1.2 Primates and Humans

Majority of the menstrual cycles are anovulatory during the last 10 months before final menstrual period, despite normal or high estrogen levels. It has been hypothesized that the sensitivity to positive estrogen feedback is attenuated with aging. This has been suggested by diminished ability of exogenous estrogen to induce an LH surge [156]. Similarly, LH response to GnRH administration is also decreased [157, 158]. On the other hand, sensitivity to estrogen-negative feedback remains intact during the menopausal transition, as shown by suppression of FSH levels with exogenous estrogen administration [159, 160]. GnRH secretion undergoes changes with aging as well. In rhesus monkeys, pulsatile GnRH release, particularly GnRH pulse amplitude, is elevated during perimenopause, consistent with the decreased peripheral estradiol levels and the removal of negative feedback [161]. In postmenopausal women, the pulse amplitude but not the frequency of GnRH is higher when compared to premenopausal women [162]. Actually, GnRH pulse frequency has been shown to decrease in postmenopausal women, as demonstrated by measurements of gonadotropin free-α subunit [163]. Similar to rodent models, LH surges are found only in half of perimenopausal women who have estrogen peaks, suggesting that sensitivity to positive estrogen feedback is diminished [164]. There are also changes in the expression of kisspeptin in postmenopausal women. For example, the number, size, and gene expression of kisspeptin-secreting neurons in the infundibular nucleus are increased in postmenopausal women when compared to premenopausal women [165]. Similarly, kisspeptin and its receptor GPR54 [165] expression are increased in the medial basal hypothalamus in postmenopausal rhesus macaques when compared to premenopausal counterparts [166] and in the arcuate nucleus-median eminence of perimenopausal macaques compared to premenopausal macaques [167]. Finally, kisspeptin, kisspeptin receptor, *TAC3* (tachynin 3, a neurotransmitter, the mutation of which is associated with normosmic hypogonadotropic hypogonadism), and *NPY2R* (neuropeptide Y2 receptor, a central mediator of food intake) gene expression are increased in ovariectomized old female rhesus macaque arcuate-median eminence of hypothalamus when compared to ovariectomized young female macaques that were supplemented with estradiol [168]. These results suggest that even at old age, arcuate-median eminence is responsive to circulating estrogen levels.

2.3.2 Anatomic and Histologic Changes in the Hypothalamic/ Pituitary Axis

The nature of GnRH neuronal activity shows changes with advancing age in all species examined. These changes may be related to alterations in the number of GnRH neurons and/or their morphology, leading to modifications in the production, transport, and secretion of GnRH. However, most studies to date reported either no change in GnRH cell number, morphology or distribution [169, 170], or slight increase in the GnRH cell numbers with aging in female rats [171]. Similarly, no alterations were observed in mice [133] or rhesus macaques [172]. However, other studies reported a decrease, albeit small (<20%), in GnRH cell numbers in mice [173] and rats [174]. Similarly, the distribution of GnRH neurons is not affected with aging neither in rats [169] nor in monkeys [172]. These studies suggest that neither the number nor the distribution of GnRH neuronal cells play a major role in determining alterations in GnRH secretion with aging. GnRH neurons have a close physical relationship with glial cells, mainly astrocytes, allowing cell-to-cell communication. Interestingly, in the preoptic area, the relationship between GnRH perikarya and astrocytes may change with advancing age [175]. The glial apposition to GnRH neurons undergoes circadian fluctuations in proestrus in young but not in middle-aged rats, suggesting that loss of plasticity may contribute to the alterations seen in GnRH secretion. Tanycytes are special ependymal cells found in the third and on the floor of the fourth ventricle of the brain, with processes extending deep into the hypothalamus. They are involved in the transport and release of estrogen and GnRH in the median eminence [176]. They may also have phagocytic actions on degenerating neurons [177, 178] and have been shown to undergo morphological changes with aging in female rats [177]. With aging, tanycytes processes become thicker and disorganized in the pericapillary zone, and they lose their perpendicular orientation [179]. Gonadotropin inhibitory neurons are localized in the dorsomedial nucleus and project axons to GnRH neurons. There is an age-related decline in the gonadotropin inhibitory cell numbers. Moreover, the apposition of gonadotropin inhibitory neurons to GnRH neurons is lessened with aging [180]. Ultrastructural changes at the cellular level have also been observed in the GnRH neurons of rats. The rough endoplasmic reticulum and Golgi volume fractions are significantly lower in the GnRH neurons of middle-aged acyclic rats when compared to young cycling rats [181], suggesting that aging is associated with changes in protein synthesis in GnRH cells. GnRH fiber staining is reduced [182], and the number, area, and immunoreactivity of GnRH axons are decreased in the median eminence in old compared to young rats [183].

2.4 Conclusion

Female reproductive aging is a complex process that involves the hypothalamus, the pituitary, and the ovaries. Genetic, epigenetic, environmental, and metabolic factors as well as mitochondrial dysfunction, telomerases, oxidative stress, and others have been implicated in ovarian aging. Although accelerated ovarian follicular depletion is a hallmark of reproductive senescence, impending ovarian failure is not the only driving force behind the transition into reproductive quiescence. Emerging data in human and nonhuman models clearly argue for a role of the HPA in female reproductive aging, mainly related to changes in the neuronal synapses and ultrastructural changes in GnRH neurons. Although evidence suggests that central alterations in the HPA contribute to reproductive senescence, minimal translational research efforts directed toward delaying ovarian aging and improving the responsiveness of the HPA to ovarian steroids have been published. Further research in this area is suggested as a potential strategy that may offer potential for extending the reproductive life span of women and postponing the negative consequences of reproductive senescence.

References

1. Arias E, Heron M, Xu J. United States life tables, 2014. Natl Vital Stat Rep. 2017;66(4):1–64.
2. Shifren JL, Gass ML, Group NRfCCoMWW. The North American Menopause Society recommendations for clinical care of midlife women. Menopause. 2014;21(10):1038–62.

3. Nichols HB, Trentham-Dietz A, Hampton JM, Titus-Ernstoff L, Egan KM, Willett WC, et al. From menarche to menopause: trends among US women born from 1912 to 1969. Am J Epidemiol. 2006;164(10):1003–11.

4. Hall JE. Neuroendocrine changes with reproductive aging in women. Semin Reprod Med. 2007;25(5):344–51.

5. Downs JL, Wise PM. The role of the brain in female reproductive aging. Mol Cell Endocrinol. 2009;299(1):32–8.

6. Martin JA, Hamilton BE, Osterman MJ, Driscoll AK, Mathews TJ. Births: final data for 2015. Natl Vital Stat Rep. 2017;66(1):1.

7. Hodes-Wertz B, Druckenmiller S, Smith M, Noyes N. What do reproductive-age women who undergo oocyte cryopreservation think about the process as a means to preserve fertility? Fertil Steril. 2013;100(5):1343–9.

8. Heck KE, Schoendorf KC, Ventura SJ, Kiely JL. Delayed childbearing by education level in the United States, 1969-1994. Matern Child Health J. 1997;1(2):81–8.

9. Hammarberg K, Clarke VE. Reasons for delaying childbearing – a survey of women aged over 35 years seeking assisted reproductive technology. Aust Fam Physician. 2005;34(3):187–8, 206.

10. Centers for Disease Control and Prevention 2005-2014. Available from: https://www.cdc.gov/art/reports/archive.html.

11. Testing and interpreting measures of ovarian reserve: a committee opinion. Fertil Steril. 2015;103(3):e9–17.

12. Zuckerman S. The number of oocytes in the mature ovary. Recent Prog Horm Res. 1951;6:63–109.

13. Zuckerman S, Baker T. The development of the ovary and the process of oogenesis. Ovary. 1977;1:41–67.

14. Peters H. Migration of gonocytes into the mammalian gonad and their differentiation. Philos Trans R Soc Lond Ser B Biol Sci. 1970;259(828):91–101.

15. Johnson J, Bagley J, Skaznik-Wikiel M, Lee HJ, Adams GB, Niikura Y, et al. Oocyte generation in adult mammalian ovaries by putative germ cells in bone marrow and peripheral blood. Cell. 2005;122(2):303–15.

16. Johnson J, Canning J, Kaneko T, Pru JK, Tilly JL. Germline stem cells and follicular renewal in the postnatal mammalian ovary. Nature. 2004;428(6979):145–50.

17. Virant-Klun I, Rozman P, Cvjeticanin B, Vrtacnik-Bokal E, Novakovic S, Rulicke T, et al. Parthenogenetic embryo-like structures in the human ovarian surface epithelium cell culture in postmenopausal women with no naturally present follicles and oocytes. Stem Cells Dev. 2009;18(1):137–49.

18. Zhang D, Fouad H, Zoma WD, Salama SA, Wentz MJ, Al-Hendy A. Expression of stem and germ cell markers within nonfollicle structures in adult mouse ovary. Reprod Sci. 2008;15(2):139–46.

19. Ye H, Zheng T, Li W, Li X, Fu X, Huang Y, et al. Ovarian stem cell nests in reproduction and ovarian aging. Cell Physiol Biochem. 2017;43(5):1917–25.

20. Parte S, Bhartiya D, Telang J, Daithankar V, Salvi V, Zaveri K, et al. Detection, characterization, and spontaneous differentiation in vitro of very small embryonic-like putative stem cells in adult mammalian ovary. Stem Cells Dev. 2011;20(8):1451–64.

21. Virant-Klun I, Skutella T, Hren M, Gruden K, Cvjeticanin B, Vogler A, et al. Isolation of small SSEA-4-positive putative stem cells from the ovarian surface epithelium of adult human ovaries by two different methods. Biomed Res Int. 2013;2013:690415.

22. White YA, Woods DC, Takai Y, Ishihara O, Seki H, Tilly JL. Oocyte formation by mitotically active germ cells purified from ovaries of reproductive-age women. Nat Med. 2012;18(3):413–21.

23. Santoro N. The menopausal transition. The American journal of medicine. 2005;118(Suppl 12B):8–13.

24. Faddy MJ, Gosden RG, Gougeon A, Richardson SJ, Nelson JF. Accelerated disappearance of ovarian follicles in mid-life: implications for forecasting menopause. Hum Reprod. 1992;7(10):1342–6.

25. Hansen KR, Knowlton NS, Thyer AC, Charleston JS, Soules MR, Klein NA. A new model of reproductive aging: the decline in ovarian non-growing follicle number from birth to menopause. Hum Reprod. 2008;23(3):699–708.
26. Wu JM, Zelinski MB, Ingram DK, Ottinger MA. Ovarian aging and menopause: current theories, hypotheses, and research models. Exp Biol Med (Maywood). 2005;230(11):818–28.
27. Lenton EA, Landgren BM, Sexton L, Harper R. Normal variation in the length of the follicular phase of the menstrual cycle: effect of chronological age. Br J Obstet Gynaecol. 1984;91(7):681–4.
28. van Montfrans JM, Hoek A, van Hooff MH, de Koning CH, Tonch N, Lambalk CB. Predictive value of basal follicle-stimulating hormone concentrations in a general subfertility population. Fertil Steril. 2000;74(1):97–103.
29. van Rooij IA, Broekmans FJ, Scheffer GJ, Looman CW, Habbema JD, de Jong FH, et al. Serum antimullerian hormone levels best reflect the reproductive decline with age in normal women with proven fertility: a longitudinal study. Fertil Steril. 2005;83(4):979–87.
30. Seifer DB, Lambert-Messerlian G, Hogan JW, Gardiner AC, Blazar AS, Berk CA. Day 3 serum inhibin-B is predictive of assisted reproductive technologies outcome. Fertil Steril. 1997;67(1):110–4.
31. Santoro N, Isaac B, Neal-Perry G, Adel T, Weingart L, Nussbaum A, et al. Impaired folliculogenesis and ovulation in older reproductive aged women. J Clin Endocrinol Metab. 2003;88(11):5502–9.
32. Pellatt L, Rice S, Dilaver N, Heshri A, Galea R, Brincat M, et al. Anti-Mullerian hormone reduces follicle sensitivity to follicle-stimulating hormone in human granulosa cells. Fertil Steril. 2011;96(5):1246–51 e1.
33. Sowers MR, Eyvazzadeh AD, McConnell D, Yosef M, Jannausch ML, Zhang D, et al. Anti-mullerian hormone and inhibin B in the definition of ovarian aging and the menopause transition. J Clin Endocrinol Metab. 2008;93(9):3478–83.
34. van Rooij IA, Tonkelaar I, Broekmans FJ, Looman CW, Scheffer GJ, de Jong FH, et al. Anti-mullerian hormone is a promising predictor for the occurrence of the menopausal transition. Menopause. 2004;11(6 Pt 1):601–6.
35. Welt CK, McNicholl DJ, Taylor AE, Hall JE. Female reproductive aging is marked by decreased secretion of dimeric inhibin. J Clin Endocrinol Metab. 1999;84(1):105–11.
36. Steiner AZ, Pritchard D, Stanczyk FZ, Kesner JS, Meadows JW, Herring AH, et al. Association between biomarkers of ovarian reserve and infertility among older women of reproductive age. JAMA. 2017;318(14):1367–76.
37. Majumder K, Gelbaya TA, Laing I, Nardo LG. The use of anti-Mullerian hormone and antral follicle count to predict the potential of oocytes and embryos. Eur J Obstet Gynecol Reprod Biol. 2010;150(2):166–70.
38. Blazar AS, Lambert-Messerlian G, Hackett R, Krotz S, Carson SA, Robins JC. Use of in-cycle antimullerian hormone levels to predict cycle outcome. Am J Obstet Gynecol. 2011;205(3):223. e1–5.
39. Anckaert E, Smitz J, Schiettecatte J, Klein BM, Arce JC. The value of anti-Mullerian hormone measurement in the long GnRH agonist protocol: association with ovarian response and gonadotrophin-dose adjustments. Hum Reprod. 2012;27(6):1829–39.
40. Kotanidis L, Nikolettos K, Petousis S, Asimakopoulos B, Chatzimitrou E, Kolios G, et al. The use of serum anti-Mullerian hormone (AMH) levels and antral follicle count (AFC) to predict the number of oocytes collected and availability of embryos for cryopreservation in IVF. J Endocrinol Investig. 2016;39(12):1459–64.
41. van Disseldorp J, Lambalk CB, Kwee J, Looman CW, Eijkemans MJ, Fauser BC, et al. Comparison of inter- and intra-cycle variability of anti-Mullerian hormone and antral follicle counts. Hum Reprod. 2010;25(1):221–7.
42. Gougeon A, Chainy GB. Morphometric studies of small follicles in ovaries of women at different ages. J Reprod Fertil. 1987;81(2):433–42.
43. Jayaprakasan K, Campbell B, Hopkisson J, Johnson I, Raine-Fenning N. A prospective, comparative analysis of anti-Mullerian hormone, inhibin-B, and three-dimensional ultrasound determinants of ovarian reserve in the prediction of poor response to controlled ovarian stimulation. Fertil Steril. 2010;93(3):855–64.

44. Jiang JY, Cheung CK, Wang Y, Tsang BK. Regulation of cell death and cell survival gene expression during ovarian follicular development and atresia. Front Biosci. 2003;8:d222–37.
45. Tilly JL, Kowalski KI, Johnson AL, Hsueh AJ. Involvement of apoptosis in ovarian follicular atresia and postovulatory regression. Endocrinology. 1991;129(5):2799–801.
46. Regan SLP, Knight PG, Yovich JL, Stanger JD, Leung Y, Arfuso F, et al. The effect of ovarian reserve and receptor signalling on granulosa cell apoptosis during human follicle development. Mol Cell Endocrinol. 2018;470:219–27.
47. Burger HG, Hale GE, Dennerstein L, Robertson DM. Cycle and hormone changes during perimenopause: the key role of ovarian function. Menopause. 2008;15(4 Pt 1):603–12.
48. Titus S, Li F, Stobezki R, Akula K, Unsal E, Jeong K, et al. Impairment of BRCA1-related DNA double-strand break repair leads to ovarian aging in mice and humans. Sci Transl Med. 2013;5(172):172ra21.
49. Ben-Aharon I, Levi M, Margel D, Yerushalmi R, Rizel S, Perry S, et al. Premature ovarian aging in BRCA carriers: a prototype of systemic precocious aging? Oncotarget. 2018;9(22):15931–41.
50. Lin W, Titus S, Moy F, Ginsburg ES, Oktay K. Ovarian aging in women with BRCA germline mutations. J Clin Endocrinol Metab. 2017;102(10):3839–47.
51. Al-Edani T, Assou S, Ferrieres A, Bringer Deutsch S, Gala A, Lecellier CH, et al. Female aging alters expression of human cumulus cells genes that are essential for oocyte quality. Biomed Res Int. 2014;2014:964614.
52. Goldmann JM, Seplyarskiy VB, Wong WSW, Vilboux T, Neerincx PB, Bodian DL, et al. Germline de novo mutation clusters arise during oocyte aging in genomic regions with high double-strand-break incidence. Nat Genet. 2018;50(4):487–92.
53. Liang X, Ma J, Schatten H, Sun Q. Epigenetic changes associated with oocyte aging. Sci China Life Sci. 2012;55(8):670–6.
54. Yue M X, Fu X W, Zhou G B, et al. Abnormal DNA methylation in oocytes could be associated with a decrease in reproductive potential in old mice. J Assist Reprod Genet, 2012;29: 643–650.
55. Bonomi M, Somigliana E, Cacciatore C, Busnelli M, Rossetti R, Bonetti S, et al. Blood cell mitochondrial DNA content and premature ovarian aging. PLoS One. 2012;7(8):e42423.
56. Babayev E, Wang T, Szigeti-Buck K, Lowther K, Taylor HS, Horvath T, et al. Reproductive aging is associated with changes in oocyte mitochondrial dynamics, function, and mtDNA quantity. Maturitas. 2016;93:121–30.
57. Wang T, Zhang M, Jiang Z, Seli E. Mitochondrial dysfunction and ovarian aging. Am J Reprod Immunol. 2017;77(5):1–9.
58. Wang T, Babayev E, Jiang Z, Li G, Zhang M, Esencan E, et al. Mitochondrial unfolded protein response gene Clpp is required to maintain ovarian follicular reserve during aging, for oocyte competence, and development of pre-implantation embryos. Aging Cell. 2018;17:e12784.
59. Bentov Y, Yavorska T, Esfandiari N, Jurisicova A, Casper RF. The contribution of mitochondrial function to reproductive aging. J Assist Reprod Genet. 2011;28(9):773–83.
60. Ben-Meir A, Burstein E, Borrego-Alvarez A, Chong J, Wong E, Yavorska T, et al. Coenzyme Q10 restores oocyte mitochondrial function and fertility during reproductive aging. Aging Cell. 2015;14(5):887–95.
61. Kansaku K, Takeo S, Itami N, Kin A, Shirasuna K, Kuwayama T, et al. Maternal aging affects oocyte resilience to carbonyl cyanide-m-chlorophenylhydrazone -induced mitochondrial dysfunction in cows. PLoS One. 2017;12(11):e0188099.
62. Bentov Y, Casper RF. The aging oocyte – can mitochondrial function be improved? Fertil Steril. 2013;99(1):18–22.
63. Liu J, Liu M, Ye X, Liu K, Huang J, Wang L, et al. Delay in oocyte aging in mice by the anti-oxidant N-acetyl-L-cysteine (NAC). Hum Reprod. 2012;27(5):1411–20.
64. Goud AP, Goud PT, Diamond MP, Gonik B, Abu-Soud HM. Reactive oxygen species and oocyte aging: role of superoxide, hydrogen peroxide, and hypochlorous acid. Free Radic Biol Med. 2008;44(7):1295–304.

65. Wang T, Gao YY, Chen L, Nie ZW, Cheng W, Liu X, et al. Melatonin prevents postovulatory oocyte aging and promotes subsequent embryonic development in the pig. Aging (Albany NY). 2017;9(6):1552–64.
66. Bogliolo L, Murrone O, Di Emidio G, Piccinini M, Ariu F, Ledda S, et al. Raman spectroscopy-based approach to detect aging-related oxidative damage in the mouse oocyte. J Assist Reprod Genet. 2013;30(7):877–82.
67. Massasa E, Costa XS, Taylor HS. Failure of the stem cell niche rather than loss of oocyte stem cells in the aging ovary. Aging (Albany NY). 2010;2(1):1–2.
68. Bhartiya D, Singh J. FSH-FSHR3-stem cells in ovary surface epithelium: basis for adult ovarian biology, failure, aging, and cancer. Reproduction. 2015;149(1):R35–48.
69. Hosni W, Bastu E. Ovarian stem cells and aging. Climacteric. 2012;15(2):125–32.
70. Li J, Zhou F, Zheng T, Pan Z, Liang X, Huang J, et al. Ovarian germline stem cells (OGSCs) and the hippo signaling pathway association with physiological and pathological ovarian aging in mice. Cell Physiol Biochem. 2015;36(5):1712–24.
71. Ding C, Li H, Wang Y, Wang F, Wu H, Chen R, et al. Different therapeutic effects of cells derived from human amniotic membrane on premature ovarian aging depend on distinct cellular biological characteristics. Stem Cell Res Ther. 2017;8(1):173.
72. Morin GB. The human telomere terminal transferase enzyme is a ribonucleoprotein that synthesizes TTAGGG repeats. Cell. 1989;59(3):521–9.
73. Bayne S, Li H, Jones ME, Pinto AR, van Sinderen M, Drummond A, et al. Estrogen deficiency reversibly induces telomere shortening in mouse granulosa cells and ovarian aging in vivo. Protein Cell. 2011;2(4):333–46.
74. Valerio D, Luddi A, De Leo V, Labella D, Longobardi S, Piomboni P. SA1/SA2 cohesion proteins and SIRT1-NAD+ deacetylase modulate telomere homeostasis in cumulus cells and are eligible biomarkers of ovarian aging. Hum Reprod. 2018;33(5):887–94.
75. Li Q, Miao DQ, Zhou P, Wu YG, Gao D, Wei DL, et al. Glucose metabolism in mouse cumulus cells prevents oocyte aging by maintaining both energy supply and the intracellular redox potential. Biol Reprod. 2011;84(6):1111–8.
76. Zhang J, Fang L, Lu Z, Xiong J, Wu M, Shi L, et al. Are sirtuins markers of ovarian aging? Gene. 2016;575(2 Pt 3):680–6.
77. Ma R, Zhang Y, Zhang L, Han J, Rui R. Sirt1 protects pig oocyte against in vitro aging. Anim Sci J. 2015;86(9):826–32.
78. Mumusoglu S, Turan V, Uckan H, Suzer A, Sokmensuer LK, Bozdag G. The impact of a long-acting oral sphingosine-1-phosphate analogue on ovarian aging in a rat model. Reprod Sci. 2018;25(9):1330–5.
79. Sharara FI, Beatse SN, Leonardi MR, Navot D, Scott RT Jr. Cigarette smoking accelerates the development of diminished ovarian reserve as evidenced by the clomiphene citrate challenge test. Fertil Steril. 1994;62(2):257–62.
80. De Bruin ML, Van Dulmen-den Broeder E, Van den Berg MH, Lambalk CB. Fertility in female childhood cancer survivors. Endocr Dev. 2009;15:135–58.
81. Vermeulen A. Environment, human reproduction, menopause, and andropause. Environ Health Perspect. 1993;101(Suppl 2):91–100.
82. Thomas-Teinturier C, Allodji RS, Svetlova E, Frey MA, Oberlin O, Millischer AE, et al. Ovarian reserve after treatment with alkylating agents during childhood. Hum Reprod. 2015;30(6):1437–46.
83. Marder W, McCune WJ, Wang L, Wing JJ, Fisseha S, McConnell DS, et al. Adjunctive GnRH-a treatment attenuates depletion of ovarian reserve associated with cyclophosphamide therapy in premenopausal SLE patients. Gynecol Endocrinol. 2012;28(8):624–7.
84. Hoyer PB, Cannady EA, Kroeger NA, Sipes IG. Mechanisms of ovotoxicity induced by environmental chemicals: 4-vinylcyclohexene diepoxide as a model chemical. Adv Exp Med Biol. 2001;500:73–81.

85. Roosa KA, Mukai M, Place NJ. 4-Vinylcyclohexene diepoxide reduces fertility in female Siberian hamsters when treated during their reproductively active and quiescent states. Reprod Toxicol. 2015;51:40–6.
86. Hsu SY, Lai RJ, Finegold M, Hsueh AJ. Targeted overexpression of Bcl-2 in ovaries of transgenic mice leads to decreased follicle apoptosis, enhanced folliculogenesis, and increased germ cell tumorigenesis. Endocrinology. 1996;137(11):4837–43.
87. Kappeler CJ, Hoyer PB. 4-vinylcyclohexene diepoxide: a model chemical for ovotoxicity. Syst Biol Reprod Med. 2012;58(1):57–62.
88. Holehan AM, Merry BJ. Lifetime breeding studies in fully fed and dietary restricted female CFY Sprague-Dawley rats. 1. Effect of age, housing conditions and diet on fecundity. Mech Ageing Dev. 1985;33(1):19–28.
89. Shi LY, Luo AY, Tian Y, Lai ZW, Zhang JJ, Wang SX. Protective effects of caloric restriction on ovarian function. Zhonghua Fu Chan Ke Za Zhi. 2013;48(10):745–9.
90. Tilly JL, Sinclair DA. Germline energetics, aging, and female infertility. Cell Metab. 2013;17(6):838–50.
91. Cordeiro FB, Montani DA, Pilau EJ, Gozzo FC, Fraietta R, Turco EGL. Ovarian environment aging: follicular fluid lipidomic and related metabolic pathways. J Assist Reprod Genet. 2018;35(8):1385–93.
92. Miao YL, Sun QY, Zhang X, Zhao JG, Zhao MT, Spate L, et al. Centrosome abnormalities during porcine oocyte aging. Environ Mol Mutagen. 2009;50(8):666–71.
93. Jiang GJ, Wang K, Miao DQ, Guo L, Hou Y, Schatten H, et al. Protein profile changes during porcine oocyte aging and effects of caffeine on protein expression patterns. PLoS One. 2011;6(12):e28996.
94. Zhang X, Liu X, Chen L, Wu DY, Nie ZW, Gao YY, et al. Caffeine delays oocyte aging and maintains the quality of aged oocytes safely in mouse. Oncotarget. 2017;8(13):20602–11.
95. Wilcox A, Weinberg C, Baird D. Caffeinated beverages and decreased fertility. Lancet. 1988;332(8626):1453–6.
96. Hatch EE, Bracken MB. Association of delayed conception with caffeine consumption. Am J Epidemiol. 1993;138(12):1082–92.
97. IS L, Jensen A, Juul KE, Kesmodel US, Frederiksen K, Kjaer SK, et al. Coffee, tea and caffeine consumption and risk of primary infertility in women: a Danish cohort study. Acta Obstet Gynecol Scand. 2018;97(5):570–6.
98. Chavarro JE, Rich-Edwards JW, Rosner BA, Willett WC. Caffeinated and alcoholic beverage intake in relation to ovulatory disorder infertility. Epidemiology. 2009;20(3):374–81.
99. Olsen J. Cigarette smoking, tea and coffee drinking, and subfecundity. Am J Epidemiol. 1991;133(7):734–9.
100. Gaskins AJ, Chavarro JE. Diet and fertility: a review. Am J Obstet Gynecol. 2018;218(4):379–89.
101. Ricci E, Noli S, Cipriani S, La Vecchia I, Chiaffarino F, Ferrari S, et al. Maternal and paternal caffeine intake and ART outcomes in couples referring to an Italian fertility clinic: a prospective cohort. Nutrients. 2018;17(8):1–9.
102. Selby CP, Sancar A. Molecular mechanisms of DNA repair inhibition by caffeine. Proc Natl Acad Sci U S A. 1990;87(9):3522–5.
103. Chen LW, Fitzgerald R, Murrin CM, Mehegan J, Kelleher CC, Phillips CM, et al. Associations of maternal caffeine intake with birth outcomes: results from the Lifeways Cross Generation Cohort Study. Am J Clin Nutr. 2018;108(6):1301–8.
104. Shen M, Qi C, Kuang YP, Yang Y, Lyu QF, Long H, et al. Observation of the influences of diosgenin on aging ovarian reserve and function in a mouse model. Eur J Med Res. 2017;22(1):42.
105. Schneider A, Matkovich SJ, Victoria B, Spinel L, Bartke A, Golusinski P, et al. Changes of ovarian microRNA profile in long-living Ames Dwarf mice during aging. PLoS One. 2017;12(1):e0169213.
106. Battaglia R, Vento ME, Ragusa M, Barbagallo D, La Ferlita A, Di Emidio G, et al. MicroRNAs are stored in human MII oocyte and their expression profile changes in reproductive aging. Biol Reprod. 2016;95(6):131.

107. Lovasco LA, Seymour KA, Zafra K, O'Brien CW, Schorl C, Freiman RN. Accelerated ovarian aging in the absence of the transcription regulator TAF4B in mice. Biol Reprod. 2010;82(1):23–34.
108. Smith ER, Yeasky T, Wei JQ, Miki RA, Cai KQ, Smedberg JL, et al. White spotting variant mouse as an experimental model for ovarian aging and menopausal biology. Menopause. 2012;19(5):588–96.
109. Chun SY, Billig H, Tilly JL, Furuta I, Tsafriri A, Hsueh AJ. Gonadotropin suppression of apoptosis in cultured preovulatory follicles: mediatory role of endogenous insulin-like growth factor I. Endocrinology. 1994;135(5):1845–53.
110. Bartke A, Chandrashekar V, Dominici F, Turyn D, Kinney B, Steger R, et al. Insulin-like growth factor 1 (IGF-1) and aging: controversies and new insights. Biogerontology. 2003;4(1):1–8.
111. Wilshire GB, Loughlin JS, Brown JR, Adel TE, Santoro N. Diminished function of the somato-tropic axis in older reproductive-aged women. J Clin Endocrinol Metab. 1995;80(2):608–13.
112. Todd BJ, Merhi ZO, Shu J, Etgen AM, Neal-Perry GS. Hypothalamic insulin-like growth factor-I receptors are necessary for hormone-dependent luteinizing hormone surges: implications for female reproductive aging. Endocrinology. 2010;151(3):1356–66.
113. Baker J, Hardy MP, Zhou J, Bondy C, Lupu F, Bellve AR, et al. Effects of an Igf1 gene null mutation on mouse reproduction. Mol Endocrinol. 1996;10(7):903–18.
114. Billig H, Furuta I, Hsueh AJ. Gonadotropin-releasing hormone directly induces apoptotic cell death in the rat ovary: biochemical and in situ detection of deoxyribonucleic acid fragmentation in granulosa cells. Endocrinology. 1994;134(1):245–52.
115. Yang Y, Balla A, Danilovich N, Sairam MR. Developmental and molecular aberrations associated with deterioration of oogenesis during complete or partial follicle-stimulating hormone receptor deficiency in mice. Biol Reprod. 2003;69(4):1294–302.
116. Hosaka T, Biggs WH 3rd, Tieu D, Boyer AD, Varki NM, Cavenee WK, et al. Disruption of forkhead transcription factor (FOXO) family members in mice reveals their functional diversification. Proc Natl Acad Sci U S A. 2004;101(9):2975–80.
117. Liu Z, Castrillon DH, Zhou W, Richards JS. FOXO1/3 depletion in granulosa cells alters follicle growth, death and regulation of pituitary FSH. Mol Endocrinol. 2013;27(2):238–52.
118. Brenkman AB, Burgering BM. FoxO3a eggs on fertility and aging. Trends Mol Med. 2003;9(11):464–7.
119. Castrillon DH, Miao L, Kollipara R, Horner JW, DePinho RA. Suppression of ovarian follicle activation in mice by the transcription factor Foxo3a. Science. 2003;301(5630):215–8.
120. Krohn PL. Ovarian homotransplantation. Ann N Y Acad Sci. 1955;59(3):443–7.
121. Huang HH, Meites J. Reproductive capacity of aging female rats. Neuroendocrinology. 1975;17(4):289–95.
122. Reame NE, Wyman TL, Phillips DJ, de Kretser DM, Padmanabhan V. Net increase in stimulatory input resulting from a decrease in inhibin B and an increase in activin A may contribute in part to the rise in follicular phase follicle-stimulating hormone of aging cycling women. J Clin Endocrinol Metab. 1998;83(9):3302–7.
123. Santoro N, Adel T, Skurnick JH. Decreased inhibin tone and increased activin A secretion characterize reproductive aging in women. Fertil Steril. 1999;71(4):658–62.
124. Klein NA, Battaglia DE, Woodruff TK, Padmanabhan V, Giudice LC, Bremner WJ, et al. Ovarian follicular concentrations of activin, follistatin, inhibin, insulin-like growth factor I (IGF-I), IGF-II, IGF-binding protein-2 (IGFBP-2), IGFBP-3, and vascular endothelial growth factor in spontaneous menstrual cycles of normal women of advanced reproductive age. J Clin Endocrinol Metab. 2000;85(12):4520–5.
125. Muttukrishna S, Fowler PA, Groome NP, Mitchell GG, Robertson WR, Knight PG. Serum concentrations of dimeric inhibin during the spontaneous human menstrual cycle and after treatment with exogenous gonadotrophin. Hum Reprod. 1994;9(9):1634–42.
126. Baccarelli A, Morpurgo PS, Corsi A, Vaghi I, Fanelli M, Cremonesi G, et al. Activin A serum levels and aging of the pituitary-gonadal axis: a cross-sectional study in middle-aged and elderly healthy subjects. Exp Gerontol. 2001;36(8):1403–12.

127. Klein NA, Battaglia DE, Fujimoto VY, Davis GS, Bremner WJ, Soules MR. Reproductive aging: accelerated ovarian follicular development associated with a monotropic follicle-stimulating hormone rise in normal older women. J Clin Endocrinol Metab. 1996;81(3):1038–45.

128. Landgren BM, Collins A, Csemiczky G, Burger HG, Baksheev L, Robertson DM. Menopause transition: annual changes in serum hormonal patterns over the menstrual cycle in women during a nine-year period prior to menopause. J Clin Endocrinol Metab. 2004;89(6):2763–9.

129. Hansen KR, Thyer AC, Sluss PM, Bremner WJ, Soules MR, Klein NA. Reproductive ageing and ovarian function: is the early follicular phase FSH rise necessary to maintain adequate secretory function in older ovulatory women? Hum Reprod. 2005;20(1):89–95.

130. Welt CK, Jimenez Y, Sluss PM, Smith PC, Hall JE. Control of estradiol secretion in reproductive ageing. Hum Reprod. 2006;21(8):2189–93.

131. Lloyd JM, Hoffman GE, Wise PM. Decline in immediate early gene expression in gonadotropin-releasing hormone neurons during proestrus in regularly cycling, middle-aged rats. Endocrinology. 1994;134(4):1800–5.

132. Gore AC, Oung T, Yung S, Flagg RA, Woller MJ. Neuroendocrine mechanisms for reproductive senescence in the female rat: gonadotropin-releasing hormone neurons. Endocrine. 2000;13(3):315–23.

133. Hoffman GE, Finch CE. LHRH neurons in the female C57BL/6J mouse brain during reproductive aging: no loss up to middle age. Neurobiol Aging. 1986;7(1):45–8.

134. Zuo Z, Mahesh VB, Zamorano PL, Brann DW. Decreased gonadotropin-releasing hormone neurosecretory response to glutamate agonists in middle-aged female rats on proestrus afternoon: a possible role in reproductive aging? Endocrinology. 1996;137(6):2334–8.

135. Rubin BS. Naloxone stimulates comparable release of luteinizing hormone-releasing hormone from tissue fragments from ovariectomized, estrogen-treated young and middle-aged female rats. Brain Res. 1993;601(1–2):246–54.

136. Le WW, Wise PM, Murphy AZ, Coolen LM, Hoffman GE. Parallel declines in Fos activation of the medial anteroventral periventricular nucleus and LHRH neurons in middle-aged rats. Endocrinology. 2001;142(11):4976–82.

137. Krajnak K, Rosewell KL, Wise PM. Fos-induction in gonadotropin-releasing hormone neurons receiving vasoactive intestinal polypeptide innervation is reduced in middle-aged female rats. Biol Reprod. 2001;64(4):1160–4.

138. Brann DW, Zamorano PL, De Sevilla L, Mahesh VB. Expression of glutamate receptor subunits in the hypothalamus of the female rat during the afternoon of the proestrous luteinizing hormone surge and effects of antiprogestin treatment and aging. Neuroendocrinology. 2005;81(2):120–8.

139. Neal-Perry GS, Zeevalk GD, Santoro NF, Etgen AM. Attenuation of preoptic area glutamate release correlates with reduced luteinizing hormone secretion in middle-aged female rats. Endocrinology. 2005;146(10):4331–9.

140. Gore AC, Yeung G, Morrison JH, Oung T. Neuroendocrine aging in the female rat: the changing relationship of hypothalamic gonadotropin-releasing hormone neurons and N-methyl-D-aspartate receptors. Endocrinology. 2000;141(12):4757–67.

141. Grove-Strawser D, Jimenez-Linan M, Rubin BS. Middle-aged female rats lack the dynamic changes in GAD(67) mRNA levels observed in young females on the day of a luteinising hormone surge. J Neuroendocrinol. 2007;19(9):708–16.

142. Khan M, De Sevilla L, Mahesh VB, Brann DW. Enhanced glutamatergic and decreased GABAergic synaptic appositions to GnRH neurons on proestrus in the rat: modulatory effect of aging. PLoS One. 2010;5(4):e10172.

143. Mohankumar PS, Thyagarajan S, Quadri SK. Tyrosine hydroxylase and DOPA decarboxylase activities in the medial preoptic area and arcuate nucleus during the estrous cycle: effects of aging. Brain Res Bull. 1997;42(4):265–71.

144. Szawka RE, Poletini MO, Leite CM, Bernuci MP, Kalil B, Mendonca LB, et al. Release of norepinephrine in the preoptic area activates anteroventral periventricular nucleus neurons and stimulates the surge of luteinizing hormone. Endocrinology. 2013;154(1):363–74.

145. Ferreira LB, de Nicola AC, Anselmo-Franci JA, Dornelles RC. Activity of neurons in the preoptic area and their participation in reproductive senescence: preliminary findings. Exp Gerontol. 2015;72:157–61.
146. Herbison AE, Pape JR. New evidence for estrogen receptors in gonadotropin-releasing hormone neurons. Front Neuroendocrinol. 2001;22(4):292–308.
147. Wilson ME, Rosewell KL, Kashon ML, Shughrue PJ, Merchenthaler I, Wise PM. Age differentially influences estrogen receptor-alpha (ERalpha) and estrogen receptor-beta (ERbeta) gene expression in specific regions of the rat brain. Mech Ageing Dev. 2002;123(6):593–601.
148. Lehman MN, Coolen LM, Goodman RL. Minireview: kisspeptin/neurokinin B/dynorphin (KNDy) cells of the arcuate nucleus: a central node in the control of gonadotropin-releasing hormone secretion. Endocrinology. 2010;151(8):3479–89.
149. Iwata K, Ikehara M, Kunimura Y, Ozawa H. Interactions between kisspeptin neurons and hypothalamic tuberoinfundibular dopaminergic neurons in aged female rats. Acta Histochem Cytochem. 2016;49(6):191–6.
150. Ishii MN, Matsumoto K, Matsui H, Seki N, Matsumoto H, Ishikawa K, et al. Reduced responsiveness of kisspeptin neurons to estrogenic positive feedback associated with age-related disappearance of LH surge in middle-age female rats. Gen Comp Endocrinol. 2013;193:121–9.
151. Ukena K, Tsutsui K. Distribution of novel RFamide-related peptide-like immunoreactivity in the mouse central nervous system. Neurosci Lett. 2001;300(3):153–6.
152. Ukena K, Iwakoshi E, Minakata H, Tsutsui K. A novel rat hypothalamic RFamide-related peptide identified by immunoaffinity chromatography and mass spectrometry. FEBS Lett. 2002;512(1–3):255–8.
153. Kriegsfeld LJ, Gibson EM, Williams WP 3rd, Zhao S, Mason AO, Bentley GE, et al. The roles of RFamide-related peptide-3 in mammalian reproductive function and behaviour. J Neuroendocrinol. 2010;22(7):692–700.
154. Geraghty AC, Muroy SE, Kriegsfeld LJ, Bentley GE, Kaufer D. The role of RFamide-related peptide-3 in age-related reproductive decline in female rats. Front Endocrinol (Lausanne). 2016;7:71.
155. DePaolo LV. Age-associated increases in serum follicle-stimulating hormone levels on estrus are accompanied by a reduction in the ovarian secretion of inhibin. Exp Aging Res. 1987;13(1–2):3–7.
156. van Look PF, Lothian H, Hunter WM, Michie EA, Baird DT. Hypothalamic-pituitary-ovarian function in perimenopausal women. Clin Endocrinol. 1977;7(1):13–31.
157. Fujimoto VY, Spencer SJ, Rabinovici J, Plosker S, Jaffe RB. Endogenous catecholamines augment the inhibitory effect of opioids on luteinizing hormone secretion during the midluteal phase. Am J Obstet Gynecol. 1993;169(6):1524–30.
158. Shaw ND, Srouji SS, Histed SN, McCurnin KE, Hall JE. Aging attenuates the pituitary response to gonadotropin-releasing hormone. J Clin Endocrinol Metab. 2009;94(9): 3259–64.
159. Shideler SE, DeVane GW, Kalra PS, Benirschke K, Lasley BL. Ovarian-pituitary hormone interactions during the perimenopause. Maturitas. 1989;11(4):331–9.
160. Santoro N, Brown JR, Adel T, Skurnick JH. Characterization of reproductive hormonal dynamics in the perimenopause. J Clin Endocrinol Metab. 1996;81(4):1495–501.
161. Gore AC, Windsor-Engnell BM, Terasawa E. Menopausal increases in pulsatile gonadotropin-releasing hormone release in a nonhuman primate (Macaca mulatta). Endocrinology. 2004;145(10):4653–9.
162. Rossmanith WG. Gonadotropin secretion during aging in women: review article. Exp Gerontol. 1995;30(3–4):369–81.
163. Hall JE, Lavoie HB, Marsh EE, Martin KA. Decrease in gonadotropin-releasing hormone (GnRH) pulse frequency with aging in postmenopausal women. J Clin Endocrinol Metab. 2000;85(5):1794–800.
164. Weiss G, Skurnick JH, Goldsmith LT, Santoro NF, Park SJ. Menopause and hypothalamic-pituitary sensitivity to estrogen. JAMA. 2004;292(24):2991–6.

165. Rance NE. Menopause and the human hypothalamus: evidence for the role of kiss-peptin/neurokinin B neurons in the regulation of estrogen negative feedback. Peptides. 2009;30(1):111–22.
166. Kim W, Jessen HM, Auger AP, Terasawa E. Postmenopausal increase in KiSS-1, GPR54, and luteinizing hormone releasing hormone (LHRH-1) mRNA in the basal hypothalamus of female rhesus monkeys. Peptides. 2009;30(1):103–10.
167. Eghlidi DH, Haley GE, Noriega NC, Kohama SG, Urbanski HF. Influence of age and 17beta-estradiol on kisspeptin, neurokinin B, and prodynorphin gene expression in the arcuate-median eminence of female rhesus macaques. Endocrinology. 2010;151(8):3783–94.
168. Eghlidi DH, Urbanski HF. Effects of age and estradiol on gene expression in the rhesus macaque hypothalamus. Neuroendocrinology. 2015;101(3):236–45.
169. Rubin BS, King JC, Bridges RS. Immunoreactive forms of luteinizing hormone-releasing hormone in the brains of aging rats exhibiting persistent vaginal estrus. Biol Reprod. 1984;31(2):343–51.
170. Miller BH, Gore AC. N-methyl-D-aspartate receptor subunit expression in GnRH neurons changes during reproductive senescence in the female rat. Endocrinology. 2002;143(9):3568–74.
171. Merchenthaler I, Lengvari I, Horvath J, Setalo G. Immunohistochemical study of the LHRH-synthesizing neuron system of aged female rats. Cell Tissue Res. 1980;209(3):499–503.
172. Witkin JW. Luteinizing hormone releasing hormone (LHRH) neurons in aging female rhesus macaques. Neurobiol Aging. 1986;7(4):259–63.
173. Miller MM, Joshi D, Billiar RB, Nelson JF. Loss of LH-RH neurons in the rostral forebrain of old female C57BL/6J mice. Neurobiol Aging. 1990;11(3):217–21.
174. Funabashi T, Kimura F. The number of luteinizing hormone-releasing hormone immunoreac-tive neurons is significantly decreased in the forebrain of old-aged female rats. Neurosci Lett. 1995;189(2):85–8.
175. Cashion AB, Smith MJ, Wise PM. The morphometry of astrocytes in the rostral preoptic area exhibits a diurnal rhythm on proestrus: relationship to the luteinizing hormone surge and effects of age. Endocrinology. 2003;144(1):274–80.
176. Akmayev IG, Fidelina OV. Tanycytes and their relation to the hypophyseal gonadotrophic function. Brain Res. 1981;210(1–2):253–60.
177. Brawer JR, Walsh RJ. Response of tanycytes to aging in the median eminence of the rat. Am J Anat. 1982;163(3):247–56.
178. Zoli M, Ferraguti F, Frasoldati A, Biagini G, Agnati LF. Age-related alterations in tanycytes of the mediobasal hypothalamus of the male rat. Neurobiol Aging. 1995;16(1):77–83.
179. Yin W, Gore AC. The hypothalamic median eminence and its role in reproductive aging. Ann N Y Acad Sci. 2010;1204:113–22.
180. Soga T, Kitahashi T, Clarke IJ, Parhar IS. Gonadotropin-inhibitory hormone promoter-driven enhanced green fluorescent protein expression decreases during aging in female rats. Endocrinology. 2014;155(5):1944–55.
181. Romero MT, Silverman AJ, Wise PM, Witkin JW. Ultrastructural changes in gonadotropin-releasing hormone neurons as a function of age and ovariectomy in rats. Neuroscience. 1994;58(1):217–25.
182. Hoffman GE, Sladek JR Jr. Age-related changes in dopamine, LHRH and somatostatin in the rat hypothalamus. Neurobiol Aging. 1980;1(1):27–37.
183. Bestetti GE, Reymond MJ, Blanc F, Boujon CE, Furrer B, Rossi GL. Functional and morpho-logical changes in the hypothalamo-pituitary-gonadal axis of aged female rats. Biol Reprod. 1991;45(2):221–8.

Chapter 3
Natural History of Diminished Ovarian Reserve

Orhan Bukulmez

3.1 Oocyte Endowment Models: Fixed Versus Stem Cell Model

There are two schools of thought about oocyte development in relevance to reproductive life span of females. The current teaching is based on the "fixed model." The alternate hypothesis is the "stem cell model."

Per the fixed model, in human females the number of oocytes in the ovaries is determined during fetal life. At around 20 weeks of gestation, the number of oocytes reaches 6–7 million. After attaining such a peak, lifelong decrease in oocytes ensues [1, 2]. At birth, this number may decline to 1–2 million and to 500,000–300,000 by puberty. The oocyte numbers decrease due to ongoing growth of primordial follicles, and most primordial follicles demise before even reaching antral follicle stage through apoptosis [3]. The oocyte or primordial follicle numbers show profound variation among females. Some models also predict that the rate of decrease in primordial follicles, rather than showing sudden increase in decline rate, shows a constantly increasing rate over the years [4].

Tilly's group postulated the stem cell model. They demonstrated the presence of ovarian stem cells (OSC) in juvenile and adult mice. These cells were mitotically active to assure oocyte production after birth [5]. This hypothesis is based on the observation that there was a conflict between the reproductive period and the follicle diminution rate. Busulfan-treated mice still showed healthy growing ovarian follicles. Also, when ovarian grafts obtained from adult wild-type mice were placed into the ovaries of green fluorescent protein (GFP)-expressing transgenic mice, the wild-type mice grafts showed GFP-positive oocytes but GFP negative granulosa

O. Bukulmez (✉)
Division of Reproductive Endocrinology and Infertility, Fertility and Advanced Reproductive Medicine Assisted Reproductive Technologies Program, Department of Obstetrics and Gynecology, University of Texas Southwestern Medical Center, Dallas, TX, USA
e-mail: Orhan.Bukulmez@UTSouthwestern.edu

© Springer Nature Switzerland AG 2020
O. Bukulmez (ed.), *Diminished Ovarian Reserve and Assisted Reproductive Technologies*, https://doi.org/10.1007/978-3-030-23235-1_3

cells. This finding suggested that OSCs from GFP-positive mice migrated into the graft developing follicles using adult mice granulosa cells. A lot of controversies followed the initial publication with some authors criticizing the methodology and presenting some other data supporting rather the fixed model in mice [6]. Then the presence of OSCs in the bone marrow of adult mice was demonstrated by germ cell markers (Oct4, MVH, Dazl, Stella, Fragilis). These cells in the bone marrow were observed to lead to the development of new ovarian follicles in mice sterilized by the alkylating agents, cyclophosphamide and busulfan. Similar experiments were also performed by transplanting the bone marrow from GFP mice to alkylating agent-sterilized mice with resulting offspring [7–9].

Female aging, however, influences both models. In fixed model, with female aging the number of primordial follicles decrease throughout the years from puberty to menopause when the number of primordial follicles with primary oocytes is estimated to be 1000–2000, while the regular ovarian follicular activity comes to a stop [10]. Per stem cell model, postnatal oocyte reserve may not be a finite entity at birth since the oogonial stem cells may constantly contribute to the ovarian reserve over the female reproductive life span. However, stem cell model also acknowledges that OSC function declines with age. In a recent paper, Tilly's group postulated that "depletion of oocyte pool in female mammals with age, which appears to result from a combination of oocyte loss through growth activation followed by ovulation or atresia coupled with a progressive decline in new oocyte input...." The same researchers believe that this process can be reversed or prevented [11].

3.2   Decline in Ovarian Reserve Over Time

There is a wide age range at which natural menopause occurs. However many years before the menopause, reproductive decline starts. After reaching peak fertility at mid-20s, reproductive decline starts and accelerates after early 30s [12]. This decline in fertility with aging happens with normal endocrine function of the ovaries, which is maintained until about 4 years before the final menstrual period. Then menstrual disturbances start, which are linked to decrease in number of follicles leading to decreased inhibin B secretion, causing luteal phase increase in FSH levels, finally resulting in early follicle growth with shortened follicular phase [13, 14] . Nevertheless, the fertility decline and endocrinologic changes with female aging are associated with the depletion of ovarian follicles. There is also mostly parallel decline in oocyte quality [15]. Primordial follicles have been thought to be the determining factor for ovarian reserve. Per clinical and histological studies, the number of primordial follicles correlates with the number of antral follicles. The decline in primordial follicle pool correlates with decrease in both FSH-sensitive antral follicles and anti-Mullerian hormone (AMH) levels [16, 17].

Currently it is believed that the nongrowing follicle pool in the ovaries eventually dictates both the ovarian reserve and the function [4, 18, 19]. Nongrowing follicles

(NGFs) include primordial, intermediate, and primary follicles. A single layer of flat granulosa cells surrounds primordial follicles. A single layer of cuboidal granulosa cells surrounds primary follicles. Intermediate follicles show single layer of both flat and cuboidal granulosa cells. Therefore, majority of the ovarian research on aging is performed by counting NGFs while always noting for primordial follicles within the cortical sections of the ovary.

3.2.1 Estimating the Age of Natural Menopause with Histological Assessment of the Ovary

There are numerous models to predict the rate of decrease in follicle pool with female aging until the final menstrual period. These models attempted to calculate individualized menopausal age and the reproductive decline. In one of these attempts, a large database was developed from eight different cohorts. The data consisted of the histologically calculated number of NGFs in human ovaries. The limitations were: it was not possible to provide an age when the NGF count became zero and, only 218 cases could be analyzed. The model providing expected ages were then compared with a population-based natural menopause database. The model used natural logarithmic transformation for NGF counts. Age range of the ovarian specimens was 0–51 years. It was noted that the decline in NGF pool showed close relationship with the observed age of menopause [20]. In this model, the threshold of 498 NGFs in a single ovary was predicting menopause. In an earlier model, the same number was calculated as 1000 follicles while assuming the mean menopausal age of 51 years [21].

The authors acknowledged the presence of excess variation of NGF while studying the age of menopause prediction using various studies. This was related to differences in NGF counting methods. These counting methods do show great variation, which brings a lot of concerns. Earlier studies manually counted NGFs in 1 slice per 200 or 100 slices or unknown number of slices with slice thicknesses ranging from 10 to 40 μm [22–24]. Studies that are more recent utilized automatic counting methods. In one such study, investigators sliced the ovaries in one 1-μm-thick and ten 100-μm-thick slices and counted NGFs in every 1-μm slice [25]. In another study, the authors sliced the total ovary into slabs of 1 mm, selected eight of them to slice them into 25-μm-thick slices while counting follicles one in every ten such slices [4]. The authors concluded that at least the model shows the correlation between the age of menopause and the number of NGFs which they call as true ovarian reserve. Although clinical utility of NGF count and prediction of menopause is very limited, it still needs to be determined if the known markers of clinical ovarian reserve like AMH and antral follicle counts (AFCs) or response to stimulation for in vitro fertilization (IVF) may serve as surrogate markers for the prediction of menopausal age [20].

3.2.2   Estimating the Age of Menopause with Anti-Mullerian Hormone

The attempts were made to predict age at menopause by using AMH by hypothesizing that AMH levels below a certain threshold or the increased rate for decline in AMH levels over time correlate with age at menopause [26–28]. It has also been suggested that AMH may become very low or undetectable about 5 years prior to the age at menopause [29]. The AMH was modeled in prediction of age at menopause with various equations [30, 31].

One large recent study used the AMH levels obtained from women seen in fertility clinics while comparing with the data of another population-based study. This study also showed that AMH decreases with female aging and it became undetectable about 5 years before menopause. Although the lower limit of detection for the AMH assay was 0.2 ng/mL, the model extrapolated that the menopause occurs at AMH threshold of 0.075 ng/mL [32]. The authors though discussed the discrepancy between the variation in age of menopause and more variation in AMH levels as important concerns. The critical AMH threshold for menopause varied in such a way that this threshold was higher for women with high AMH for their age and lower for women with low AMH for their age. The authors brought two speculations to explain this phenomenon noted in their model. Women with higher AMH level would be having menopause at a later age, but due to other factors playing roles in ovarian aging, they still reach natural menopause while there are still having many follicles left in their ovaries. In women with low AMH per their ages, due to some compensatory mechanisms, these ovaries show decreased threshold for remaining primordial follicles to go into menopause to prevent very early menopause. Therefore, not only the initial endowment of the primordial follicles but the rate of decline of these follicles may also be important, which should be regulated by complex factors. The number of primordial or nongrowing follicle lost may be slowed down in women with low AMH levels. Others and we have recognized that quite few women continue to have regular cyclic menses while having undetectable AMH levels [33, 34]. Therefore, the natural history of diminished ovarian reserve detected by AMH levels may also show wide variation among women, which may be explained by alternative models of ovarian aging. In addition, varying AMH measurement consistency among the centers and the laboratories is another concern hindering the development of clinically useful models of AMH in ovarian aging or in age at menopause predictions [35].

3.2.3   Past and Current Models for Ovarian Aging

As discussed above, the NGF decline with aging was studied with updated methods of ovarian tissue processing and counting. Past models have suggested that the decline rate of NGFs is exponential and biphasic, which predict about one million NGFs at birth, with acceleration of NGF loss at or after age of 38 years when about

25,000 NGFs remain (Fig. 3.1a). Then at around the NGF number of 1000, women reach menopause [36]. Due to the many limitations of this model, a new model was developed from ovaries obtained from 122 females between the ages of 0 and 51 years [4]. This cohort was larger than the studies published prior to this study. By using more refined sampling as mentioned above and automated counting techniques, the range of NGFs was between 0 and 916,500. This power model suggests that the decline of NGFs is constantly accelerating rather than suddenly increasing at the age of 38 years as suggested by exponential and biphasic model (Fig. 3.1b).

3.2.4 Stages of Reproductive Aging Workshop (STRAW) and the Ovarian Aging Model

After defining the new NGF decay model with aging as discussed above, the same group examined the correlation between the stages of reproductive aging workshop (STRAW) [37] and the number of NGFs.

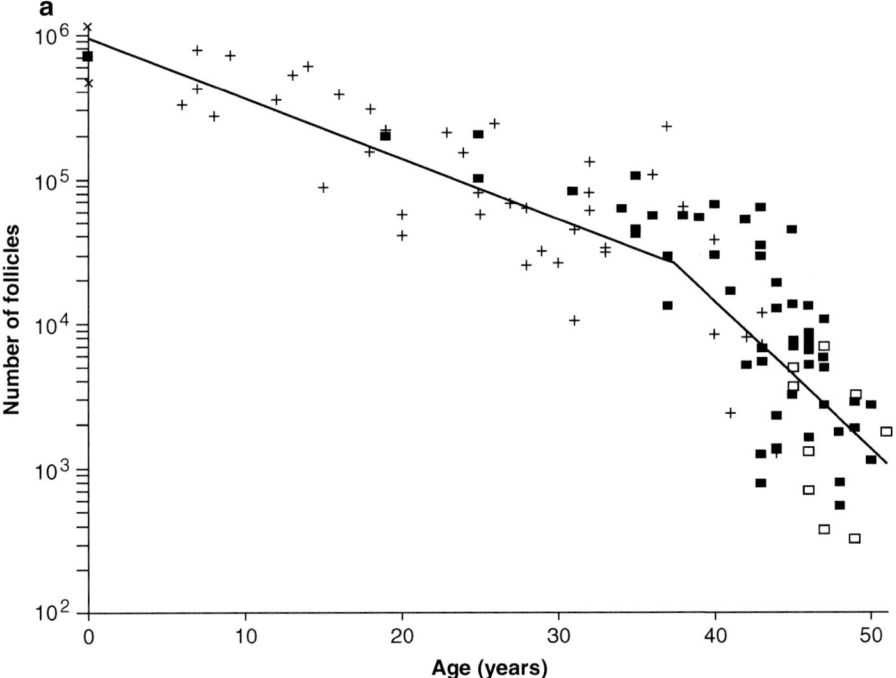

Fig. 3.1 (a) Decrease in ovarian follicles of <0.1 mm in size with female aging per bi-exponential model. After about 25,000 follicles are reached at the age of 37.5 ± 1.2 years the rate of follicle loss accelerates. Combination of studies 1952–1992. (b) Decrease in non-growing ovarian follicles per power model with 95% confidence intervals. The decrease in follicles is constantly accelerating suggesting a more smooth decline. Age accounts for the 84% of the variation in follicles counts at different ages

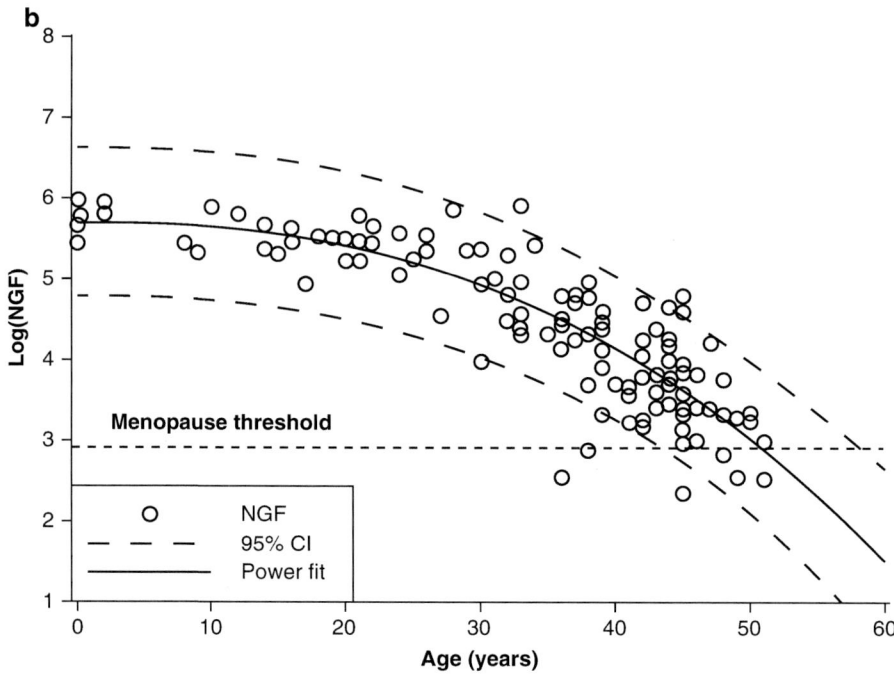

Fig. 3.1 (continued)

STRAW stages before "0" (the final menstrual period) involve late menopausal transition with amenorrhea episodes, increased FSH ≥ 25 IU/L, low AMH, and low AFC and vasomotor symptoms, which was designated as -1. In early menopausal transition or stage -2, menstrual cycle lengths vary by at least 7 days or above in association with variable FSH levels but low AMH and AFC with no vasomotor symptoms. Stage -3 represents the late reproductive period which is characterized by women with either regular (-3a) or subtle changes in menstrual bleeding pattern (-3b). In -3b FSH levels may vary, but other markers of ovarian reserve would be low. In stage -3a, still AMH and AFC would be low but FSH stays normal.

This study demonstrated that although mean female age which was at about mid-40s was not significantly different among groups, advancing STRAW stages from -3 to -1 was associated with decrease in both NGFs and primordial follicles in ovarian cortical specimen collected from patients undergoing hysterectomy with oophorectomy [38]. Therefore, regardless of age, going through stages -3 to -1 was associated with decrease in NGFs. Therefore, the decrease in primordial follicle and NGFs is associated with impending menopausal state. It is still not clear if this progression would also be correct for young women with DOR, younger than ≤ 35 or ≤ 40 years of age, since the study considered all women with regular menses (which many young DOR patients have) and age ≤ 35 years as -4 meaning peak reproductive stage. The authors considered females ≥ 40 years of age with regular cycles as stage -3. The study was able to be performed from 60 women with 43 women having transvaginal ultrasound and blood work.

3.2.5   The Latest Ovarian Aging Model for NGF Loss

Another study from the group presented the power model of NGF decay, analyzed the ovaries of 52 women between the ages of 28 and 51 years to validate their power model [39]. These patients were undergoing oophorectomy for benign gynecologic indications as well. The authors again challenged the conclusion from the earlier studies stating that the rate of oocyte decline should show a biphasic pattern with an acceleration at about the age of 38 years, while the women were progressing toward menopause [36, 40].

The authors studied NGF decline with female aging and came up with their latest validated power model of NGF decrease. This model suggests that by age of 33 years, about 90% of NGFs are depleted. The model predicts peak rate of NGF loss of about 1821 per month at about 19 years of age, while the youngest patient included was 28 years old. Average follicle loss increases from birth to about 20 years of age, and then the average number of follicles lost decreases with the lowest level as close to as menopause. Otherwise, if a female continues to lose the same high number of follicles that they have been losing in their late teens, then the natural menopause would occur at much younger ages than early 50s. Hence, absolute number of follicles lost should decrease with aging through 2nd, 3rd, and 4th decades of life. It seems that as compared to the prior studies and models, there is no sudden decrease of ovarian reserve after certain age, but rather decline is more gradual over time [39].

This recent validation of the power model still predicts that there are still 750 NGFs at the age at the time of menopause. It is more reasonable to consider that the decline in ovarian reserve should be more smooth and gradual rather than showing drastic changes after a certain age. This model may also be applicable to DOR women at any age, except one can consider the NGF decay graph may be skewed to earlier ages in such women. Therefore, although more prospective longitudinal studies are required, these younger women with spontaneous DOR may progress to menopause at earlier ages as proposed before [18].

3.2.6   Experience from Ovarian Autotransplantation

Ovarian cortical autotransplantation experience suggests a different paradigm than above. Massive recruitment of primordial follicles after autotransplantation is followed by extremely low recruitment rate later, resulting in prolonged endocrine function of the ovarian cortical graft even with limited number of primordial follicles [41, 42]. As we discuss in the activation of ovarian cortex chapter, ovarian stroma may also influence primordial follicle activation. The rate of primordial follicle recruitment and demise may actually be decreasing with further decrease in primordial follicle pool [42]. This may explain our observations that in especially younger women with DOR defined by low AFC and AMH criteria, these values may stay stable for a long time. However, some women still show profound decline in ovarian reserve markers in a very short time. Hence, wide individual variation in the natural progression of DOR exists, and this may be related to differing etiologies.

3.3 Decline in Oocyte Quality

Apart from decline in quantity of NGFs, oocyte quality is also affected adversely by aging. It has been estimated that female fecundity decline starts by the early 30s [43]. Earlier studies suggested that women who postpone their first live birth beyond the age of 30 years might increase their chances of involuntary childlessness [44–46]. Then approximately 10 years before the natural menopause at the ages of 40–41 years, almost the end of fertility is reached in populations that did not use contraception. This occurs though with the presence of comparably regular menstrual cycles until the age of 45 or so. Then about 5 years later, natural menopause is reached [47]. It was also shown that in women with diminished ovarian reserve younger than 37 years of age undergoing IVF with classic long agonist protocol, similar number of oocytes can be obtained as compared to the women with DOR at or older than 37 years of age. However, in women younger than 37 years, the clinical pregnancy rate was significantly higher, and miscarriage rates were significantly lower than the women at or older than 37 years [48]. Therefore, oocyte quality, the most important variable of fecundity, should be primarily associated with chronological age. There are many proposed reasons for decline in oocyte quality with aging which shows individual variation as well. Hence ovarian aging pattern is considered as complex polygenic and multifactorial trait shaped by genetic, epigenetic, and environmental factors [15].

Most of the genetic studies were performed in women with premature ovarian insufficiency (POI). Most of POI genome-wide studies do not have power to detect genes with small effect sizes. In addition, unlike natural menopause, POI patients may have occasional ovarian function. Although 90% of POI is still considered idiopathic, spontaneous POI has been associated with genetic factors like abnormal karyotypes, fragile X mental retardation (FMR)-1 premutation, single-gene mutations (bone morphogenic protein 15-BMP15, diaphanous homolog 2-DIAPH2, inhibin alpha subunit-INHA, and others), familial presentation, or autoimmune diseases [49]; most patients with DOR and earlier than expected natural menopause may simply lack such factors [50–52]. Therefore, DOR may not simply be one of the phenotypes eventually progressing to POI. We still need real population-based data rather than inferential data from measurements of ovarian reserve markers. As we will discuss in the definitions, DOR is considered a clinical entity when it is associated with decreased fecundity (live birth per menstrual cycle) or when the response to controlled ovarian stimulation for assisted reproductive technologies (ART) was reduced as compared to women of similar age [53]. The progression rate of DOR may vary among women. It is still not clear if DOR is simply an acceleration of aging or if it is due to factors related to initial oocyte endowment and/or the varying rates of oocyte depletion.

It is well known that pregnancy outcomes are much better in younger DOR patients as compared to the older women with DOR. A retrospective cohort study of 1957 DOR patients showed that maternal age was one of the independent factors of live birth after treatment with ART. Live birth rates were higher in DOR patients <35 years of age as compared those at or above the age of 35 years [54]. In another retrospective study conducted in women undergoing IVF for preimplantation genetic testing for aneuploidy (PGT-A) due to unexplained recurrent spontaneous miscarriage, low AMH level was associated with significantly increased risk of embryonic aneuploidy only in women ≥35 years of age. Low AMH (<1.5 ng/mL) level was not associated with increased embryonic aneuploidy rates in women younger than 35 years of age as compared to the same age groups with normal (1.5 ng/mL – <5.6 ng/mL) and high AMH levels [55]. These data suggest that age alone still dictates oocyte quality regardless of the ovarian reserve. Declining oocyte quality may be associated with the frequency of meiotic non-disjunction of the chromosomes, granulosa cell dysfunction, DNA repair dysfunction, mitochondrial defects, increased protein synthesis, increased metabolic demands, short telomeres, and epigenetic factors [56–58]. Such factors are also main factors associated with aging in general.

3.4 Fertility Decline as Reflection of General Aging

Due to decreased rate of childbearing in modern societies, age at first pregnancy increased as addressed in this book. Some population-based studies suggest that mothers having babies late in reproductive life like after age of 33 years may live longer [59]. There is also some data suggesting that long-lived people are more likely born to young mothers [60]. Making it more complex, age at first reproduction could not be associated with longevity [60]. Another study suggested that women who had their last children later than their sisters did not live any longer [61]. Although this historical sibling study from European royalty did not show any advantage of childbearing at later years, having a baby later in the reproductive years has been correlated with prolongation of life span within the context of natural fertility. Some studies connected somatic senescence to the last age of reproductive performance. Women who delivered their last offspring at advanced age lived longest, while neither the age at first child birth nor the total fecundity was related to longevity of the women [62]. Inspired from animal data, some researchers suggested the rejuvenating effects of pregnancy, childbirth, and breastfeeding on women. This hypothesis suggests that having a childbirth at later years of life may trigger some sort of somatic self-renewal [63, 64]. However, the potential relevance of any of these hypotheses to the pregnancies at late ages, which resulted from assisted reproductive technologies, requires more studies and biological justification.

Some studies linked diminished ovarian reserve to aging-associated disorders like cardiovascular disease. In a small study investigating urinary gonadotropins and urinary estrogen and progesterone metabolites in regularly cycling women with diminished ovarian reserve, as compared to age-matched control women, higher FSH levels, LH surge at somewhat lower levels of estradiol, prolonged LH and FSH surge, and lower luteal phase levels for progesterone and estrogen metabolites were observed. However, all women with DOR had basal FSH levels >10 IU/L with history of suboptimal response to high-dose stimulation with a regular menstrual cycle duration of 21–35 days. These findings were found similar to women in menopausal transition [65]. It is not clear if these findings would be applicable to DOR patients with normal menstrual cycles at or above 28 days of duration with normal basal FSH levels below 10 IU/L.

Menstrual cycle duration mostly decreases with female chronologic aging, which is associated with decline in fecundity as discussed above. The menstrual cycle length may also be a predictor of ART outcomes. Menstrual cycle length shorter than 26 days was reported to result in lower rates of live birth than the women with the cycle lengths of over 34 days, independent of female age as reported from an ART program [66]. After the age of 40 but before menopause, shorter follicular phase is the reason for shorter cycle length. This was shown to be due to advanced follicle growth due to increased FSH levels during the luteal phase of the preceding cycle, which may also result in follicle asynchrony in the beginning of the follicular phase [13]. Luteal phase selection and growth of follicle(s) toward the early follicular phase were blamed to have some endocrinologic effects in terms of serum estradiol levels which might result in increased cardiovascular risk in women with DOR, similar to those women with menopause [67]. It is still not clear if this hypothetical increased risk of cardiovascular disease in women with DOR is solely related to ovarian follicular dysfunction or a reflection of somatic aging. The strong direct clinical correlations are also needed. The issue is that such women may actually present with high estradiol levels throughout the follicular phase due to both advanced dominant follicle growth and due to growth of other follicles unlike estradiol-deficient state of menopause. In addition, the optimal levels of estradiol and progesterone are not clearly defined to assure a conception cycle. It was reported that ovulation of a 13-mm follicle resulted in a normal pregnancy [68]. Although the range of ovulatory follicle diameter is considered to be between 17 and 25 mm, ovulation can occur at <17 mm in both women younger than 34 and older than 40 years, with varying estradiol and luteal phase progesterone levels [13, 69, 70]. Therefore, fertility decline and proposed increased in general morbidity in women with DOR may not be merely because of presumed endocrine disturbances due to changes in follicle growth dynamics. Therefore, more longitudinal and patient outcome-based data are needed.

Another aspect of reproductive aging was linked to telomere lengths as discussed in this book. A study reported shorter telomere length in peripheral leukocytes, granulosa cells, and lower telomerase (terminal transferase) activity from granulosa cells in women biochemically within POI spectrum as compared to controls when adjusted for age [71]. All patients were younger than 40 years of age and having regular menstrual cycles between 23 and 35 days but having basal FSH ≥10 IU/L, and unilateral antral follicle count was <5. Therefore, these women were rather with DOR. An earlier study on overt POI diagnosed with cessation of menses and FSH > 40 IU/L demonstrated that the age adjusted telomere length studied from peripheral leukocytes were longer as compared to controls [72]. Although the differences in results between two studies can be discussed in various ways, the association between the telomere length and morbidity is rather complex. A Mendelian randomization study analyzed genome-wide association studies published until 2015. Per study results, longer telomeres may increase the risk for several cancers (ovarian, endometrial, testicular, brain) but may reduce the risk for some non-neoplastic diseases like, cardiovascular disease, Alzheimer's disease, type I diabetes mellitus, celiac disease, and interstitial lung disease [73].

3.5 Conclusion

Natural history of diminished ovarian reserve shows great variation among the patients. The rate of further decline in ovarian reserve with further aging in women with DOR may follow recently proposed model of primordial and/or nongrowing follicle depletion by aging. In many patients with DOR, this graph perhaps just shifted toward a younger age. Some DOR patients though end up with profound depletion of oocyte pool at a faster rate than others do. It seems that still younger DOR patients show higher pregnancy and live birth rates than older DOR patients. Therefore, age may still dictate oocyte quality. Variations in the rate of oocyte depletion and decline in oocyte quality may be related to many genetic, epigenetic, and environmental factors, which are yet to be determined.

References

1. Baker TG. A quantitative and cytological study of germ cells in human ovaries. Proc R Soc Lond B Biol Sci. 1963;158:417–33.
2. McGee EA, Hsueh AJ. Initial and cyclic recruitment of ovarian follicles. Endocr Rev. 2000;21(2):200–14.
3. Fortune JE, Cushman RA, Wahl CM, Kito S. The primordial to primary follicle transition. Mol Cell Endocrinol. 2000;163(1–2):53–60.
4. Hansen KR, Knowlton NS, Thyer AC, Charleston JS, Soules MR, Klein NA. A new model of reproductive aging: the decline in ovarian non-growing follicle number from birth to menopause. Hum Reprod. 2008;23(3):699–708.
5. Johnson J, Canning J, Kaneko T, Pru JK, Tilly JL. Germline stem cells and follicular renewal in the postnatal mammalian ovary. Nature. 2004;428(6979):145–50.
6. Bristol-Gould SK, Kreeger PK, Selkirk CG, Kilen SM, Mayo KE, Shea LD, et al. Fate of the initial follicle pool: empirical and mathematical evidence supporting its sufficiency for adult fertility. Dev Biol. 2006;298(1):149–54.
7. Johnson J, Bagley J, Skaznik-Wikiel M, Lee HJ, Adams GB, Niikura Y, et al. Oocyte generation in adult mammalian ovaries by putative germ cells in bone marrow and peripheral blood. Cell. 2005;122(2):303–15.
8. Lee HJ, Selesniemi K, Niikura Y, Niikura T, Klein R, Dombkowski DM, et al. Bone marrow transplantation generates immature oocytes and rescues long-term fertility in a preclinical mouse model of chemotherapy-induced premature ovarian failure. J Clin Oncol. 2007;25(22):3198–204.

9. Zou K, Yuan Z, Yang Z, Luo H, Sun K, Zhou L, et al. Production of offspring from a germline stem cell line derived from neonatal ovaries. Nat Cell Biol. 2009;11(5):631–6.

10. Gougeon A. Regulation of ovarian follicular development in primates: facts and hypotheses. Endocr Rev. 1996;17(2):121–55.

11. Wang N, Satirapod C, Ohguchi Y, Park ES, Woods DC, Tilly JL. Genetic studies in mice directly link oocytes produced during adulthood to ovarian function and natural fertility. Sci Rep. 2017;7(1):10011.

12. Practice Committee of the American Society for Reproductive Medicine in collaboration with the Society for Reproductive Endocrinology, Infertility. Electronic address ASRM@asrm.org. Practice Committee of the American Society for Reproductive Medicine in collaboration with the Society for Reproductive Endocrinology, Infertility. Optimizing natural fertility: a committee opinion. Fertil Steril. 2017;107(1):52–8.

13. van Zonneveld P, Scheffer GJ, Broekmans FJ, Blankenstein MA, de Jong FH, Looman CW, et al. Do cycle disturbances explain the age-related decline of female fertility? Cycle characteristics of women aged over 40 years compared with a reference population of young women. Hum Reprod. 2003;18(3):495–501.

14. Burger HG, Hale GE, Dennerstein L, Robertson DM. Cycle and hormone changes during perimenopause: the key role of ovarian function. Menopause. 2008;15(4 Pt 1):603–12.

15. Broekmans FJ, Soules MR, Fauser BC. Ovarian aging: mechanisms and clinical consequences. Endocr Rev. 2009;30(5):465–93.

16. Scheffer GJ, Broekmans FJ, Dorland M, Habbema JD, Looman CW, te Velde ER. Antral follicle counts by transvaginal ultrasonography are related to age in women with proven natural fertility. Fertil Steril. 1999;72(5):845–51.

17. Hansen KR, Hodnett GM, Knowlton N, Craig LB. Correlation of ovarian reserve tests with histologically determined primordial follicle number. Fertil Steril. 2011;95(1):170–5.

18. Lambalk CB, van Disseldorp J, de Koning CH, Broekmans FJ. Testing ovarian reserve to predict age at menopause. Maturitas. 2009;63(4):280–91.

19. Charleston JS, Hansen KR, Thyer AC, Charleston LB, Gougeon A, Siebert JR, et al. Estimating human ovarian non-growing follicle number: the application of modern stereology techniques to an old problem. Hum Reprod. 2007;22(8):2103–10.

20. Depmann M, Faddy MJ, van der Schouw YT, Peeters PH, Broer SL, Kelsey TW, et al. The relationship between variation in size of the primordial follicle pool and age at natural menopause. J Clin Endocrinol Metab. 2015;100(6):E845–51.

21. Wallace WH, Kelsey TW. Human ovarian reserve from conception to the menopause. PLoS One. 2010;5(1):e8772.

22. Block E. A quantitative morphological investigation of the follicular system in newborn female infants. Acta Anat (Basel). 1953;17(3):201–6.

23. Gougeon A, Chainy GB. Morphometric studies of small follicles in ovaries of women at different ages. J Reprod Fertil. 1987;81(2):433–42.

24. Richardson SJ, Senikas V, Nelson JF. Follicular depletion during the menopausal transition: evidence for accelerated loss and ultimate exhaustion. J Clin Endocrinol Metab. 1987;65(6):1231–7.

25. Forabosco A, Sforza C. Establishment of ovarian reserve: a quantitative morphometric study of the developing human ovary. Fertil Steril. 2007;88(3):675–83.

26. Broer SL, Eijkemans MJ, Scheffer GJ, van Rooij IA, de Vet A, Themmen AP, et al. Antimullerian hormone predicts menopause: a long-term follow-up study in normoovulatory women. J Clin Endocrinol Metab. 2011;96(8):2532–9.

27. Freeman EW, Sammel MD, Lin H, Boorman DW, Gracia CR. Contribution of the rate of change of antimullerian hormone in estimating time to menopause for late reproductive-age women. Fertil Steril. 2012;98(5):1254–9.e1–2.

28. Freeman EW, Sammel MD, Lin H, Gracia CR. Anti-mullerian hormone as a predictor of time to menopause in late reproductive age women. J Clin Endocrinol Metab. 2012;97(5):1673–80.

29. Sowers MR, Eyvazzadeh AD, McConnell D, Yosef M, Jannausch ML, Zhang D, et al. Antimullerian hormone and inhibin B in the definition of ovarian aging and the menopause transition. J Clin Endocrinol Metab. 2008;93(9):3478–83.
30. Nelson SM, Messow MC, McConnachie A, Wallace H, Kelsey T, Fleming R, et al. External validation of nomogram for the decline in serum anti-Mullerian hormone in women: a population study of 15,834 infertility patients. Reprod Biomed Online. 2011;23(2):204–6.
31. Nelson SM, Messow MC, Wallace AM, Fleming R, McConnachie A. Nomogram for the decline in serum antimullerian hormone: a population study of 9,601 infertility patients. Fertil Steril. 2011;95(2):736–41.e1–3.
32. Dolleman M, Faddy MJ, van Disseldorp J, van der Schouw YT, Messow CM, Leader B, et al. The relationship between anti-Mullerian hormone in women receiving fertility assessments and age at menopause in subfertile women: evidence from large population studies. J Clin Endocrinol Metab. 2013;98(5):1946–53.
33. Overbeek A, Broekmans FJ, Hehenkamp WJ, Wijdeveld ME, van Disseldorp J, van Dulmen-den Broeder E, et al. Intra-cycle fluctuations of anti-Mullerian hormone in normal women with a regular cycle: a re-analysis. Reprod Biomed Online. 2012;24(6):664–9.
34. La Marca A, Spada E, Grisendi V, Argento C, Papaleo E, Milani S, et al. Normal serum anti-Mullerian hormone levels in the general female population and the relationship with reproductive history. Eur J Obstet Gynecol Reprod Biol. 2012;163(2):180–4.
35. Kumar A, Kalra B, Patel A, McDavid L, Roudebush WE. Development of a second generation anti-Mullerian hormone (AMH) ELISA. J Immunol Methods. 2010;362(1–2):51–9.
36. Faddy MJ, Gosden RG, Gougeon A, Richardson SJ, Nelson JF. Accelerated disappearance of ovarian follicles in mid-life: implications for forecasting menopause. Hum Reprod. 1992;7(10):1342–6.
37. Soules MR, Sherman S, Parrott E, Rebar R, Santoro N, Utian W, et al. Executive summary: Stages of Reproductive Aging Workshop (STRAW). Fertil Steril. 2001;76(5):874–8.
38. Hansen KR, Craig LB, Zavy MT, Klein NA, Soules MR. Ovarian primordial and nongrowing follicle counts according to the Stages of Reproductive Aging Workshop (STRAW) staging system. Menopause. 2012;19(2):164–71.
39. Knowlton NS, Craig LB, Zavy MT, Hansen KR. Validation of the power model of ovarian nongrowing follicle depletion associated with aging in women. Fertil Steril. 2014;101(3):851–6.
40. Faddy MJ, Gosden RG. A model conforming the decline in follicle numbers to the age of menopause in women. Hum Reprod. 1996;11(7):1484–6.
41. Ayuandari S, Winkler-Crepaz K, Paulitsch M, Wagner C, Zavadil C, Manzl C, et al. Follicular growth after xenotransplantation of cryopreserved/thawed human ovarian tissue in SCID mice: dynamics and molecular aspects. J Assist Reprod Genet. 2016;33(12):1585–93.
42. Silber S. Ovarian tissue cryopreservation and transplantation: scientific implications. J Assist Reprod Genet. 2016;33(12):1595–603.
43. van Noord-Zaadstra BM, Looman CW, Alsbach H, Habbema JD, te Velde ER, Karbaat J. Delaying childbearing: effect of age on fecundity and outcome of pregnancy. BMJ. 1991;302(6789):1361–5.
44. Bongaarts J. Involuntary childlessness with increasing age. Res Reprod. 1982;14(4):1–2.
45. Bongaarts J. Infertility and age: not so unresolved: a reply. Fam Plann Perspect. 1982;14(5):289–90.
46. Bongaarts J. Infertility after age 30: a false alarm. Fam Plann Perspect. 1982;14(2):75–8.
47. Treloar AE. Menstrual cyclicity and the pre-menopause. Maturitas. 1981;3(3–4):249–64.
48. Chang Y, Li J, Li X, Liu H, Liang X. Egg quality and pregnancy outcome in young infertile women with diminished ovarian reserve. Med Sci Monit. 2018;24:7279–84.
49. Nelson LM. Clinical practice. Primary ovarian insufficiency. N Engl J Med. 2009;360(6):606–14.
50. Voorhuis M, Onland-Moret NC, Fauser BC, Ploos van Amstel HK, van der Schouw YT, Broekmans FJ. The association of CGG repeats in the FMR1 gene and timing of natural menopause. Hum Reprod. 2013;28(2):496–501.

51. Murray A, Schoemaker MJ, Bennett CE, Ennis S, Macpherson JN, Jones M, et al. Population-based estimates of the prevalence of FMR1 expansion mutations in women with early menopause and primary ovarian insufficiency. Genet Med. 2014;16(1):19–24.
52. Pastore LM, Young SL, Manichaikul A, Baker VL, Wang XQ, Finkelstein JS. Distribution of the FMR1 gene in females by race/ethnicity: women with diminished ovarian reserve versus women with normal fertility (SWAN study). Fertil Steril. 2017;107(1):205–11.e1.
53. Practice Committee of the American Society for Reproductive Medicine. Testing and interpreting measures of ovarian reserve: a committee opinion. Fertil Steril. 2015;103(3):e9–e17.
54. Huang Y, Li J, Zhang F, Liu Y, Xu G, Guo J, et al. Factors affecting the live-birth rate in women with diminished ovarian reserve undergoing IVF-ET. Arch Gynecol Obstet. 2018;298(5):1017–27.
55. Jiang X, Yan J, Sheng Y, Sun M, Cui L, Chen ZJ. Low anti-Mullerian hormone concentration is associated with increased risk of embryonic aneuploidy in women of advanced age. Reprod Biomed Online. 2018;37(2):178–83.
56. Ben-Meir A, Yahalomi S, Moshe B, Shufaro Y, Reubinoff B, Saada A. Coenzyme Q-dependent mitochondrial respiratory chain activity in granulosa cells is reduced with aging. Fertil Steril. 2015;104(3):724–7.
57. Duncan FE, Jasti S, Paulson A, Kelsh JM, Fegley B, Gerton JL. Age-associated dysregulation of protein metabolism in the mammalian oocyte. Aging Cell. 2017;16(6):1381–93.
58. Nguyen AL, Drutovic D, Vazquez BN, El Yakoubi W, Gentilello AS, Malumbres M, et al. Genetic Interactions between the Aurora Kinases Reveal New Requirements for AURKB and AURKC during Oocyte Meiosis. Curr Biol. 2018;28(21):3458–68. e5
59. Sun F, Sebastiani P, Schupf N, Bae H, Andersen SL, McIntosh A, et al. Extended maternal age at birth of last child and women's longevity in the Long Life Family Study. Menopause. 2015;22(1):26–31.
60. Gagnon A. Natural fertility and longevity. Fertil Steril. 2015;103(5):1109–16.
61. Mueller U. Does late reproduction extend the life span? Findings from European royalty. Popul Dev Rev. 2004;30(3):449–+.
62. Helle S, Lummaa V, Jokela J. Are reproductive and somatic senescence coupled in humans? Late, but not early, reproduction correlated with longevity in historical Sami women. Proc Biol Sci. 2005;272(1558):29–37.
63. Gielchinsky Y, Laufer N, Weitman E, Abramovitch R, Granot Z, Bergman Y, et al. Pregnancy restores the regenerative capacity of the aged liver via activation of an mTORC1-controlled hyperplasia/hypertrophy switch. Genes Dev. 2010;24(6):543–8.
64. Yi Z, Vaupel J. Association of late childbearing with healthy longevity among the oldest-old in China. Popul Stud (Camb). 2004;58(1):37–53.
65. Pal L, Zhang K, Zeitlian G, Santoro N. Characterizing the reproductive hormone milieu in infertile women with diminished ovarian reserve. Fertil Steril. 2010;93(4):1074–9.
66. Brodin T, Bergh T, Berglund L, Hadziosmanovic N, Holte J. Menstrual cycle length is an age-independent marker of female fertility: results from 6271 treatment cycles of in vitro fertilization. Fertil Steril. 2008;90(5):1656–61.
67. Quinn MM, Cedars MI. Cardiovascular health and ovarian aging. Fertil Steril. 2018;110(5):790–3.
68. van Zonneveld P, te Velde ER, Koppeschaar HP. Low luteal phase serum progesterone levels in regularly cycling women are predictive of subtle ovulation disorders. Gynecol Endocrinol. 1994;8(3):169–74.
69. Eissa MK, Obhrai MS, Docker MF, Lynch SS, Sawers RS, Newton JR. Follicular growth and endocrine profiles in spontaneous and induced conception cycles. Fertil Steril. 1986;45(2):191–5.
70. Zegers-Hochschild F, Gomez Lira C, Parada M, Altieri Lorenzini E. A comparative study of the follicular growth profile in conception and nonconception cycles. Fertil Steril. 1984;41(2):244–7.

71. Xu X, Chen X, Zhang X, Liu Y, Wang Z, Wang P, et al. Impaired telomere length and telom-erase activity in peripheral blood leukocytes and granulosa cells in patients with biochemical primary ovarian insufficiency. Hum Reprod. 2017;32(1):201–7.
72. Hanna CW, Bretherick KL, Gair JL, Fluker MR, Stephenson MD, Robinson WP. Telomere length and reproductive aging. Hum Reprod. 2009;24(5):1206–11.
73. Telomeres Mendelian Randomization Collaboration, Haycock PC, Burgess S, Nounu A, Zheng J, Okoli GN, et al. Association between telomere length and risk of cancer and non-neoplastic diseases: a Mendelian randomization study. JAMA Oncol. 2017;3(5):636–51.

Chapter 4
Definitions and Relevance: Diminished Ovarian Reserve, Poor Ovarian Response, Advanced Reproductive Age, and Premature Ovarian Insufficiency

Orhan Bukulmez

4.1 Introduction

The robust discussions about the definition of poor ovarian response (POR) and its most common cause, diminished ovarian reserve (DOR), reflect the heterogeneity of their presentation in each patient and even the heterogeneity of each natural or stimulated cycle in each patient. In assisted reproductive technology (ART), this type of presentation may require rather personalized approaches for each patient and for each treatment cycle of the same patient. For instance, in some patients, poor ovarian response may be noted during the first controlled ovarian stimulation cycle for in vitro fertilization (IVF), which may not be repetitive in a subsequent cycle. In addition, ovarian reserve assessment per se may not predict live birth outcome in natural cycles or with ART treatment.

4.2 Different Definition of Diminished Ovarian Reserve

There is another discussion that, since we measure antral follicle count (AFC) and anti-Mullerian hormone (AMH) levels as the reflection of ovarian reserve, we just measure the FSH-sensitive pool of follicles. Primordial follicles and intermediate and primary follicles are in general considered as the non-growing follicle (NGF) pool. Hence one particular group suggests that we do not assess total ovarian reserve (TOR) which should include NGFs, but rather we assess functional ovarian reserve (FOR) [1–3]. It has been shown that tests of ovarian reserve, namely, both AFC and

O. Bukulmez (✉)
Division of Reproductive Endocrinology and Infertility, Fertility and Advanced Reproductive Medicine Assisted Reproductive Technologies Program, Department of Obstetrics and Gynecology, University of Texas Southwestern Medical Center, Dallas, TX, USA
e-mail: Orhan.Bukulmez@UTSouthwestern.edu

© Springer Nature Switzerland AG 2020
O. Bukulmez (ed.), *Diminished Ovarian Reserve and Assisted Reproductive Technologies*, https://doi.org/10.1007/978-3-030-23235-1_4

AMH, correlate strongly with the number of the primordial follicles [4–6] and the NGFs, which are included in what is defined as total ovarian reserve. It is currently elusive if renaming DOR as low FOR (LFOR) would make any difference in identification and treatment of such patients.

4.3   Advanced Reproductive Age, Poor Ovarian Response, and Gonadotropin Dose

Many practitioners have observed that the younger women with POR can have better outcomes with IVF [7, 8]. It is also reported that young women with POR still show low success rates with IVF [9]. Advanced reproductive age definitions show profound variation in relevant studies. Per American Society for Reproductive Medicine, fertility evaluation is recommended after 6 months rather than 12 months of trying if the female age is over 35 years [10]. Although the age cutoff is mostly considered as at or above 35 years of age, >37 years or ≥40 years are frequently used threshold levels for advanced reproductive age (ARA) for women.

In one of these studies, the authors reviewed the IVF cycles resulted in fresh transfer. The women with predicted POR were defined as mean AFC ≤4 per ovary, who were treated with a high-dose gonadotropin protocol. The authors defined POR as ≤5 follicles at oocyte retrieval [11]. Hence, the definition is different from Bologna criteria, but at the same time, the protocol decisions were made solely relying on AFC. Then the authors only included those cycles reaching the oocyte retrieval with at least 1 follicle development, i.e., 1706 of 1803 started cycles, and reported the prevalence of POR as 17%. Good responders were younger and had higher number of top-grade, cleavage-stage embryos than the poor responders. Median age of 290 poor responders were 37 years, and therefore, the authors compared the IVF outcomes according to this cutoff age, while the maximum number of embryos transferred were kept at a maximum of 2. Among poor responders >37 years of age, the total FSH doses required were significantly higher, and the mean number of oocytes obtained were lower, and the number of patients undergoing single embryo transfer were lower than the group ≤37 years of age. In those with POR, women older than 37 years showed much lower live birth rates per embryo transfer than those with younger age (4% vs 19.1%, respectively). Univariate logistic regression including 290 women with POR revealed that total FSH dose along with age and the number of oocytes were associated with treatment outcome. In a bivariate model, mean FSH dose was significantly negatively associated with pregnancy, but the age was not significantly associated with the pregnancy. Further models revealed that women older than 37 years of age who received high doses of FSH had a significantly poorer outcome than explained by either age or FSH dose alone [11]. In poor responders between the ages of 30 and 40 years, the probability of pregnancy decreased with increasing mean doses of FSH, and as the age advances, the decrease in pregnancy rates was somewhat more intense than 30 years of age. Therefore, both advancing age and the increasing FSH dose used for stimulation were associated with poor IVF outcomes.

In a prospective randomized trial which included 52 women with predicted POR per AFC of <5 follicles of 2–5 mm diameters prior to starting their first IVF cycles, administering either 150 IU (group I) or 300 IU (group II) of recombinant FSH did not change median number of oocytes obtained and pregnancy rates achieved (Group I 8% vs group II 4%, $p = 0.55$) [12].

In older women with DOR, those with predicted POR may not show any advantages from high starting doses of FSH. High doses of FSH may even be detrimental for IVF outcome in such women, and milder approaches may be more beneficial [13–15].

4.4 Premature Ovarian Insufficiency

Premature ovarian insufficiency (POI) is a form of extreme spectrum of an impaired ovarian function associated with amenorrhea, low estradiol (E2) levels, and high menopausal levels of FSH in women younger than 40 years of age. Prior to 2008, mostly premature ovarian failure (POF) terminology was used. Literature review shows that both POF and PIO terms were used interchangeably. Because it was noted that such patients might ovulate and conceive after getting such diagnosis, POI became the preferred terminology. Per the European Society of Human Reproduction and Embryology (ESHRE) consensus, it was decided that "insufficiency" more accurately describes the fluctuating nature of the condition and does not carry the negative connotation of "failure" (https://www. eshre.eu/Guidelines-and-Legal/Guidelines/Management-of-premature-ovarian-insufficiency.aspx) [16]. This condition is also named as primary ovarian insufficiency especially in the United States, honoring the first-time use of the term in 1942 by Albright [17–19]. POI is not premature menopause since the resumption of ovarian function can be observed in more than 25% of such women. The condition is noted in 1% of females [17].

It was postulated that POI may represent a continuum ovarian functional decline from occult state with reduced fecundity with regular menstrual cycles and normal FSH levels, transitioning to an overt state presenting as menopause [20]. Hence a broadened criteria for POI was defined as cycle irregularities persisting more than 4 consecutive months and two recordings of postmenopausal FSH levels (FSH > 40 IU/L) at least 1 month apart in a woman younger than 40 years of age. However, it has not been documented that such continuum exists, and it is generally acknowledged that DOR and POI are different entities [17]. DOR is expected at or after the age of 40 unlike POI. DOR patients mostly have regular periods. Although it is suggested that DOR should not be associated with postmenopausal ovarian test results like basal or day 3 FSH > 40 with low E2 levels and undetectable AMH levels, occasionally such results are possible in DOR patients as well. DOR patients continue with their cyclic menstrual function, while cycle length may vary.

Since there is no strong evidence that DOR is a precursor to POI, DOR and POI patients have different needs for their medical management and for fertility treatment. POI and DOR may have some common or genetic etiologies like ovarian surgery, chemotherapy, fragile X mental retardation 1 (FMR-1) gene premutation (expansion of CGG repeats within the 5' untranslated region of the gene to 55–199, mostly due to repeats between 70 and 100), and mosaic Turner's Syndrome (45X/45XX) [17]. However, all these entities are more frequently associated with POI rather than DOR.

4.5 Majority of the Poor Ovarian Response Is Due to Diminished Ovarian Reserve Albeit Ovarian Reserve Assessment in General Population May Not Predict Fertility

Diminished ovarian reserve actually does not have a uniformly accepted definition as also noted in the Bologna criteria for POR. The diagnosis does require clinical judgment. Ovarian reserve in general is determined by female age, genetics, and environmental influences. At any ovarian reserve, each woman of same age shows different reproductive potential and variable response to ovarian stimulation for IVF. Ovarian reserve, although should only implicate the quantity but not quality of the remaining oocytes, definitions usually include both quantity and quality [21]. In that respect, DOR is relevant to women of reproductive age with regular menstrual cycles showing poor response to ovarian stimulation for IVF or solely presenting with low fecundity as compared to an age-matched group.

With the current definitions in mind, the ovarian reserve tests are expected to provide information about fecundity and on both oocyte quantity and quality. This brings though many controversies in such a way that these tests were often regarded as "fertility tests." If ovarian reserve were synonymous for fertility and fecundity, then many women with "abnormal" ovarian reserve tests would be excluded from fertility treatment options with their own oocytes.

The findings of a recent prospective time-to-pregnancy cohort study suggest that the results of the ovarian reserve tests which included serum AMH, serum FSH, serum inhibin B, and urinary FSH in women aged 30–44 years without infertility, the level of these markers were not associated with natural reproductive potential per general definition of fecundability [22]. Women with low AMH levels showed 84% predicted cumulative probability of conception by 12 menstrual cycles of pregnancy attempt as compared with 75% in women with normal AMH levels (Fig. 4.1). Although this was the first study of its kind, possible concerns for the study, as the authors also admitted, included the following: primary outcome did not include live

Fig. 4.1 Adjusted Kaplan-Meier curve with 95% confidence intervals for time to pregnancy by AMH. Model adjusted for age, body mass index and race groups, and also for smoking status and history of contraceptive use in the preceding year. All confidence intervals overlap [22] (with permission)

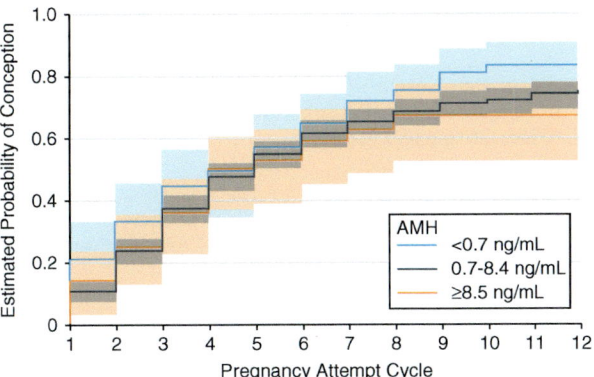

birth and fecundity cannot be calculated, and since ovulation was not assessed, the strict definition of fecundability could not be achieved.

It is now clearer that DOR anticipated by AMH does not necessarily predict fertility. Therefore, fertility can only be tested and confirmed by attempting to conceive. If this attempt is not successful and the infertility diagnosis is actually made per the described definitions and the IVF treatment is decided on, then AMH is considered a great marker to predict oocyte yield [23]. In that respect, some women can be diagnosed with DOR. Then this assessment would be invaluable to select the best-controlled ovarian stimulation protocols for women with DOR.

4.6   Closing Remarks and Conclusion

Diminished ovarian reserve is a physiological phenomenon through reproductive aging and becomes more frequent with advanced reproductive age, mostly defined as the female age of at or above 35 years. It is considered that at or above the age of 40, many women will present with DOR. During an IVF cycle, such women may have no follicles developed or no oocytes retrieved, or the retrieved oocytes may not become an embryo. At times, even with acceptable follicle growth and endocrine response during the ovarian stimulation, the oocyte retrieval may not be successful even with high-pressure follicle aspiration or multiple flushing of the follicles [24]. Patients with DOR also show high cycle cancellation and lower pregnancy rates with assisted reproductive technologies [25]. Younger DOR patients have better ART pregnancy outcomes than those with ARA. POI and DOR may have different pathogenesis although the recent POI definition includes some women with profound DOR. Ovarian reserve tests may not predict fertility in the general population.

The management of patients with DOR has become a relentless quest for success. In the upcoming pages of this book, our team of authors will provide a comprehensive information about the known physiology, research and clinical management strategies, and imminent developments to assure reproductive success in patients with diminished ovarian reserve.

References

1. Barad DH, Kushnir VA, Gleicher N. The importance of redundancy of functional ovarian reserve when investigating potential genetic effects on ovarian function. J Assist Reprod Genet. 2016;33(9):1157–60.
2. Gleicher N, Kushnir VA, Weghofer A, Barad DH. The importance of adrenal hypoandrogenism in infertile women with low functional ovarian reserve: a case study of associated adrenal insufficiency. Reprod Biol Endocrinol. 2016;14:23.
3. Gleicher N, Weghofer A, Barad DH. Defining ovarian reserve to better understand ovarian aging. Reprod Biol Endocrinol. 2011;9:23.
4. Kevenaar ME, Meerasahib MF, Kramer P, van de Lang-Born BM, de Jong FH, Groome NP, et al. Serum anti-mullerian hormone levels reflect the size of the primordial follicle pool in mice. Endocrinology. 2006;147(7):3228–34.
5. Hansen KR, Craig LB, Zavy MT, Klein NA, Soules MR. Ovarian primordial and nongrowing follicle counts according to the Stages of Reproductive Aging Workshop (STRAW) staging system. Menopause. 2012;19(2):164–71.
6. Hansen KR, Hodnett GM, Knowlton N, Craig LB. Correlation of ovarian reserve tests with histologically determined primordial follicle number. Fertil Steril. 2011;95(1):170–5.
7. Biljan MM, Buckett WM, Dean N, Phillips SJ, Tan SL. The outcome of IVF-embryo transfer treatment in patients who develop three follicles or less. Hum Reprod. 2000;15(10):2140–4.
8. Check JH, Nazari P, Check ML, Choe JK, Liss JR. Prognosis following in vitro fertilization-embryo transfer (IVF-ET) in patients with elevated day 2 or 3 serum follicle stimulating hormone (FSH) is better in younger vs older patients. Clin Exp Obstet Gynecol. 2002;29(1):42–4.
9. El-Toukhy T, Khalaf Y, Hart R, Taylor A, Braude P. Young age does not protect against the adverse effects of reduced ovarian reserve – an eight year study. Hum Reprod. 2002;17(6):1519–24.
10. Practice Committee of American Society for Reproductive Medicine. Definitions of infertility and recurrent pregnancy loss: a committee opinion. Fertil Steril. 2013;99(1):63.
11. Saldeen P, Kallen K, Sundstrom P. The probability of successful IVF outcome after poor ovarian response. Acta Obstet Gynecol Scand. 2007;86(4):457–61.
12. Klinkert ER, Broekmans FJ, Looman CW, Habbema JD, te Velde ER. Expected poor responders on the basis of an antral follicle count do not benefit from a higher starting dose of gonadotrophins in IVF treatment: a randomized controlled trial. Hum Reprod. 2005;20(3):611–5.
13. Check JH, Choe JK, Katsoff D, Summers-Chase D, Wilson C. Controlled ovarian hyperstimulation adversely affects implantation following in vitro fertilization-embryo transfer. J Assist Reprod Genet. 1999;16(8):416–20.
14. Check ML, Check JH, Wilson C, Choe JK, Krotec J. Outcome of in vitro fertilization-embryo transfer according to age in poor responders with elevated baseline serum follicle stimulation hormone using minimal or no gonadotropin stimulation. Clin Exp Obstet Gynecol. 2004;31(3):183–4.
15. Check JH. Mild ovarian stimulation. J Assist Reprod Genet. 2007;24(12):621–7.
16. Webber L, Davies M, Anderson R, et al. ESHRE guideline: management of women with premature ovarian insufficiency. Grimbergen: European Society of Human Reproduction and Embryology; 2015.
17. Tucker EJ, Grover SR, Bachelot A, Touraine P, Sinclair AH. Premature ovarian insufficiency: new perspectives on genetic cause and phenotypic spectrum. Endocr Rev. 2016;37(6):609–35.
18. Nelson LM. Clinical practice. Primary ovarian insufficiency. N Engl J Med. 2009;360(6):606–14.
19. Cooper AR, Baker VL, Sterling EW, Ryan ME, Woodruff TK, Nelson LM. The time is now for a new approach to primary ovarian insufficiency. Fertil Steril. 2011;95(6):1890–7.
20. Welt CK. Primary ovarian insufficiency: a more accurate term for premature ovarian failure. Clin Endocrinol (Oxf). 2008;68(4):499–509.

21. Practice Committee of the American Society for Reproductive Medicine. Testing and interpreting measures of ovarian reserve: a committee opinion. Fertil Steril. 2015;103(3):e9–e17.
22. Steiner AZ, Pritchard D, Stanczyk FZ, Kesner JS, Meadows JW, Herring AH, et al. Association between biomarkers of ovarian reserve and infertility among older women of reproductive age. JAMA. 2017;318(14):1367–76.
23. Wu CH, Chen YC, Wu HH, Yang JG, Chang YJ, Tsai HD. Serum anti-Mullerian hormone predicts ovarian response and cycle outcome in IVF patients. J Assist Reprod Genet. 2009;26(7):383–9.
24. Kumaran A, Narayan PK, Pai PJ, Ramachandran A, Mathews B, Adiga SK. Oocyte retrieval at 140-mmHg negative aspiration pressure: a promising alternative to flushing and aspiration in assisted reproduction in women with low ovarian reserve. J Hum Reprod Sci. 2015;8(2):98–102.
25. Reed BG, Babayev SN, Bukulmez O. Shifting paradigms in diminished ovarian reserve and advanced reproductive age in assisted reproduction: customization instead of conformity. Semin Reprod Med. 2015;33(3):169–78.

Chapter 5
Food Supplements and Hormonal Products to Improve Assisted Reproductive Technology Outcomes in Patients with Diminished Ovarian Reserve

Volkan Turan, Melis Bozan, and Gurkan Bozdag

5.1 Introduction

Poor ovarian response (POR) represents a common problem in assisted reproduction. Women with POR reflects a group of women mostly with diminished ovarian reserve (DOR) who do not respond to adequate dose of gonadotropins during ovarian stimulation (OS). Although there is a lack of consensus on the definition of POR, the European Society of Human Reproduction and Embryology (ESHRE) group standardized the definition under the name of Bologna criteria as discussed in this book [1]. Since cumulative live birth rate per initiated cycle decreases with the number of oocytes retrieved, definitions of POR and DOR and their management are crucial in clinical practice.

Historically, there has been several attempts to increase the number of available oocytes including modifications in gonadotropin-releasing hormone analog, increasing gonadotropin doses, and last utilization of adjuvant therapies such as growth hormone, dehydroepiandrosterone, coenzyme Q10, transdermal testosterone, and others. Herein, we will discuss the effects of potential hormonal supplements and dietary adjuvants to improve assisted reproductive technology (ART) outcomes in women with proven or expected poor ovarian response.

V. Turan
Department of Obstetrics and Gynecology, Yeni Yuzyil University School of Medicine, GOP Hospital, Istanbul, Turkey

M. Bozan
Hacettepe University School of Medicine, Ankara, Turkey

G. Bozdag (✉)
Department of Obstetrics and Gynecology, Hacettepe University School of Medicine, Ankara, Turkey
e-mail: gbozdag@hacettepe.edu.tr

© Springer Nature Switzerland AG 2020
O. Bukulmez (ed.), *Diminished Ovarian Reserve and Assisted Reproductive Technologies*, https://doi.org/10.1007/978-3-030-23235-1_5

5.2   Hormonal Supplementation in Women with POR

5.2.1   Growth Hormone

Growth hormone (GH) is a polypeptide hormone secreted by somatotropic cells of the anterior pituitary gland that stimulates cell growth and proliferation. It was previously demonstrated that GH may play a crucial role in follicular development and oocyte maturation via regulating the synthesis of insulin growth factor-1 (IGF-1) in granulosa cells and increase follicular sensitivity to gonadotropins [2]. There are IGF-1 receptors within oocytes, granulosa, and theca cells. In women undergoing IVF, IGF-1 concentrations are directly related to the number of developing follicles due to the suppressive effect of IGF-1 on follicular apoptosis. GH itself is also required for follicular development and inhibition of follicular apoptosis.

Several studies have been conducted to evaluate the effect of GH supplementation in women with POR undergoing ART. The main success parameters considered in those studies are the number of oocytes retrieved and clinical pregnancy/live birth rates. One of the largest studies performed on the supplementation of GH was the LIGHT (live birth rate in vitro fertilization and growth hormone treatment) trial from Australia and New Zealand in 2016 [3]. When patients were prospectively randomized to study arm (12 IU/day GH beginning on the day of stimulation) or controls, although there were some improvements in response to ovarian stimulation, the authors did not notice any benefit with regard to live birth rate in the study arm. However, one should be cautious that this study has not been published as a full paper.

In spite of prospective trials, a recent retrospective study including 400 women in which 161 had been treated with GH (average of 1.5 IU per day), Keane et al. [4] reported that GH supplementation significantly increased clinical pregnancy rate by 3.42-fold (95% CI 1.82–6.44, $p < 0.0005$) and live birth rate by 6.16-fold (95% CI 2.83–13.39 $p < 0.0005$). When the data were scrutinized based on female age, the authors noticed that the effect of GH was mainly related to patient's age. Whereas between 35 and 40 years, it was 4.50 more likely to get pregnant in GH cycles, it did not have a significant effect on the chance of clinical pregnancy in those aged <35 years or ≥40 years.

In a recent meta-analysis including only randomized controlled trials (RCTs), although none of the seven studies showed improvement in clinical pregnancy rates, clinical pregnancy and live birth rates were found to significantly increase (OR 2.13; 95% CI 1.06–4.28 and OR 2.96; 95% CI 1.17–7.52, respectively) after analyzing pooled data [5]. In another meta-analysis including all types of trials ($n = 12$ studies), although authors presented significantly higher numbers of retrieved oocytes (OR 1.94; 95% CI 1.19–2.69) and obtained more available embryos (OR 1.72; 95% CI 1.13–2.31) under the GH therapy, clinical pregnancy and live birth rates were similar with or without GH treatment [12]. The subgroup analysis indicated that clinical pregnancy and live birth rates were significantly increased when GH was co-treated with gonadotropin; however, there were no significant differences found as for the clinical pregnancy and live birth rates when it was supplemented during the preceding luteal phase of the cycle [6].

To sum up, considering all the studies performed to date, there is some evidence that supports an improvement with regard to the number of oocytes retrieved and clinical pregnancy/live birth rates when GH supplementation was preferred. However, for more definitive results, further studies with larger sample size are needed to confirm the effects of GH supplementation and to define the optimal dose and schema in women with POR undergoing ART.

5.2.2   Dehydroepiandrosterone

Dehydroepiandrosterone (DHEA) is an endogenous steroid and originates from the adrenal zona reticularis (%85) and ovarian theca cells (%15) [7]. It improves steroidogenesis as a precursor for estradiol and testosterone and enhances follicular development [8]. It can also boost the level of IGF-1, which in turn promotes folliculogenesis by enhancing the effect of gonadotropin and reducing follicular arrest [9]. Furthermore, DHEA might decrease the level of hypoxic inducible factor-1 when compared with the controls (0.50 ± 0.52 vs. 0.08 ± 0.29, $p = 0.018$), which has crucial role in immunological responses, homeostasis, vascularization, and anaerobic metabolism [10].

In spite of preclinical data supporting its utilization, the clinical relevance during OS in women with POR or DOR undergoing in vitro fertilization (IVF) cycle is still controversial. In a recent meta-analysis including 5 studies with a total of 910 patients, although the use of DHEA did not change the number of retrieved oocytes, there was a higher likelihood of pregnancy (OR 1.8, 95% CI 1.29–2.51) [11]. Notably, DHEA was used for 12 weeks with a dose of 75 mg/day before OS in most of the studies. When the authors analyzed the association between DHEA use and the likelihood of abortion, they reported low heterogeneity between studies (I2 = 0.0%), and the use of DHEA was associated with a significant reduction in the likelihood of abortion (OR 0.25, CI 0.07–0.95; $p = 0.045$) [11].

Unlike other studies, Chern et al. investigated the effect of DHEA whose DHEA-sulphate level was less than 180 μg/dL [12] among poor ovarian responders. The authors reported that DHEA therapy might be beneficial in women with lower DHEA-sulphate level and raise the possibility of attaining more than three oocytes [12]. Another recent prospective case-control study [13] revealed that there were statistically significant differences between the groups with and without DHEA supplementation for oocyte yield (6.35 ± 2.41 vs. 3.98 ± 3.2), Grade I embryos generated (55% vs. 30%), positive pregnancy rate (21/34 vs. 10/28), and live birth rate (18/34 vs. 4/28). The beneficial effect was obvious especially in women <30 years old [13].

In conclusion, one should assume that DHEA treatment might enhance clinical pregnancy and live birth rates according to limited data. However, lack of large-scale RCTs, unknown long-term health risks, and cosmetic concerns are the main factors that limit its utilization in clinical practice.

5.2.3   Transdermal Testosterone

The rationale behind the testosterone intervention is based on the fact that androgens appear to play an important role in early follicular development and granulosa cell proliferation as well as in increasing the number of small antral follicles [14]. In a meta-analysis published in 2012, three RCTs were included to evaluate the effects of transdermal testosterone on ovarian stimulation outcomes in women with POR [15]. When a total of 113 women treated with transdermal testosterone were compared with a total of 112 controls, both clinical pregnancy (RR 2.07, 95% CI 1.13–3.78) and live birth (RR, 1.91, 95% CI 1.01–3.63) rates were significantly improved. However, a following RCT including 50 women with POR failed to note any significant difference with regard to live birth rate when patients were stratified to transdermal testosterone pretreated and no pretreatment groups (7.7% versus 8.3%, respectively) [16].

In summary, although available data support utilization of testosterone during OS, more research with larger sample size is needed in the future to confirm the efficacy and optimal treatment schema in women with POR.

5.2.4   Letrozole

Letrozole is a nonsteroidal competitive inhibitor of the aromatase enzyme system and inhibits the conversion of androgens to estrogens. It is commonly used in women with polycystic ovary syndrome for ovulation induction and in women with hormone-dependent cancers such as breast cancer to decrease the blood level of estrogen during ovarian stimulation for fertility preservation [17, 18]. The biological rationale for the possible augmentative benefit of aromatase inhibitors in ovarian stimulation is the positive effect of intraovarian androgens on development of small follicles and proliferation of granulosa and theca cells to augment follicular sensitivity to FSH [19].

Initial attempt to evaluate the efficacy of letrozole was done by comparing microdose flare-up (MF) protocol. In a retrospective case-control study including 1383 consecutive cycles predicted to have or with a history of poor ovarian response, MF protocol was used in 673 patients (1026 cycles), and the antagonist/letrozole (AL) protocol was used in the remaining 212 patients (357 cycles) [20]. Whereas the total gonadotropin consumption, duration of stimulation, estradiol level on the day of hCG administration, number of oocytes retrieved were significantly lower, and the rate of at least one top-quality embryo transferred were higher with the AL protocol, the clinical pregnancy rates were comparable between the two groups [20].

Other than case-control studies, a systematic review has been published recently including 4 studies and 223 women. The authors reported that letrozole supplementation does not improve the number of oocytes retrieved or clinical pregnancy rates (OR 1.28; 95% CI 0.60–2.73) [5]. In a following RCT [21], which had not been included in previous meta-analysis, the authors aimed to investigate whether IVF outcomes would differ between patients with POR according to Bologna criteria who received three different gonadotropin doses with or without the addition of letrozole during ovulation stimulation. Whereas 31 patients were treated with 450 IU gonadotropins, another cohort of 31 women was treated with 300 IU gonadotropins. The last group comprising 33 patients was treated with 150 IU gonadotropins in combination with letrozole. The authors reported that the total dose of gonadotropin was significantly less when letrozole was supplemented, but number of retrieved oocytes, implantation, and ongoing pregnancy rates were comparable among all groups [21]. It is not clear if mild stimulation group benefited from letrozole or the low-dose gonadotropin use per se to have comparable outcomes to high-dose gonadotropin groups. The data strongly suggested that increasing the gonadotropin doses in women with POR did not improve the outcome -in assisted reproductive technologies.

5.2.5   Luteinizing Hormone

Luteinizing hormone (LH) has crucial role during the early folliculogenesis by increasing FSH-receptor expression in granulosa cells, acting synergistically with IGF-1, and increasing recruitment of preantral and antral follicles. During the late follicular phase, its function is mandatory for optimization of steroidogenesis, regulation of final folliculogenesis, and oocyte maturation.

Based on theoretical advantages, there have been various conditions in which LH supplementation was tested. In patients with hypo-response, as defined by unexpected poor ovarian response in spite of apparently normal ovarian reserve, LH supplementation from stimulation days 7–10 might be more efficient with regard to number of oocytes retrieved, implantation and pregnancy rates when compared with increasing FSH dose only [22–24]. In a randomized, open-label, controlled trial performed in two age subgroups, impact of LH administration on GnRH antagonist cycles was evaluated [25]. In women ≤35 years old, they were randomized either FSH (225 IU/day) or FSH (150 IU/day) + LH (75 IU/day) arms [25]. With a similar design, women with an age of 36–39 years old were randomized as (300 IU/day) or FSH (225 IU/day) + LH (75 IU/day) arms. Whereas there was no significant difference between the two protocols in terms of implantation and pregnancy rates in women ≤35 years old, there was statistically higher implantation and ongoing pregnancy rate per cycle in LH supplemented group for women 36–39 years old [25]. Besides those particular cohorts of patients, unfortunately, available data ($n = 7$ studies) does not support adding LH to FSH with the aim of improving success rates in patients with POR or DOR when compared with women treated with FSH alone [26].

5.2.6   Melatonin

Melatonin is a hormone secreted by the pineal gland that aids sleep process as well as serves as an antioxidant [27]. It was reported that melatonin levels are higher in follicular fluid of preovulatory follicles suggesting that it has a potential role in follicular development and maturation [28]. Melatonin levels of the patients were also positively correlated with antral follicle count and serum anti-Müllerian hormone concentrations [29].

Although there are several studies aiming to assess the role of melatonin treatment in animal models, there is paucity of data for its role in women with POR or DOR during an IVF cycle. In a double-blinded RCT [28], the authors investigated the effect of melatonin on the outcome of ART cycles in women with diminished ovarian reserve by administering 3 mg daily from the fifth day of the preceding cycle before OS. Although higher serum estradiol levels on the trigger day and better-quality embryos were obtained compared to controls, overall pregnancy rate did not differ from the control group [28]. In spite of those encouraging results, we need more data to obtain conclusive results for the efficacy of melatonin supplementation.

5.3   Dietary Supplementation in Women with POR

5.3.1   Coenzyme Q10

The underlying molecular mechanisms of ovarian aging are not fully understood; however, one of the hypothesis is a breakage of DNA strand due to increased oxidative stress [30]. Since mitochondria and nucleus have their own DNA, the accumulation of reactive oxygen species may lead to oxidative damage in both of them. In this respect, coenzyme Q10 (CoQ10) might be a potential source of adjuvant to enhance OS outcome and pregnancy rate in patients with diminished ovarian reserve given to its antioxidant feature. Together with its antioxidative property, CoQ10 also plays a role in the production of cellular energy and adenosine triphosphate.

CoQ10 supplementation was previously tested in normal-responder women to improve cycle outcomes. The available data suggested that CoQ10 concentration within the follicular fluid was positively correlated with embryo quality and pregnancy rate [31, 32]. However, particularly for low-prognosis young women, there is only one RCT investigating the effect of CoQ10 on ovarian response and embryo quality [33]. In this trial, a total of 186 consecutive young patients (age < 35) with low ovarian reserve parameters were randomized to CoQ10 pretreatment for 60 days before IVF cycle or to no pretreatment arm. Although baseline demographic and clinical characteristics were comparable between the two groups, CoQ10 pretreatment arm required significantly lower gonadotropin dose with gained increased number of oocytes and high-quality embryos [33]. Although there was numerically higher clinical pregnancy and live births per embryo transfer and initiated cycle in favor of CoQ10 group, it did not reach statistical significance [33].

Although CoQ10 appears to be a promising supplement particularly for young women but with low ovarian reserve markers, further research is required with larger sample size to conclude its efficacy. Timing, duration, and dose of CoQ10 also need attention to be defined for future investigations.

5.3.2 Vitamin D

Previous studies demonstrated that vitamin D might play a role in ovarian steroidogenesis, but the mechanism underlying the relationship between deficiency and reproduction is still unclear [34]. Those assumptions are mainly due to the fact that gonadal function may be influenced when there is obvious vitamin D deficiency, as observed by the expression of vitamin D receptor mRNA in human ovaries, mixed ovarian cell cultures, and granulosa cell cultures [35]. Although there is no study showing the effects of vitamin D supplementation on ovarian stimulation outcomes particularly in women with POR, the association between vitamin D and ovarian reserve was investigated in some studies with conflicting results. According to the largest cross-sectional study including 388 premenopausal women with regular menstrual cycles, a relationship exists between circulating 25-hydroxyvitamin D (25 OH-D) and AMH in women $\geq$40 years old. The authors emphasized that 25 OH-D deficiency might be associated with lower ovarian reserve in late reproductive-aged women [36]. In contrast, a prospective cross-sectional study including 283 consecutive infertile women younger than 42 years old revealed that the mean AMH (3.9 ± 3.8 ng/mL vs. 4.3 ± 4.8 ng/mL) and AFC (13.9 ± 13.3 vs. 12.7 ± 11.4) levels did not differ significantly between patients with 25 OH-D deficiency or not [35]. In multiple linear regression analysis, after adjusting for potential confounders (age, body mass index, smoking status, infertility cause, and season of blood sampling), the regression slope in all participants for total 25 OH-D predicting log10 AMH was 0.006 (standard error = 0.07, $P = 0.9$).

To sum up, we can underline the need for further research for the possible effect of vitamin D on ovarian reserve and fertility not only for poor responders but also for the whole infertile population.

5.3.3 Weight Loss and IVF

Understanding the correlation between female body mass index (BMI) and IVF outcomes is very important since approximately half of reproductive-aged women in the USA is overweight [37]. In the context of Nurses' Health Study-3 (2010–2014), in which 1950 women has been prospectively followed and attempting pregnancy, the authors tested whether a weight change since age 18 years, current BMI, and BMI at age 18 years were associated with fecundity [38]. The authors noticed that for every 5-kg increase in body weight from age 18 years, current duration of pregnancy attempt increased by 5% (95% CI, 3–7%). Compared with women who maintained weight, the adjusted median current duration was 0.5 months shorter in those who lost weight, 0.3 months longer for those who gained 4–9.9 kg and 10–19.9 kg, and 1.4 months longer for those who gained 20 kg or more (p trend <0.001). The adjusted time ratio (95% CI) for a 5-kg/m^2 increase in current BMI was 1.08 (95% CI, 1.04–1.12). Overall, gaining weight in adulthood, being overweight or obese in adulthood, and being underweight at age 18 years were associated with a modest reduction in fecundity [38].

Other than natural conception, studies investigating the potential impact of elevated BMI on fertility treatment outcomes are conflicting. Although some studies are reporting no significant adverse effect of elevated BMI on IVF outcomes [39, 40], there are other studies associating elevated BMI with fewer retrieved oocytes and reduced rates of pregnancy and live birth [41]. In the most recent study, from 2018, 51,198 women who initiated their first autologous IVF cycle in 13 different fertility centers were examined for the impact of BMI on IVF cycle outcomes [42]. Women who are overweight (BMI = 25–29.9 kg/m^2) or obese (BMI >30 kg/m^2) experienced greater odds of cycle cancellation, fewer retrieved oocytes, fewer usable embryos, and lower odds of ongoing clinical pregnancy. In concordance, a meta-analysis including 33 studies including 47,967 treatment cycles [43], overweight or obese women undergoing IVF were observed to have a lower relative risk of clinical pregnancy (RR = 0.90, $P < 0.0001$) and live birth (RR = 0.84, $P = 0.0002$), with a higher miscarriage rate (RR = 1.31, $P < 0.0001$).

Although there is enough number of studies to conclude against obesity with respect to IVF outcome, it is interesting to note that there are no conclusive data that indicate if weight reduction can rectify success rates. In a multicenter randomized controlled trial including 317 women, intensive weight reduction prior to IVF revealed that the live birth rate was 29.6% (45/152) in the weight reduction and IVF group and 27.5% (42/153) in the IVF-only group [44]. The difference was not statistically significant (difference 2.2%, 95% CI, 12.9 to −8.6, $P = 0.77$). The mean (SD) weight change was −9.44 (6.57) kg in the weight reduction and IVF group as compared to +1.19 (1.95) kg in the IVF-only group, being highly significant ($p < 0.0001$). Notably, significantly more live births were achieved through spontaneous pregnancies in the weight reduction and IVF group, at 10.5%, as compared to the IVF-only group, at 2.6% ($P = 0.009$). Miscarriage rates and gonadotropin dose used for IVF stimulation did not differ between groups (29.6% vs. 27.5%) [44].

Since there is no direct assessment of patients with high BMI and POR, we can assume that obesity might further decrease the chance of live birth based on available studies conducted among the whole population. However, as is in the case of whole population, there are no data suggesting that losing weight during or immediately before IVF makes any benefit with regard to live birth rate beyond some improvements on ovarian stimulation parameters.

5.3.4 Dietary Context and IVF

The dietary context and its effect on fertility treatment have been a matter of debate between physicians and patients. However, there are only a few prospective and longitudinal studies looking into this issue. In the context of EARTH (Environment and Reproductive Health) study, which is an ongoing prospective cohort started in 2006 aiming at identifying determinants of fertility, the effect of pretreatment whole-grain intake on IVF outcomes were assessed [45]. The authors reported that higher pretreatment whole-grain intake was associated with higher probability implantation and live birth. The adjusted percentage of cycles resulting in live birth for women in the highest quartile of whole-grain intake (>52.4 g/day) was 53% (95% CI, 41–65%) compared with 35% (95% CI, 25–46%) for women in the lowest quartile (<21.4 g/day) [45].

Other than grains, EARTH study group has also investigated association between protein intake and fertility. In two consecutive studies, the authors reported that whereas women with higher pretreatment intakes of fish had a higher probability of live birth following an ART cycle [46], a higher dairy protein intake ($\geq$5.24% of energy) was associated with lower AFC among women presenting for infertility treatment [47]. The authors also confirmed that serum polyunsaturated fatty acids concentrations, including omega-3 but not omega-6 were positively associated with probability of live birth among women undergoing ART [48]. For the folate and vitamin B-12 intake, the authors noticed that women in the highest quartile of serum folate (>26.3 ng/mL) had 1.62 (95% CI, 0.99–2.65) times the probability of live birth compared with women in the lowest quartile (<16.6 ng/mL) [49]. Women in the highest quartile of serum vitamin B-12 (>701 pg/mL) had 2.04 (95%; CI, 1.14–3.62) times the probability of live birth compared with women in the lowest quartile (<439 pg/mL). Of interest, women with serum folate and vitamin B-12 concentrations greater than the median had 1.92 (95% CI, 1.12–3.29) times the probability of live birth compared with women with folate and vitamin B-12 concentrations less than or equal to the median. This translated into an adjusted difference in live birth rates of 26% (95% CI, 10–48%; $p = 0.02$) [49].

The optimal dietary setting that should be warranted during fertility treatment needs further evaluation with RCTs, because available studies suggesting positive effects of various products on treatment outcome have not been validated. Until that time, specifically for patients with POR and/or DOR, physicians might offer general recommendations for the ingredients of the diet based on aforementioned studies and findings.

5.4 Conclusion

To manage women with POR and/or DOR, many dietary and hormonal supplements have been tested during an IVF cycle to obtain higher number of oocytes retrieved and/or pregnancy rates. However, as mentioned above, very few of the available data might be gained from large RCTs, and there is no uniform approach for their utilization among studies. Just depending on limited data, one can claim that GH, DHEA, and transdermal testosterone might influence IVF outcomes to some extent. But neither the optimal time to commence and to cease nor the ideal dose and duration to apply are not clear. By extrapolating the data retrieved from the general population, we can assume that maintenance of normal weight beginning from the very early years of adulthood and the presence of a balanced diet context might be additional factors that can be considered in such cases.

References

1. Ferraretti AP, La Marca A, Fauser BC, et al. ESHRE consensus on the definition of 'poor response' to ovarian stimulation for in vitro fertilization: the Bologna criteria. Hum Reprod. 2011;26:1616–24.
2. Tapanainen J, Martikainen H, Voutilainen R, et al. Effect of growth hormone administration on human ovarian function and steroidogenic gene expression in granulosa-luteal cells. Fertil Steril. 1992;58:726–32.
3. Norman R, Alvino H, Hart R, et al. A randomised double blind placebo controlled study of recombinant human growth hormone (h-GH) on live birth rates in women who are poor responders. Hum Reprod. 2016;31:i37.
4. Keane KN, Yovich JL, Hamidi A, et al. Single-centre retrospective analysis of growth hormone supplementation in IVF patients classified as poor-prognosis. BMJ Open. 2017;7:e018107.
5. Jeve YB, Bhandari HM. Effective treatment protocol for poor ovarian response: a systematic review and meta-analysis. J Hum Reprod Sci. 2016;9:70–81.
6. Li XL, Wang L, Lv F, et al. The influence of different growth hormone addition protocols to poor ovarian responders on clinical outcomes in controlled ovary stimulation cycles: a systematic review and meta-analysis. Medicine (Baltimore). 2017;96:e6443.
7. Li J, Yuan H, Chen Y, et al. A meta-analysis of dehydroepiandrosterone supplementation among women with diminished ovarian reserve undergoing in vitro fertilization or intracytoplasmic sperm injection. Int J Gynaecol Obstet. 2015;131:240–5.
8. Dorrington JH, Moon YS, Armstrong DT. Estradiol-17beta biosynthesis in cultured granulosa cells from hypophysectomized immature rats; stimulation by follicle-stimulating hormone. Endocrinology. 1975;97:1328–31.
9. Zhang M, Niu W, Wang Y, et al. Dehydroepiandrosterone treatment in women with poor ovarian response undergoing IVF or ICSI: a systematic review and meta-analysis. J Assist Reprod Genet. 2016;33:981–91.
10. Artini PG, Simi G, Ruggiero M, et al. DHEA supplementation improves follicular microenviroment in poor responder patients. Gynecol Endocrinol. 2012;28:669–73.
11. Schwarze JE, Canales J, Crosby J, et al. DHEA use to improve likelihood of IVF/ICSI success in patients with diminished ovarian reserve: a systematic review and meta-analysis. JBRA Assist Reprod. 2018;22:369–74.
12. Chern CU, Tsui KH, Vitale SG, et al. Dehydroepiandrosterone (DHEA) supplementation improves in vitro fertilization outcomes of poor ovarian responders, especially in women with low serum concentration of DHEA-S: a retrospective cohort study. Reprod Biol Endocrinol. 2018;16:90.
13. Al-Turki HA. Dehydroepiandrosterone supplementation in women undergoing assisted reproductive technology with poor ovarian response. A prospective case-control study. J Int Med Res. 2018;46:143–9.

14. Weil S, Vendola K, Zhou J, et al. Androgen and follicle-stimulating hormone interactions in primate ovarian follicle development. J Clin Endocrinol Metab. 1999;84:2951–6.
15. Gonzalez-Comadran M, Duran M, Sola I, et al. Effects of transdermal testosterone in poor responders undergoing IVF: systematic review and meta-analysis. Reprod Biomed Online. 2012;25:450–9.
16. Bosdou JK, Venetis CA, Dafopoulos K, et al. Transdermal testosterone pretreatment in poor responders undergoing ICSI: a randomized clinical trial. Hum Reprod. 2016;31:977–85.
17. Guang HJ, Li F, Shi J. Letrozole for patients with polycystic ovary syndrome: a retrospective study. Medicine (Baltimore). 2018;97:e13038.
18. Turan V, Bedoschi G, Emirdar V, et al. Ovarian stimulation in patients with cancer: impact of letrozole and BRCA mutations on fertility preservation cycle outcomes. Reprod Sci. 2018;25:26–32.
19. Garcia-Velasco JA, Moreno L, Pacheco A, et al. The aromatase inhibitor letrozole increases the concentration of intraovarian androgens and improves in vitro fertilization outcome in low responder patients: a pilot study. Fertil Steril. 2005;84:82–7.
20. Yarali H, Esinler I, Polat M, et al. Antagonist/letrozole protocol in poor ovarian responders for intracytoplasmic sperm injection: a comparative study with the microdose flare-up protocol. Fertil Steril. 2009;92:231–5.
21. Bastu E, Buyru F, Ozsurmeli M, et al. A randomized, single-blind, prospective trial comparing three different gonadotropin doses with or without addition of letrozole during ovulation stimulation in patients with poor ovarian response. Eur J Obstet Gynecol Reprod Biol. 2016;203:30–4.
22. De Placido G, Alviggi C, Perino A, et al. Recombinant human LH supplementation versus recombinant human FSH (rFSH) step-up protocol during controlled ovarian stimulation in normogonadotrophic women with initial inadequate ovarian response to rFSH. A multicentre, prospective, randomized controlled trial. Hum Reprod. 2005;20:390–6.
23. De Placido G, Mollo A, Alviggi C, et al. Rescue of IVF cycles by HMG in pituitary down-regulated normogonadotrophic young women characterized by a poor initial response to recombinant FSH. Hum Reprod. 2001;16:1875–9.
24. Ferraretti AP, Gianaroli L, Magli MC, et al. Exogenous luteinizing hormone in controlled ovarian hyperstimulation for assisted reproduction techniques. Fertil Steril. 2004;82:1521–6.
25. Bosch E, Labarta E, Crespo J, et al. Impact of luteinizing hormone administration on gonadotropin-releasing hormone antagonist cycles: an age-adjusted analysis. Fertil Steril. 2011;95:1031–6.
26. Alviggi C, Conforti A, Esteves SC, et al. Recombinant luteinizing hormone supplementation in assisted reproductive technology: a systematic review. Fertil Steril. 2018;109:644–64.
27. Tomas-Zapico C, Coto-Montes A. A proposed mechanism to explain the stimulatory effect of melatonin on antioxidative enzymes. J Pineal Res. 2005;39:99–104.
28. Jahromi BN, Sadeghi S, Alipour S, et al. Effect of melatonin on the outcome of assisted reproductive technique cycles in women with diminished ovarian reserve: a double-blinded randomized clinical trial. Iran J Med Sci. 2017;42:73–8.
29. Zheng M, Tong J, Li WP, et al. Melatonin concentration in follicular fluid is correlated with antral follicle count (AFC) and in vitro fertilization (IVF) outcomes in women undergoing assisted reproductive technology (ART) procedures. Gynecol Endocrinol. 2018;34:446–50.
30. Tanaka T, Huang X, Halicka HD, et al. Cytometry of ATM activation and histone H2AX phosphorylation to estimate extent of DNA damage induced by exogenous agents. Cytometry A. 2007;71:648–61.
31. Akarsu S, Gode F, Isik AZ, et al. The association between coenzyme Q10 concentrations in follicular fluid with embryo morphokinetics and pregnancy rate in assisted reproductive techniques. J Assist Reprod Genet. 2017;34:599–605.
32. Turi A, Giannubilo SR, Bruge F, et al. Coenzyme Q10 content in follicular fluid and its relationship with oocyte fertilization and embryo grading. Arch Gynecol Obstet. 2012;285:1173–6.

33. Xu Y, Nisenblat V, Lu C, et al. Pretreatment with coenzyme Q10 improves ovarian response and embryo quality in low-prognosis young women with decreased ovarian reserve: a randomized controlled trial. Reprod Biol Endocrinol. 2018;16:29.
34. Parikh G, Varadinova M, Suwandhi P, et al. Vitamin D regulates steroidogenesis and insulin-like growth factor binding protein-1 (IGFBP-1) production in human ovarian cells. Horm Metab Res. 2010;42:754–7.
35. Drakopoulos P, van de Vijver A, Schutyser V, et al. The effect of serum vitamin D levels on ovarian reserve markers: a prospective cross-sectional study. Hum Reprod. 2017;32:208–14.
36. Merhi ZO, Seifer DB, Weedon J, et al. Circulating vitamin D correlates with serum antimullerian hormone levels in late-reproductive-aged women: Women's Interagency HIV Study. Fertil Steril. 2012;98:228–34.
37. Practice Committee of the American Society for Reproductive M. Obesity and reproduction: a committee opinion. Fertil Steril. 2015;104:1116–26.
38. Gaskins AJ, Rich-Edwards JW, Missmer SA, et al. Association of fecundity with changes in adult female weight. Obstet Gynecol. 2015;126:850–8.
39. Dechaud H, Anahory T, Reyftmann L, et al. Obesity does not adversely affect results in patients who are undergoing in vitro fertilization and embryo transfer. Eur J Obstet Gynecol Reprod Biol. 2006;127:88–93.
40. Legge A, Bouzayen R, Hamilton L, et al. The impact of maternal body mass index on in vitro fertilization outcomes. J Obstet Gynaecol Can. 2014;36:613–9.
41. Comstock IA, Kim S, Behr B, et al. Increased body mass index negatively impacts blastocyst formation rate in normal responders undergoing in vitro fertilization. J Assist Reprod Genet. 2015;32:1299–304.
42. Kudesia R, Wu H, Hunter Cohn K, et al. The effect of female body mass index on in vitro fertilization cycle outcomes: a multi-center analysis. J Assist Reprod Genet. 2018;35:2013–23.
43. Rittenberg V, Seshadri S, Sunkara SK, et al. Effect of body mass index on IVF treatment outcome: an updated systematic review and meta-analysis. Reprod Biomed Online. 2011;23:421–39.
44. Einarsson S, Bergh C, Friberg B, et al. Weight reduction intervention for obese infertile women prior to IVF: a randomized controlled trial. Hum Reprod. 2017;32:1621–30.
45. Gaskins AJ, Chiu YH, Williams PL, et al. Maternal whole grain intake and outcomes of in vitro fertilization. Fertil Steril. 2016;105:1503–10.e4.
46. Nassan FL, Chiu YH, Vanegas JC, et al. Intake of protein-rich foods in relation to outcomes of infertility treatment with assisted reproductive technologies. Am J Clin Nutr. 2018;108:1104–12.
47. Souter I, Chiu YH, Batsis M, et al. The association of protein intake (amount and type) with ovarian antral follicle counts among infertile women: results from the EARTH prospective study cohort. BJOG. 2017;124:1547–55.
48. Chiu YH, Karmon AE, Gaskins AJ, et al. Serum omega-3 fatty acids and treatment outcomes among women undergoing assisted reproduction. Hum Reprod. 2018;33:156–65.
49. Gaskins AJ, Chiu YH, Williams PL, et al. Association between serum folate and vitamin B-12 and outcomes of assisted reproductive technologies. Am J Clin Nutr. 2015;102:943–50.

Chapter 6
Traditional Chinese Medicine for Assisted Reproductive Technology

Wei Shang

6.1 Introduction

In 1978, Dr. Patrick Steptoe, an expert in gynecology and laparoscopic surgery, and embryologist Dr. Robert Edwards successfully applied in vitro fertilization–embryo transfer (IVF–ET) technology resulting in and the first case of test-tube baby in the world, which was a big milestone and opened up a new way to treat infertile couples with assisted reproductive technology (ART). At present, ART has been expanded significantly in its clinical applications, incorporating various advances in ovarian physiology, reproductive endocrinology cryobiology, genetics, embryo culture, and transfer techniques [1].

However, there are still many challenges in ART. Currently, the average global clinical pregnancy rates with ART is running between 30% and 40%, and the take-home baby rates are even much lower [2]. Some patients are still unable to achieve successful pregnancy outcomes after repetitive trials at various ART practices. Therefore, they may face with the serious consequences of lifelong infertility [3]. There are many other problems needed to be solved, such as poor ovarian response, advanced reproductive age, diminished ovarian reserve (DOR), and recurrent implantation failure, all of which should be overcome in order to boost live birth rates with ART.

Traditional Chinese medical science (TCMS) has a long and extensive history. Traditional Chinese medical science has applied methods for curing infertility, and its efficacies have been clinically affirmed. This chapter reviews TCMS approaches for fertility treatment or to support ART success.

W. Shang (✉)
Reproductive Medicine Center, Department of Obstetrics and Gynecology, Sixth Medical Center, Chinese PLA General Hospital, Beijing, China

© Springer Nature Switzerland AG 2020
O. Bukulmez (ed.), *Diminished Ovarian Reserve and Assisted Reproductive Technologies*, https://doi.org/10.1007/978-3-030-23235-1_6

6.2   Traditional Chinese Medicine Science

6.2.1   Reproduction

Per TCMS "kidneys control reproduction," "menstruation is based on kidneys," and "menstruation is from kidneys." With abundant and vigorous kidney energy, full kidney essence, unblocked Ren and Chong channels, and harmonious vital energy and blood, the menstruation will be symphonious, and women can get pregnant. However, with insufficient kidney energy and insufficient kidney essence, women may suffer from the disorder of vital energy and blood and cannot get pregnant. Therefore, tonifying the kidney and regulating menstruation are important treatment approaches for infertility in TCMS.

Many studies have shown that the use of TCMS in IVF can enhance clinical pregnancy rate [4, 5]. TCMS already has rich record of accomplishment and perfect theoretical system in gynecology and obstetrics. Theories such as "regulating menstruation before infertility treatment" and "two kinds of essences should be met to achieve pregnancy" play important roles for guiding modern medical treatment [5].

6.2.2   Assisted Reproductive Technology

The aspects of ART where TCMS found its applications include the following:

1. Controlled ovarian stimulation (COS): Tonifying the kidney, invigorating the spleen, and draining dampness can significantly reduce the risk of ovarian hyperstimulation syndrome (OHSS), alleviate the severity of OHSS, and increase the chance of fresh embryo transfer in patients at high risk for OHSS [6]. Periodic traditional Chinese medicine (TCM) treatment before COS by tonifying the kidney and regulating menstrual cycles in women with predicted poor ovarian response can improve ovarian response, which may involve the regulation of the hypothalamus–pituitary–ovary axis and ovarian microenvironment [7]. The combination of kidney-tonifying TCM can significantly reduce the dose of gonadotropins (Gn), improve the ovarian response, increase the number of oocytes retrieved, and improve oocyte quality, which result in increased pregnancy rates [8]. The mechanism of action of tonifying the kidney and activating blood circulation in diminished ovarian reserve patients is intended to regulate reproductive hormones, inhibit the apoptosis of ovarian granulosa cells, and promote ovarian angiogenesis [9].
2. Embryo transfer: It is very important to improve endometrial receptivity, and therefore TCMS believes that viscera, menstruation, vital energy and blood, and uterus and Chong, Ren, Du, and Dai channels are the physiological bases of female reproductive system. Among them, the kidney, menstruation, uterus, and Chong and Ren channels are the central lines. According to TCM theory, kidney

vacuity and essence depletion cause reproductive problems. In addition, liver dysfunction leads to inability of storing and regulating blood; dysfunction of spleen in transportation causes inability of producing blood and absorbing blood. All of these components are involved in the main pathogenesis of low endometrial receptivity. We should apply vital energy-enhancing, blood-replenishing, and liver and kidney-tonifying TCM in ART to optimize endometrial receptivity, to improve embryo implantation and pregnancy rates [10].

3. Prevention of miscarriages: TCMS emphasizes that the pathogenesis of miscarriage is due to the damage to Chong and Ren channels and instability of embryo due to various causes of disease. Therefore, tonifying the spleen and kidney is the key to prevent miscarriage [11]. It is found that the Modified An Dian Laing Tian Tang has a significant effect in treatment of threatened abortion due to spleen and kidney deficiency in ART patients. It can promote embryo development and reduce excitability of myometrium by regulating the endocrine system and result in strengthen vigor and prevent miscarriage [12]. The research showed that TCM, such as using Gu Tai Tang and Sheng Qi Shou Tai Wan, is effective treatment for late threatened abortion in ART patients [13].

In short, further studies are needed regarding how to standardize and expand the TCM in every aspect of IVF–ET. It is necessary to make further efforts and research on combining the theory of TCMS and the research methodology of Western medicine to provide new and cost-effective treatment alternatives for women undergoing ART cycles.

6.3 Traditional Chinese Medicine

Traditional Chinese medicine is also known as Han medicine. It is considered a valuable treasure of Chinese culture, and TCM has made great contributions to the prosperity of the Chinese nation. The treatment concepts of TCM are finding more acceptance worldwide. Traditional medicine has attracted more and more attention from the international community. Traditional Chinese medicine is mentioned as "Chinese materia medica" in ancient Chinese books. The earliest Chinese monograph on science of Chinese pharmacology is Sheng Nong's *Herbal Classic* written during the Han Dynasty. *Tang Materia Medica* issued by the government in the Tang Dynasty is the earliest pharmacopoeia in the world. *Valuable Prescriptions for Emergency* and *Supplement to Valuable Prescriptions for Emergency* compiled by Sun Simiao in the Tang Dynasty are the culmination of experience in diagnosis and treatment before the Tang Dynasty and have great influence on doctors of later ages. *Compendium of Materia Medica* written by Li Shizhen in the Ming Dynasty summarizes the drug experience before the sixteenth century and makes great contributions to the development of pharmacology in later ages.

6.3.1 Infertility

Traditional Chinese medicine and pharmacology have a long history in infertility treatment. According traditional Chinese medicine theory, the pathogenesis of infertility is the deficiency of the kidney [14]. In this section, we will present TCM formulas for infertility.

6.3.1.1 ART

Among infertile women receiving treatment of ART, 53.9% of them were diagnosed with kidney–Yang deficiency by doctors of TCM [15]. Wenshen'antai Decoction, including prepared *Rehmannia* root, pulp of *Cornus*, seed of Chinese dodder, Sichuan teasel, fried *Eucommia ulmoides*, *Loranthus parasiticus*, *Morinda officinalis*, glossy privet fruit, *Angelica sinensis*, root of red-rooted *Salvia*, Scutellaria baicalensis, and some others should be decocted in water for oral intake one dose twice per day. The decoction should be commenced on the second day after embryo transfer and continued for 5–7 days. Then the components which will nourish the blood and promote the blood circulation, such as root of red-rooted *Salvia. Angelica sinensis* should be removed from the decoction, and the decoction should be taken for another 5–7 consecutive days. In a relevant study, progesterone or human chorionic gonadotropin (HCG) was also administered to 40 patients with history of IVF–ET failure after the embryo transfer. Compared with the control group only taking Western medicine, the result shows Wenshen'antai Decoction can enhance the pregnancy rate of the second embryo transfer of patients who experienced embryo implantation failure ($P < 0.05$); moreover, it can increase the pregnancy rate of patients who experienced multiple implantation failures ($P < 0.01$) [16]. Li et al. [16] found that Wenshen'antai Decoction with prepared *Rehmannia* root, pulp of *Cornus*, glossy privet fruit, and *Angelica sinensis* can nourish blood and Yin and tonify the liver and kidney; seed of Chinese dodder, Sichuan teasel, fried *Eucommia ulmoides*, *Loranthus parasiticus*, and *Morinda officinalis* can warm the uterus and kidney, nourish the bone marrow, strengthen Chong and Ren channels, promote pregnancy, and prevent miscarriage; largehead *Atractylodes rhizome* can tonify the spleen and prevent miscarriage; *Scutellaria baicalensis* can clear heat, relieve fidgetiness, and prevent miscarriage; and root of red-rooted *Salvia* can promote blood circulation, remove blood stasis, cool blood, and calm the nerves, which not only improves blood circulation of endometrium but also relieves mental anxiety and tension. Cooperation of the medicinal materials can strengthen Chong and Ren channels, warm the kidney, and promote pregnancy, which will create a good internal environment for the uterus and enhance the affinity between embryo and the uterus.

6.3.1.2 Tubal Factor

Damaged or blocked fallopian tubes is a main cause of female infertility. Feng et al. [17] utilized triple treatment, including TCM, Western medicine, and laparoscopy for woman with hydrosalpinx. They found that the pregnancy rate was 66.67%; the recovery rate was 66.67%; and the hydrosalpinx recurrence rate was 6.67% 1 year after triple treatments. In the triple treatments, TCM and Western medicine included the following steps:

1. Enema with TCM and Western medicine: Use 20 ml normal saline to dissolve 4000 units of chymotrypsin; then draw 16 units of gentamicin, 10 mg dexamethasone injection, and 20 ml red-rooted salvia injection to inject into rectum. Then inject metronidazole sodium chloride injection in the same way.
2. Application of hot compresses of TCM on abdomen: Hot compress of TCM consists of monkshood 15 g, cassia Twig 10 g, Sichuan pepper 10 g, green Chinese onion 3, *Ephedra* 5 g, ginger 10 g, garden balsam stem 15 g, *Impatiens* 15 g, *Angelica sinensis* 10 g, *Sanguis draconis* 3 g, frankincense 3 g, myrrh 3 g, borneol 1 g, camphor 1 g, and appropriate amount of vinegar.
3. Prescriptions of TCM as an oral medication: *Angelica sinensis* 10 g, root of red-rooted *Salvia* 10 g, Chinese honey locust spine 10 g, *Leonurus japonicus houtt* 10 g, *Fructus liquidambaris* 10 g, *Herba lycopi* 10 g, seed of cowherb 10 g, *Fructus aurantii* 10 g, red peony root 10 g, medicinal *Cyathula* root 10 g, *Akebia quinata* 5 g, *Angelica Sinensis* 5 g, and sliced *Cornus cervi* 5 g.

For patients with severe hydrosalpinx, the following medicinal materials shall be added: Rhizoma Sparganii treated with vinegar 5 g, *Curcuma zedoaria* treated with vinegar 5 g, and endothelium corneum gigeriae galli 5 g.

For patients with severe heat and dampness, the following medicinal materials shall be added: Shuteria pampaniniana 5 g, Herba Patriniae 5 g, and raw *Coix* seed 5 g.

For patients with kidney–Qi deficiency, the following medicinal materials shall be added: seed of Chinese dodder 10 g and teasel 10 g; for patients with kidney–Yang deficiency, the following medicinal materials shall be added: *Fluoritum* 5 g, *Morinda officinalis* 5 g, and raspberry 5 g.

6.3.1.3 Ovarian Factor

Ovarian follicular development disorders, such as polycystic ovary syndrome, luteinized unruptured follicle syndrome, anovulation, and others, are common causes of infertility. In TCM, treatment for ovarian follicular development disorder mainly focuses on treating "kidney deficiency." Deficiency of kidney essence is the key pathogenesis of ovarian follicular development disorder. Kidney deficiency causes blood stasis, which blocks Chong and Ren channels and the uterus. Without adequate nutrition, oocytes cannot be matured and excreted. Therefore, kidney nourishing and essence replenishing should be emphasized in the treatment. Yin nourishing and supporting Yang should be carried out at the same time. Both Yin and Yang should be nourished. Meanwhile, the right amount of blood nourishing and blood circulation-activating and blood stasis-removing medicines with appropriate compatibility should be used to treat both symptoms and root causes of disease [18]. In a study by Zhang et al. [19], PCOS patients receiving IVF–ET were randomly allocated to TCM group and control group, with 30 patients in each group. Compared to the control group, the patients in TCM arm took TCM formula (*Fluoritum* 30 g, seed of Chinese dodder 30 g, fruit of Chinese wolfberry 15 g, *Eucommia ulmoides* 15 g, *Angelica sinensis* 12 g, root of red-rooted *Salvia* 15 g, *Radix Achyranthis Bidentatae* 15 g, white peony root 12 g, Rhizoma Cyperi 12 g, and licorice 6 g) to tonify kidney and activate blood circulation in the process of COS. Their results showed that there was significantly higher rates of fertilization and embryo cleavage and greater high-quality embryo rate and clinical pregnancy rate in TCM arm as compared to those in the control group (*P* < 0.05). However, there was no significant difference in the number of eggs retrieved between the two groups (*P* > 0. 05).

6.3.1.4 Prevention of Ovarian Hyperstimulation Syndrome

Ovarian hyperstimulation syndrome (OHSS) is a dreaded complication of ART. Patients with severe OHSS present with hemoconcentration, hydrothorax and ascites, liver and kidney function damage, thrombosis, adult respiratory distress syndrome, and even death. In the view of TCM, the mechanism of OHSS is a large amount of kidney essence lost, which results in the emptiness of the uterus and loss of nourishment in Chong and Ren channels. Disorder of vital energy and blood and disorder of viscera function result in the occurrence of pathological products such as blood stasis and phlegm. The two disorders can interact with each other, which causes vicious circle and results in severe disorder of viscera function, vital energy, and blood, finally causing abdominal distention and edema [20]. Niu et al. [21] used kidney-tonifying and blood circulation-activating prescription to induce ovulation in 56 PCOS patients with clomiphene citrate. Control group only used HCG to induce ovulation. Their results demonstrated that kidney-tonifying and blood circulation-activating TCM (prepared *Rehmannia* root 10 g, monkshood 5 g, seed of Chinese dodder 15 g, fruit of Chinese wolfberry 15 g, *Poria cocos* 15 g, longspur *Epimedium* 15 g, *Ligusticum wallichii* 10 g, *Angelica sinensis* 10 g, peach kernel 10 g, safflower *Carthamus* 10 g, *Gleditsia sinensis* 15 g, pangolin 10 g) can significantly reduce the incidence of OHSS without affecting the ovulation rate and the pregnancy rate. For OHSS treatment, Zhao Rong et al. [22] used luteinizing granules (prepared *Rehmannia* root, Chinese yam, fruit of Chinese wolfberry, pulp of *Cornus*, seed of Chinese dodder, deer horn glue, tortoise plastron, *Codonopsis pilosula*, largehead Atractylodes rhizome, hyacinth bean, *Coix* seed, *Poria cocos*, and some others) combined with conventional luteal support treatment, which is compared with using luteal support treatment only. The cure rate of the test group was 90.9%, and the total effective rate was 100%; the cure rate and total effective rate in the control group were 61.5% and 80.8%. These differences were statistically significant favoring TCM co-treatment (*P* < 0.05). The authors mentioned that largehead Atractylodes rhizome and *Poria cocos* can invigorate the spleen and drain dampness; Chinese yam can strengthen the spleen and tonify the kidney; hyacinth bean and *Coix* seed can clear damp and promote diuresis and be helpful in treating the symptoms; seed of Chinese dodder and deer horn glue can warm and tonify kidney Yang; prepared *Rehmannia* root, fruit of Chinese wolfberry, tortoise plastron, and pulp of *Cornus* can nourish kidney Yin, which achieves the purpose of reinforcing Yang from Yin. The prescription treats both symptoms and root causes of OHSS.

6.3.1.5 Western Medicine

Supplementing modern ART with diagnosis and treatment of TCM plays an affirmative role in areas such as ovarian stimulation, increasing IVF success rate, increasing endometrial receptivity, and preventing complications of ART like OHSS. However, TCM is not standardized, lacking unified and objective diagnosis and treatment standards and also lacking evidence-based medicine research, poor theoretical repeatability, and insufficient theoretical depth. These aspects of TCM may lead to some concerns regarding its clinical applications. At present, the research on TCMS and TCM in ART is developing rapidly. It is believed that the combined treatment of TCM and Western medicine can be used widely. Traditional Chinese and Western medicines can complement each other advantages, to improve the treatment efficiency and quality of ART.

6.4 Acupuncture and Moxibustion

6.4.1 Definitions and Types

Acupuncture and moxibustion are the general designation of acupuncture therapy and moxibustion therapy. These are important components of TCMS, which include acupuncture theory, acupoints, acupuncture and moxibustion technology, and related instruments. These are the result of a valuable heritage developed on the basis of the cultural and scientific tradition of Chinese nation.

Acupuncture therapy refers to stabbing needling instruments (acupuncture needles in general) into patient's body in a certain angle with the guidance of TCMS and stimulates the specific parts of the human body by using acupuncture manipulation techniques, such as twirling needles and lifting and thrusting needles, to achieve the purpose of treating diseases.

Moxibustion therapy is intended to cauterize, smoke, and press certain acupoints on the surface of the human body with prefabricated moxibustion cones and moxibustion herbs through thermal stimulation to prevent and treat diseases. There are many types of acupuncture and moxibustion, and the most common types are acupuncture therapy, electroacupuncture therapy, and moxibustion therapy

6.4.2 Mechanism of Action

6.4.2.1 Dredging the Channels

The fundamental and direct therapeutic effect of acupuncture and moxibustion is to treat or prevent main and collateral channel block so that they can play their normal physiological functions. The main and collateral channels are "distributed in viscera, limbs, and joints." One of its main physiological functions is to enable vital energy and blood circulation. Blocked main and collateral channels will block vital energy and blood circulation, which clinically manifest as pain, numbness, swelling, and ecchymosis. Acupuncture and moxibustion can unblock main and collateral channels and recover normal vital energy and blood circulation by corresponding acupoints and acupuncture manipulation techniques, and by also inducing bleeding by pricking with three-edged needles.

6.4.2.2   Regulating the Balance Between Yin and Yang

The ultimate purpose of acupuncture and moxibustion treatment is to keep the balanced status of Yin and Yang. The mechanism of disease can be summarized as the imbalance of Yin and Yang. The acupuncture and moxibustion regulate the balance between Yin and Yang through Yin and Yang attributes of the main and collateral channels, compatibility of channels and acupoints, and acupuncture manipulation techniques.

6.4.2.3   Strengthening the Body Immunity to Eliminate Pathogenic Factors

The mechanism of acupuncture and moxibustion in strengthening the body immunity to eliminate pathogenic factors is to strengthen the human body's vital energy and eliminate pathogenic factors. The occurrence, development, and prognosis of disease are the process of the battle between the vital energy and the pathogenic factor. Acupuncture and moxibustion treatment play their roles in strengthening the body immunity to eliminate pathogenic factors.

6.4.3   Clinical Applications in ART and Infertility

6.4.3.1   Acupuncture and Moxibustion to Improve Ovarian Function

Improving Ovarian Endocrine Function

Wu et al. [23] found that 3-month electroacupuncture treatment was ineffective in patients with premature ovarian insufficiency. This treatment consisted of acupoint prescription I, UB33 (bilateral); acupoint prescription II, REN4; ST25 (bilateral); and ST29 (bilateral). The two acupoint prescriptions were acupunctured alternately every other day. The results suggested that acupuncture and moxibustion may significantly improve the endocrinologic function of patients with premature ovarian insufficiency by reducing FSH and LH levels while increasing estradiol (E2) levels ($P < 0.01$). FSH, LH, and E2 levels were not statistically significant between the month that the acupuncture and moxibustion treatment ended and the third-month follow-up visit. Therefore, the potential treatment effects were temporary. Mi et al. [24] treated 30 patients with poor ovarian response with transcutaneous electrical nerve stimulation (TENS). The main acupoints selected were REN4, REN3, SP6, EX-CA1, ST25, UB23, DU3, and DU4. After 3 months of treatment, patients' serum levels of FSH, LH, and E2 were significantly different from those before treatment.

Xu Yin et al., [25] treated 40 patients with ovulatory infertility by using electroacupuncture and moxa moxibustion on acupoints such as EX-CA1, REN4, and REN3 combined with activating acupoints with eight methods of intelligent turtle once a day for 3 months. They found that FSH and LH levels significantly decreased, and E2 levels significantly increased after treatment compared with the levels before treatment.

Promoting Follicular Development

Zhou et al. [26] randomly divided 63 DOR patients into treatment group and control group before they received IVF–ET treatment. The treatment group was treated with acupuncture and moxibustion sequential therapy according to menstrual cycle by stages. Acupoints selected for premenopausal period were REN6, REN4, GB34, and LIV3; acupoints selected for menstrual period were EX-B8 and DU4; acupoints selected for postmenopausal period were SP6, KID3, UB23, and UB17; and acupoints selected for ovulatory period were REN6, REN4, EX-CA1, ST36, and KID7. They found that the number of oocytes retrieved, the number of fertilized oocytes, the number of high-quality embryos, the embryo implantation rate, and the clinical pregnancy rate significantly increased in treatment group compared with control group.

Cui et al. [27] randomly divided 66 PCOS patients who were about to receive IVF–ET treatment into observation group and control group. Both groups used GnRH agonist long protocol for COS. The observation group received additional electroacupuncture intervention. The main acupoints selected were REN4, REN3, SP6, EX-CA1, and KID3. The authors noted that fertilization rate, cleavage rate, and high-quality embryo rate were significantly higher in observation group than the control group.

Lian et al. [28] randomly divided 66 IVF–ET patients diagnosed with kidney deficiency with the age 35 to 42 years old into observation group and control group. All patients received GnRH agonist long protocol. The observation group started with electroacupuncture treatment on the fifth day of menstruation, and the acupoints selected were SP6, EX-CA1, REN3, and REN4. For the control group, the same acupoints were selected for fake acupuncture. Electroacupuncture treatment was carried out every other day until the day of oocyte retrieval. High-quality oocyte rate and high-quality embryo rate were higher in observation group than in the control group.

Ovulation Induction

Yin et al. [29] treated 40 patients with anovulatory infertility with electroacupuncture, and the selected acupoints were DU4, REN4, SP6, EX-CA1, and ST36. After treatment, the ovulation rate was 45%. Total pregnancy rate within the first year after the treatment was 22.5%.

Zhang et al. [30] selected 50 patients with anovulatory disorder and randomly divided them into study group and control group. The study group was treated with acupuncture on ovarian acupoints by handle-twisting and lifting–thrusting method. Patients of the control group were given basic clinical treatment. They found that the rate of successful ovulation in the study group was 80%, which was significantly higher than the control group, in which the rate of successful ovulation was 40%.

Sheng et al. [31] randomly divided 138 infertile patients into treatment and control groups. The control group adopted long-term ovulation induction schedule. The treatment group added acupuncture and moxibustion therapy. The acupoints selected were REN8, REN3, REN4, EX-CA1, ST36, PC6, and SP6. Their results demonstrated that the ovulation rate and the pregnancy rate of the treatment group were significantly higher than those of the control group.

Improving Endometrial Receptivity

Xu et al. [32] randomly divided 176 patients undergoing frozen-thawed embryo transfer (FET) with history of recurrent implantation failure into observation group and control group. Both groups received conventional endometrial preparation before FET. The observation group was also given TENS from the tenth day of menstruation. There were significant differences in endometrial thickness, biochemical pregnancy rate, clinical pregnancy rate, and embryo implantation rate between the two groups, favoring TENS addition to conventional FET preparation. This study suggests that TENS can improve endometrial receptivity of patients with recurrent implantation failure.

Li et al. [33] randomly divided 90 patients suffering from failed IVF–ET cycles due to poor endometrial development of unknown reasons into observation group and control group. The observation group was intervened with transcutaneous electrical nerve stimulation from the fifth day of menstruation, and the acupoints selected were ST25, KID12, EX-CA1, and SP6. The observation and control groups both treated by GnRH agonist long protocol. By comparing the endometrial thickness, endometrial pattern, and blood flow parameters of the two groups, they suggest that transcutaneous electrical nerve stimulation can promote endometrial growth, improve endometrial receptivity, promote embryo implantation, and enhance clinical pregnancy rate.

Yan et al. [34] randomly divided 108 patients undergoing IVF/ICSI treatment into three groups: acupuncture group, placebo acupuncture group, and control group. Patients received acupuncture treatment 24 hours before embryo transfer and 30 minutes after embryo transfer in acupuncture group, and the acupoints selected were Group I, ST29, SP8, EX-CA1, and SP10 and Group II, ST36, KID3, UB23, and REN4. Patients receive acupuncture treatment on acupoints unrelated to embryo transfer in placebo acupuncture group. There is no acupuncture treatment in control group. They found that acupuncture can improve the endometrial blood flow and improve pregnancy rates in IVF patients.

The Analgesic Effect of Acupuncture and Moxibustion During the Oocyte Retrieval Process

Kou et al. [35] selected 462 patients receiving IVF–ET and divided them into three groups, meperidine alone, acupuncture-combined anesthesia, and intravenous anesthesia, and compared the analgesic effect and adverse reaction among the three groups. For the group of acupuncture-combined anesthesia, patients received intramuscular injection of meperidine in 50 mg 30 minutes before the operation and then received acupuncture. The acupoints selected were DU20, EX-CA1 (ear), SJ8 (ipsilateral), PC6, ST36, and SP6. The needles were retained until the end of the operation. Acupuncture-combined anesthesia and intravenous anesthesia could both alleviate patients' degree of pain and adverse reaction during the oocyte retrieval, reduce the need for other sedatives, and enhance the oocyte retrieval rate without direct effects on pregnancy results.

Chen et al. [36] randomly divided 106 IVF–ET patients into meperidine group, ear acupuncture group 1, and ear acupuncture group 2, to compare the analgesic effects of the three groups. The acupoints selected were Shen Men point and internal genitalia point in ear acupuncture group 1 and were heart point and subcortex point in ear acupuncture group 2. The electroacupuncture stimulation was applied to both groups, and the needles were retained until the end of operation. Finally, it was reported that electroacupuncture on ear acupoints is safe and effective for analgesia during the oocyte retrieval procedure. Analgesic effects were not significantly different between electroacupuncture stimulation on Shen Men point and internal genitalia point and electro acupuncture stimulation on heart point and subcortex point.

Acupuncture and Moxibustion to Reduce IVF-Associated Complications

He et al. [37] randomly divided 304 infertile ART patients into study group and control groups. GnRH-agonist long protocol was used for COS. Patients in study group were treated with acupuncture from the first day of COS until the day of embryo transfer. The control group did not receive acupuncture treatment. The main acupoints selected were REN4, REN3, EX-CA1, ST29, PC6, LI4, ST36, SP8, and SP6. The OHSS incidence rate of the study group was lower than that of the control group, and the difference was statistically significant ($P < 0.05$).

Yang [38] selected 102 patients with high risk of OHSS and randomly assigned them into acupuncture ovulation induction group (study group) and ovulation induction group (control group). COS was achieved with GnRH agonist long proto-col in both groups. The study group started receiving assisted traditional acupunc-ture treatment from the first day of COS to the day of oocyte retrieval. The main acupoints selected were Zhongyuan, REN3, REN4, EX-CA1, ST29, LI4, ST36, SP9, SP6, and KID3. The results show that the traditional acupuncture-assisted treatment can reduce the incidence of severe OHSS during the IVF–ET treatment. It may improve local microenvironment and metabolism of the ovary by reducing inflammatory response of human body and secretion of inflammatory factors.

6.4.4   Expectations and Concerns

In recent years, more research has focused on the application of acupuncture and moxibustion in reproductive medicine. These techniques may have unique advan-tages in improving ovarian response and endometrial receptivity and also in reduc-tion of COS complications and in decreasing the dose of gonadotropins. However, there are still some concerns, which need to be addressed: First, most of the researchers only pay attention to the follicular development, oocyte retrieval, and embryo implantation but ignore preconceptional care. Secondly, there are few fol-low-up studies to investigate the long-term efficacies of acupuncture and moxibus-tion, such as clinical pregnancy rate and live birth rate. Thirdly, there is a lack of high-quality, multicenter randomized controlled trials with a large sample size with a unified inclusion, exclusion, and efficacy determination criteria. In addition, therapeutic protocols reported in most clinical studies are the combinations of acu-puncture and modern therapy, which cannot well-reflect the characteristics of tra-ditional acupuncture and moxibustion. In recent years, most of the research is focused on applications of acupuncture and moxibustion to affect clinical out-comes of IVF-ET, but there are no efforts to investigate the real mechanisms of action of these technologies. This will limit the further clinical applications of acupuncture and moxibustion since they are still not justified for Western clinical practice. At present, animal testing is the main route of the exploring the mecha-nisms of acupuncture and moxibustion, although the related animal studies are very few. Moreover, the most common animal model selected is mouse, which is quite different from human beings in terms of reproduction. Exploring the mecha-nism of acupuncture and moxibustion is a unique significance for further effec-tively applying it in IVF–ET or for infertility.

6.5   Other Traditional Chinese Medicine Approaches

Besides TCMS, TCM, acupuncture, and moxibustion, there are other TCM-assisted treatments which can be used in the field of ART, such as naprapathy, cupping ther-apy, chiropractic, ear acupuncture therapy, enema therapy, navel paste made of

TCM, and music therapy of five elements of TCMS. The treatment for female infertility includes five aspects: kidney deficiency, disorder of liver and kidney, liver stagnation, internal retention of phlegm and dampness, and kidney deficiency and blood stasis.

Among them, naprapathy is a therapy, which combines modern medical theory and applies naprapathy manipulation to act on specific parts and acupoints of human body under the guidance of traditional Chinese medical theory, in order to prevent and treat diseases. From the perspective of traditional medicine, naprapathy can regulate the balance between Yin and Yang, unblock main and collateral channels, activate vital energy and blood circulation, nourish muscles and bones, and improve viscera functions. Viscera naprapathy takes effect by adjusting nerves and body fluid and can dilate blood vessels, promote blood flow, and improve the microcirculation.

The basic function of naprapathy manipulation are as follows: (1) unblock main and collateral channels and activate vital energy and blood circulation; (2) adjust viscera; (3) regulate tendons and remove stasis; and (4) bone setting and restoration.

Naprapathy therapy can promote the recovery of ovarian function and adjust endocrine disorders and basal body temperature abnormalities [39]. Naprapathy therapy can stimulate the main and collateral channels and regulate vital energy, blood circulation, and viscera functions, which result in abundant kidney essence, normal dredging function of the liver, unblocked vital energy and blood circulation, and symphonious Chong and Ren channels. Moxibustion can also stimulate Ren channel to connect to Sanyin channel, which will enhance the uterus' ability of gestating fetus [40].

Zhang et al. [41] reported that abdominal naprapathy may promote ovarian function by regulating vital energy and blood circulation, tonifying the liver and kidney, conditioning Chong and Ren channels, soothing the liver, and relieving depression. Therefore, it is significantly effective in the treatment of patients with corpus luteum maldevelopment, thin and weak body, and spleen–kidney deficiency.

Cupping therapy is a method that removes air in cups by burning and air exhaustion to create negative pressure in the cups, which can make cups adhere to acupoints or body surface of locations needing cupping therapy. This method makes congestion and blood stasis form on local skin, in order to prevent and treat diseases.

It is stated in *Plain Questions: On Dermal Parts*, "Since twelve channels are part of the skin, incidence of every disease is certainly shown on skin." Twelve dermal parts are closely related to main and collateral channels and viscera. Cupping therapy acts on the skin surface and then reaches the muscle, which can activate vital energy and blood circulation, promote blood circulation, and remove blood stasis. Modern medicine believes that cupping therapy causes a series of neuroendocrine changes and regulates the permeability of blood vessel wall, and influences diastolic and retractile function of blood vessels, which result in improved local blood circulation [42]. The main function of cupping therapy is to activate vital energy and blood circulation, to dispel pathogenic cold, to relieve pain, and to reduce swelling.

Chiropractic is a method of acting on the spine and surrounding muscles with various manipulations by physicians to achieve treatment purpose [43]. The chiropractic treatment keeps the spinal cord stage of lumbar vertebra consistent with that of pelvic organs, which makes the uterus prepared for pregnancy [44]. Some researchers believe slight anatomical position changes in the spine can cause pain in the neck, shoulders, waist, and legs and result in muscle spasm and poor blood and lymphatic circulation. Chiropractic treatment can restore normal physiological and anatomical position, thus alleviating muscle spasm, regulating nerve reflex, strengthening blood and lymphatic circulation, enhancing metabolism of tissue, relieving swelling and pain, and promoting rapid repair of damaged tissue [45, 46]. This method mainly treats infertility caused by lumbar vertebral bone injuries or lumbar vertebral diseases.

Ear acupuncture refers to the method of stimulating auricle acupoints by acupuncture to prevent and treat diseases and diagnosing diseases by observing and touching ears, preventing and treating diseases by stimulating auricle. In addition to traditional acupuncture carried out with acupuncture needles, there are more than 20 ear acupoint-stimulating methods, such as electric stimulating method, needle imbedding method, bloodletting method, injection method, magnet therapy method, ear clip method, drug application method, plaster application method, pellet pressing method, and laser method. Egyptian paleontologists documented that women used needles and braids on auricle to practice contraception in ancient Egypt. Hippocrates, an ancient Greek physician, reported that the bloodletting method was used to alleviate impotence and activate ejaculation [47].

Zhang et al. [48] used body acupuncture and ear acupuncture intervention before and after embryo transfer. With respect to body acupuncture, the acupoints selected before transplantation were PC6, SP8, LIV3, DU20, and ST29; the acupoints selected after embryo transfer were ST36, SP6, SP10, and LI4. Mild reinforcing and attenuating manipulation were used. With respect to ear acupuncture, ear acupoints, namely, HT7, EX-CA1, endocrine acupoint, and brain point, were acupunctured without twirling needle before and after embryo transfer. The non-acupuncture control group was the same as the normal treatment cycle. The results showed the pregnancy rate of the acupuncture group (46%) was significantly higher than that of the control group (26%).

Enema with traditional Chinese medicine including solution can be absorbed directly by the rectum and then act on pelvic organs, which may have benefits in endometriosis and chronic pelvic inflammatory disease treatment.

Wu [49] claimed that enema with TCM as an assisted treatment for endometriosis patients after laparoscopic operation is safe and effective, with high pregnancy rate. For infertile patients with tubal obstruction, enema therapy reduces the drug's gastrointestinal reaction, makes drug locally and directly absorbed, promotes blood circulation, increases tubal peristalsis, improves internal pelvic environment, causes tubal adhesions to release, and enhances the pregnancy rates.

Lu et al. [50] achieved good results in treating tubal obstruction by enema with TCM. For patients with chronic pelvic inflammation, they are often diagnosed with stagnation of vital energy and blood stasis and dampness–heat type by TCM. It means dampness and heat are retained in the lower energizer and block main and collateral channels of the uterus and vital energy and blood of the uterus, which form vital energy and blood stasis and obstruction in main and collateral channels and finally develop adhesions and masses. Combining enema therapy of TCM can effectively promote blood circulation to remove blood stasis, unblocking main and collateral channels, softening hardness to dissipate stagnation, and clearing heat and promoting diuresis with laparoscopic surgery. Pregnancy rate of infertile patients with chronic pelvic inflammation can be further enhanced [51].

Navel compressing with traditional Chinese medicine, including *Eucommia ulmoides*, Fennel fruit, China berry fruit, monkshood root, Radix Achyranthis Bidentatae, teasel, licorice, *Illicium verum*, tall *Gastrodia* fruit, freshwater sponge, Fructus Psoraleae, desert-living *Cistanche*, prepared Rhizome of adhesive *Rehmannia*, *Herba cynomorii*, fossil fragments, hippocampus, Chinese eaglewood, frankincense, *Fructus caryophylli*, myrrh, *Radix aucklandiae*, *Cervi cornu pantotrichum*, is also practiced. The herbal medicines should be decocted into ointment, dissolved into liquid by heat, and pasted to the navel. The ointment should be changed every 3–5 days. It can nourish the liver, kidney, and blood and warm channels, in order to treat infertility caused by deficiency of the liver and kidney.

The traditional music therapy in China takes the "harmony of music and human" and "unity of nature and human" as an ideal state. It emphasizes the balance of Yin and Yang and the inter-promoting relation among the heart, liver, spleen, lungs, and kidneys and promotes the balance of Yin and Yang in the human body, harmonization of vital energy and blood, and emotional comfort by orthodox and gentle five musical sounds and six tonalities in traditional music to treat diseases. The theory is pointed out in *The Yellow Emperor's Canon of Internal Medicine*, including that there are five elements (wood, fire, earth, metal, and water) in the world and they generate five musical sounds (Jue, Zhi, Gong, Shang, and Yu). There are five seasons (spring, summer, long summer, autumn, and winter) on the earth, and they produce five stages (birth, growth, change, collection, and store). Human has five internal organs (liver, heart, spleen, lungs, and kidneys) and five kinds of emotions (anger, joy, thought, worry, and fear). All of these reflect the organic connection between human and nature. It is also recorded that "Jue" is the sound of wood which is connected to the liver; "Zhi" is the sound of fire which is connected to the heart; "Gong" is the sound of earth which is connected to the spleen; "Shang" is the sound of metal which is connected to the lungs; and "Yu" is the sound of water which is connected to the kidneys. This is the principle of five-sound therapy. Therefore, according to the theory of five-sound therapy, the mode of motion of vital energy inside the living body is influenced by acoustic oscillations of different musical modes to comply with spreading of vital energy of wood, rising of vital energy of fire, placidity of vital energy of earth, adduction of vital energy of metal, and decline of vital energy of water, respectively. All of these result in harmonious and orderly circulation of vital energy and blood and steady state of viscera function operation [52].

The clinical diagnoses of patients with recurrent spontaneous abortion are mainly due to deficiency of spleen and kidney. "Gong" is the sound of earth, which is connected to the spleen; "Yu" is the sound of water which is connected to the kidneys.

According to the theory of midnight–midday ebb flow, vital energy and blood of spleen channel are vigorous at 10:00 a.m. (Sishi) every day. In order to enhance the efficacy of treatment, the patients should listen to music of Gong at 10 a.m. Vital energy and blood of kidney channel are vigorous at 5:00 p.m. (Youshi) every day, so the patients should listen to music of Yu at 5 p.m. Many research results show that anxiety is the only emotional factor that can cause pregnancy complications. The evidences suggest that complications of pregnancy, such as recurrent abortion, pregnancy-induced hypertension, premature delivery, and prolonged labor, may be associated with emotional factors during pregnancy, at least related to the stressful emotional conditions, which indicates that emotional stress in pregnant women can affect the fetal development and labor and delivery [53].

6.6   Conclusion

Traditional Chinese medicine is based on thousands of years of tradition and experience. There should be mechanistic and outcome-based studies in many applications and techniques we discussed in this chapter. In order to assure their real-life applications and their combination with Western medicine, more studies are required. We provide a supplemental file listing the English and Chinese names of the herbal substances, most of which are mentioned in this chapter.

Supplement

The Name of Chinese Herbal Medicine in Chinese and English

- Earthworm 地龙
- East Asian Tree Fern Rhizome 狗脊
- Elecampane Inula Root 土木香
- English Walnut Seed 胡桃仁
- Ephedra Herb 麻黄
- Epimedium Herb 淫羊藿
- Erect St. John'swort Herb 小连翘
- Eucommia Bark 杜仲
- European Verbena 马鞭草
- False Chinese Swertia Herb 当药
- Falsehellebore Root and Rhizome 藜芦
- Fennel Fruit 小茴香
- Fermented Soybean 淡豆豉
- Figwort Root 玄参

- Figwortflower Picrorhiza Rhizome 胡黄连
- Fineleaf Schizonepeta Herb 荆芥
- Finger Citron 佛手
- Fiveleaf Gynostemma Herb 绞股蓝
- Flos Caryophyllata 丁香
- Fortune Eupatorium Herb 佩兰
- Fortune's Drynaria Rhizome 骨碎补
- Fourstamen Stephania Root 粉防己/汉防己
- Fragrant Solomonseal Rhizome 玉竹
- Frankincense 乳香
- Freshwater Sponge 紫梢花

- Akebia Stem 木通
- Aloes 芦荟
- American Ginseng 西洋参
- Amur Ampelopsis Stem 山葡萄
- Amur Barberry Root 大叶小檗
- Amur Corktree Bark 黄柏
- Anemone Clematis Stem / Armand Clematis Stem 川木通
- Antelope Horn 羚羊角
- Arabian Jasmine Flower 茉莉花
- Argy Wormwood Leaf 艾叶
- Ash Bark 秦皮
- Asiatic Moonseed Rhizome 北豆根
- Asiatic Pennywort Herb 积雪草
- Baical Skullcap Root 黄芩
- Barbary Wolfberry Fruit 枸杞子
- Barbed Skullcap Herb 半枝莲
- Bear Gall 熊胆
- Beautiful Sweetgum Fruit 路路通
- Belladonna Herb 颠茄草
- Belvedere Fruit 地肤子
- Benzoin 安息香
- Bezoar 牛黄
- Biond Magnolia Flower 辛夷
- Bitter Apricot Seed 苦杏仁
- Bitter Orange 枳壳
- Black Nightshade Herb 龙葵
- Black Sesame 黑芝麻
- Blackend Swallowwort Root 白薇
- Blister Beetle 斑蝥
- Boat-fruited Scaphium Seed 胖大海
- Borax 硼砂
- Borneol 冰片

- Bottle Brush Herb 问荆
- Bottle Gourd Peel 葫芦
- Buffalo Horn 水牛角
- Bunge Auriculate Root 白首乌
- Cablin Potchouli Herb 广藿香
- Calamine 炉甘石
- Camphor 樟脑
- Camphorwood 香樟木
- Canton Ampelopsis Root 无刺根
- Cape Jasmine Fruit 栀子
- Carbonized Human Hair 血余炭
- Cassia Bark 肉桂
- Cassia Seed 决明子
- Cassia Twig 桂枝
- Castor Bean 蓖麻子
- Cattail Pollen 蒲黄
- Centipede 蜈蚣
- Chicken's Gizzard-membrane 鸡内金
- Chinaroot Greenbier Rhizome 菝契
- Chinese Angelica 当归
- Chinese Arborvitae Twig 侧柏叶
- Chinese Caterpillar Fungus 冬虫夏草
- Chinese Cricket 蟋蟀
- Chinese Date 大枣
- Chinese Dwarf Cherry Seed / 郁李仁
- Chinese Eaglewood 沉香
- Chinese Forgetmenot Root 接骨草
- Chinese Gall 五倍子
- Chinese Gentian 龙胆
- Chinese Globeflower Flower 金莲花
- Chinese Hibisci Rosae-Sinensis Flower 扶桑花
- Chinese Holly Leaf 枸骨叶
- Chinese Honeylocust Fruit 皂角
- Chinese Honeylocust Spine 皂角刺
- Chinese Ivy Stem 常春藤
- Chinese Knotweed Herb 火炭母
- Chinese Ladiestresses Root or Herb 盘龙参
- Chinese Ligusticum Rhizome / Jehol Ligusticum Rhizome 藁本
- Chinese Magnoliavine Fruit 五味子
- Chinese Mosla Herb 香薷
- Chinese Pulsatilla Root 白头翁
- Chinese Rose Flower 月季花
- Chinese Silkvine Root-bark 香加皮
- Chinese Siphonostegia Herb 铃茵陈

- Chinese Taxillus Twig 桑寄生
- Chinese Thorowax Root / 柴胡
- Chinese Trumpetcreeper Flower Common TrumpetcreeperFlower 凌霄花
- Chinese Waxgourd Peel 冬瓜皮
- Chinese Waxgourd Semen 冬瓜子
- Chinese Waxmyrtle Bark 杨梅
- Chinese Wolfberry Root-bark 地骨皮
- Cholla Stem 仙人掌
- Chrysanthemum 菊花
- Cicada Slough 蝉蜕
- Ciliatenerve Knotweed Root 朱砂莲
- Cinnabar 朱砂
- Clam Shell 蛤壳
- Clematis Root 威灵仙
- Coastal Glehnia Root 北沙参
- Cochinchina Momordica Seed 木鳖子
- Cochinchnese Asparagus Root 天门冬
- Cockscomb Flower 鸡冠花
- Coix Seed 薏苡仁
- Coloed Mistletoe Herb 槲寄生
- Colophony 松香
- Combined Spicebush Root 乌药
- Common Andrographis Herb 穿心莲
- Common Anemarrhena Rhizome 知母
- Common Bletilla Pseudobulb 白及
- Common Burreed Rhizome 三棱
- Common Cephalanoplos Herb 小蓟
- Common Cnidium Fruit 蛇床子
- Common Coltsfoot Flower 款冬花
- Common Curculigo Rhizome 仙茅
- Common Dysosmatis Rhizome and Root / Sixangular Dysosmatis Rhizome and Root 八角莲
- Common Fenugreek Seed 葫芦巴
- Common Fibraurea Stem 黄藤
- Common Floweringquince Fruit 木瓜
- Common Four-o'clock Root 紫茉莉根
- Common Foxglove Leaf 洋地黄叶
- Common Lophatherum Herb 淡竹叶
- Common Macrocarpium Fruit 山茱萸
- Common Monkshood Mother Root 川乌
- Common Nandina 天竺子

- Common Scouring Rush Herb 木贼
- Common Selfheal Fruit-Spike 夏枯草
- Common Threewingnut Root 雷公藤

- Common Vladimiria Root 川木香
- Common wedgelet Fern Leaf 乌韭
- Common Yam Rhizome / Wingde Yan Rhizome 山药
- Copperleaf Herb 铁苋菜
- Coral Ardisia Root 朱砂根
- Coralhead Plant Seed 相思子
- Coriander Fruit 芫荽子

- Costustoot 木香
- Cowherb Seed 王不留行
- Croton Seed 巴豆
- Cushaw Seed 南瓜子
- Cuttlebone 海螵蛸
- Dahurian Angelica Root/Taiwan Angelica Root 白芷
- Dahurian Rhododendron Leaf 满山红
- Danshen Root 丹参
- Dark Plum fruit 乌梅
- Decumbent Bugle Herb 筋骨草
- Dendrobium 石斛
- Densefruit Pittany Root-bark 白鲜皮
- Desertliving Cistanche 肉苁蓉
- Devil's Rush Herb 龙须草
- Digitalis Lanata Leaf 毛花洋地黄叶
- Divaricate Saposhnikovia Root 防风
- Dock Root 土大黄
- Doederlein's Spikemoss Herb 石上柏
- Donkey-hide Glue 阿胶
- DoubleteethPubescentAngilicaRoot/Pubescent Angelica Root 独活
- Dragon's Blood 血竭
- Dragon's Tongue Leaf 龙利叶
- Drgon's Bones , Fossilizid 龙骨
- Dried Ginger 干姜
- Dried Lacquer 干漆
- Dried Longan Pulp 龙眼肉
- Drug Sweetflag Rhizome 菖蒲
- Dutchmanspipe Fruit 马兜铃

- Epimedium Herb 淫羊藿
- Erect St. John'swort Herb 小连翘

- Eucommia Bark 杜仲
- Falsehellebore Root and Rhizome 藜芦
- Fennel Fruit 小茴香
- Fermented Soybean 淡豆豉
- Figwort Root 玄参
- FigwortflowerPicrorhizaRhizome 胡黄连

- Fineleaf Schizonepeta Herb 荆芥
- Finger Citron 佛手
- Fistular Onion Stalk 葱白
- Fiveleaf Gynostemma Herb 绞股蓝
- Flastem Milkvetch Seed 沙苑子
- Flos Caryophyllata 丁香
- Fluorite 紫石英
- Forest Frog's Oviduct 蛤蟆油
- Fortune Eupatorium Herb 佩兰
- Fortune Meadowrue Herb 白蓬草
- Fortune's Drynaria Rhizome 骨碎补
- Fragrant Solomonseal Rhizome 玉竹
- Frankincense 乳香
- Freshwater Sponge 紫梢花
- Galanga Galangal Seed 红豆蔻
- Gambir Plant 钩藤
- Garden Balsam Stem 透骨草
- Garden Burnet Root 地榆
- Garlic 大蒜
- Garter Snake 乌梢蛇
- Gecko 壁虎
- Giant St. John'swort Herb 红旱莲
- Giant Typhonium Rhizome 白附子
- Ginkgo Leaf 银杏叶
- Ginkgo Seed 白果

- Glabrous Greenbrier Rhizome 土茯苓
- Glossy Privet Fruit 女贞子
- Golden Larch Bark 土荆皮
- Golden Thread 黄连
- Gordon Euryale Seed 芡实
- Graceful Jessamine Herb 断肠草
- Grand Torreya Seed 榧子
- Grassleaf Sweelflag Rhizome 石菖蒲
- Great Burdock Achene 牛蒡子
- Great Willowherb Herb 柳兰
- Grosvener Siraitia 罗汉果
- Ground Beeltle 土鳖虫
- Guava Leaf 番石榴叶
- Gynura Root 红背三七
- Gypsum 石膏
- Gypsum 玄精石
- Hairy Antler 鹿茸
- Hairyvein Agrimonia Herb and Bud 仙鹤草
- Hawksbill Carapace 玳瑁

- Hawthorn Fruit 山楂
- Heartleaf Houttuynia Herb 鱼腥草
- Hedge Prinsepia Nut 蕤仁
- Hematite 赭石
- Hemp Fruit 火麻仁
- Hempleaf Negundo Chastetree Leaf 牡荆叶
- Henbane Leaf 莨菪叶
- Heterophylly Falsestarwort Root 太子参
- Himalayan Teasel Root 续断
- Hiraute Shiny Bugleweed Herb 泽兰
- Honey 蜂蜜
- Honeycomb 蜂房
- Honeysuckle Flower 金银花
- Horseweed Herb 小飞蓬
- Hot Pepper 辣椒
- Human Placenta 紫河车
- Hupeh Fritillary Bulb 湖北贝母
- Immature Bitter Orange 枳实
- Incised Notopterygium Rhizome /Forbes Notopterygium Rhizome 羌活
- India Canna Rhizome 美人蕉根
- India Madder Root 茜草
- India Mustard Seed 芥子
- Indian Buead 茯苓
- Indian Epimeredi Herb 防风草
- Indian Kalimeris Herb 马兰
- Indigowoad Leaf 大青叶
- Indigowoad Root 板蓝根
- Inula Flower 旋覆花
- Japanese Ampelopsis Root 白蔹
- Japanese Buttercup Herb 毛茛
- Japanese Climbing Fern Spore 海金沙
- Japanese Honeysuckle Stem 忍冬藤
- Japanese Hop Herb 葎草
- Japanese Snailseed Root 木防己
- Japanese Thistle Herb or Root 大蓟
- Japanese Wormwood Herb 牡蒿
- Kadsura Root-bark 紫荆皮
- Katsumade Galangal Seed 草豆蔻
- Kelp 昆布
- Knoxia Root 红大戟
- Kudzuvine Root 葛根
- Kusnezoff Monkshood Root 草乌
- Ladybell Root 南沙参
- Lalang Grass Rhizome 白茅根

- Lancelesf Lily Bulb / Greenish Lily Bulb / Low Lily Bulb 百合
- Largehead AtractylodesRhizome 白术
- Largetrifoliolious Bugbane Rhizome 升麻
- Leech 水蛭
- Lemonfragrant Angelica Root 香白芷
- Lemongrass Herb 香茅
- Lepidogrammitis Herb 鱼鳖草
- Lesser Galangal Rhizome 高良姜
- Levant Cotton Root 棉花根
- Lightyellow Sophora Root 苦参
- Lilac Daphne Flower Bud 芫花
- Lilyofthevalley Herb 铃兰
- Liquoric Root 甘草
- Little Multibanded Krait 金钱白花蛇
- Longhairy Antenoron Herb 金钱草
- Longstamen Onion Bulb 薤白
- Loquat Leaf 枇杷叶
- Lotus Leaf 荷叶
- Lotus Plumule 莲子心
- Lotus Rhizome Node 藕节
- Lotus Seed Pot 莲房
- Lotus Stamen 莲须
- Lovely Hemsleya Root 雪胆
- Lowdaphne Stringbush Flower and Leaf 黄芫花

- Lucid Ganoderma 灵芝
- Magnetite 磁石
- Malaytea Scurfpea Fruit 补骨脂
- Malt 麦芽
- Manchurian Wildginger 细辛
- Manshurian Dutchmanspipe Stem 关木通
- Mantis Egg-case 桑螵蛸
- Manyflower Gueldenstaedtid Herb 甜地丁
- ManyflowerSolomonsealRhizome / Siberian Solomonseal Rhizome / King Solomonseal Rhizome 黄精
- Manyprickle Acanto-Panax Root 刺五加

- Medcinal Evodia Fruit 吴茱萸
- Medicated Leaven 六神曲
- Medicinal Changium Root 明党参
- Medicinal Cyathula Root 川牛膝
- Medicinal Indianmulberry Root 巴戟天
- Medicine Terminalia Fruit 诃子
- Membranous Milkvetch Root / 黄芪
- Mexican Tea Herb 土荆芥

- Mirabilite 芒硝
- Moellendorf's Spidemoss Herb 地柏枝
- Mongolian Dandelion Herb 蒲公英
- Mongolian Snakegourd Root 天花粉
- Motherwort Herb 益母草
- Mountain Dragon 古山龙
- Mulberry Fruit 桑椹
- Mulberry Leaf 桑叶
- Mulberry Twig 桑枝
- Mus Covite 云母
- Musk 麝香
- Muskroot-like Semiaquilegia Root 天葵子
- Myrrh 没药
- Nacre 珍珠母
- Nakedflower Beautyberry Leaf 裸花紫珠
- Natural Indigo 青黛
- Ningpo Yam Rhizome 穿山龙
- Nutgrass Galingale Rhizome 香附
- Nutmeg 肉豆蔻
- Nux Vomica 马钱子
- Officinal Magnolia Bark 厚朴
- Opium 阿片
- Oriental Waterplantain Rhizome 泽泻
- Orpiment 雌黄
- Oyster Shell 牡蛎
- Pagodatree Pod 槐角
- Pale Butterflybush Flower 密蒙花
- Palmleaf Raspberry Fruit 覆盆子
- Pangolin Scales 穿山甲
- Panicled Fameflower Root 土人参
- Paniculate Swallowwort Root 徐长卿
- Papaya 番木瓜
- Papermulberry Fruit 楮实子
- Parslane Herb 马齿苋
- Peach Seed 桃仁
- Pearl 珍珠
- Pedate Pinallia Jackinthepulpit Rhizome 天南星
- Peking Euphorbia Root 京大戟
- Pepper 胡椒
- Peppermint 薄荷
- Pepperweed Seed / Tansymustard Seed 葶苈子
- Perilla Fruit 紫苏子
- Perilla Leaf 紫苏叶
- Perilla Stem 紫苏梗

- Pharbitis Seed 牵牛子
- Philippine Violet Herb 紫花地丁
- Phoenix Tree Seed 梧桐子
- Pilose Asiabell Root /Moderate Asiabell Root/Szechwon Tangshen Root 党参
- Pinellia Tuber 半夏
- Pipe fish 海龙
- Plant Soot 百草霜
- Plantain Herb 车前草
- Plantain Seed 车前子
- Platycladi Seed 柏子仁
- Platycodon Root 桔梗
- Pokeberry Root 商陆
- Pomegranate Rind 石榴皮
- Prepared Common Monkshood Daughter Root 附子
- Pricklyash Peel 花椒
- Pubescent Holly Root 毛冬青
- Puff-ball 马勃
- Pummelo Peel 化橘红
- Puncturevine Caltrop Fruit 蒺藜
- Purpleflower Holly Leaf 四季青
- Pyrrosia Leaf 石韦
- Quartz 白石英
- Radde Anemone Rhizome 竹节香附
- Radish Seed 莱菔子
- Ramie Root 苎麻根
- Rangooncreeper Fruit 使君子
- Realgar 雄黄
- Red Ochre 代赭石
- Red Paeony Root 赤芍
- Reed Rhizome 芦根
- Rehmannia Root 地黄
- Rhubarb 大黄
- Rice Bean 赤小豆
- Rice-grain Sprout 谷芽
- Ricepaperplant Pith 通草
- Romanet Grape Root 野葡萄
- Rose 玫瑰花
- Round Cardamom Fruit /Java Amomum Fruit 白豆蔻
- Rush 灯心草
- Rust-coloured Crotalaria Herb 假地兰
- Safflower 红花
- Saffron 西红花
- Sanchi 三七
- Sandalwood 檀香

- Scorpion 全蝎
- Sea Horse 海马
- Sea-ear Shell 石决明
- Seaweed 海藻
- Semen Nelumbinis 莲子
- Senna Leaf 番泻叶
- Sessile Stemona Root/Japanese Stemona Root/Tuber Stemona Root 百部
- Sharpleaf Galangal Fruit 益智仁
- Shepherdspurse Herb 荠菜
- Shinyleaf Pricklyash Root 两面针
- Shortleaf Kyllinga Herb 水蜈蚣
- Shortstalk Monkshood Root/Pendulous Monkshood Root 雪上一只蒿
- Shorttube Lycoris Bulb 石蒜
- Shouliang Yam Rhizome 薯莨
- Shrubalthea Bark 川槿皮
- Siberian Cocklour Fruit 苍耳子
- Silktree Albizzia Bark 合欢皮
- Sinkiang Arnebia Root /Redroot Gromwell Root 紫草
- Sinkiang Fritillary Bulb 伊贝母
- Skyblue Broomrape Herb 列当
- Slender Dutchmanspipe Root 青木香
- Slenderstyle Acanthopanax Bark 五加皮/南
- Snakegourd Fruit 瓜蒌
- Snakegourd Seed 瓜蒌仁
- Snow Lotus Herb 雪莲花
- Snowbell-leaf Tickclover Herb 广金钱草
- Songaria Cynomorium Herb 锁阳
- South Dodder Seed / Chinese Dodder Seed 菟丝子
- Spina Date Seed 酸枣仁
- Spreading Hedyotis Herb 白花蛇舌草
- Star Anise 八角茴香
- Starwort Root 银柴胡
- Stiff Silkworm 僵蚕
- Suberect Spatholobus Stem 鸡血藤
- Sulphur 硫黄
- Sun Euphorbia Herb 泽漆
- Sunflower Receptacle 向日葵
- Sweet Osmanthus Flower 桂花
- Sweet Wormwood Herb 青蒿
- Swordlike Atractylodes Rhizome / Chinese Atractylodes Rhizome 苍术
- Szechuan Lovage Rhizome 川芎
- Szechwan Chinaberry Fruit 川楝子
- Tabasheer 天竺黄
- Talc 滑石

- Tall Gastrodia Tuber 天麻
- Tamarind Pulp 酸角
- Tamariskoid Spikemoss Herb 卷柏
- Tangerine Peel 陈皮
- Tangerine Seed 橘核
- Tangut Anisodus Radix 山莨菪
- Tatarian Aster Root 紫菀
- Thinleaf Milkwort Root-bark 远志
- Thunberg Fritillary Bulb 浙贝母
- Toad Skin 蟾蜍皮
- Toad Venom 蟾酥
- Tokay 蛤蚧
- Tortoise Shell 龟甲
- Towel Gourd Stem 丝瓜藤
- Towel Gourd Vegetable Sponge 丝瓜络
- Tree Peony Bark 牡丹皮
- Tree-of-heaven Ailanthus Bark 椿皮
- Trifoliate Jewelvine Root or Stem 鱼藤
- Trifoliate-orange Immature Fruit 枸橘
- Triquetrous Tadehagi Herb 葫芦茶
- Trogopterus Dung 五灵脂
- Tsaoko Amomum Fruit 草果
- Tuber Fleeceflower Root 何首乌
- Tuber Fleeceflower Stem 夜交藤
- Tuber Onion Seed 韭菜子
- Tuberous Sword Fern Rhizome 肾蕨
- Turmeric 姜黄
- Turmeric Root-tuber 郁金
- Turtle Shell 鳖甲
- Twotooth Achyranthes Root 牛膝
- Unibract Fritillary Bulb 川贝母
- Ussuriensis Fritillary Bulb 平贝母
- Valerian Root 缬草
- Vietnamese Sophora Root 山豆根
- Villous Amomum Fruit / Cocklebur-like Amomum Fruit 砂仁
- Virgate Wormwood Herb / Capillary Wormwood Herb 茵陈
- Watermeion Peel 西瓜皮
- Waternut Herb 通天草
- Weeping Forsythiae Capsule 连翘
- White Mulberry Root-bark 桑白皮
- White Mustard Seed 白芥子
- White Paeony Root 白芍
- Whiteflower Hogfennel Root/Common Hongfennel Root 前胡
- Wild Chrysanthemum 野菊花

- Williams Elder Twig 接骨木
- Wrinkled Gianthyssop Herb 藿香
- Yanhusuo 延胡索
- Yellow Croaker Ear-stone 鱼脑石
- Yellowmouth Dutchmanspipe Root 汉中防已
- Yerbadetajo Herb 墨旱莲
- Yunnan Manyleaf Paris Rhizome / Chinese Paris Rhizome 重楼
- Zedoary 莪术
- Chinese Trumpetcreeper Flower Common TrumpetcreeperFlower 凌霄花
- Chinese Usnea 松萝

References

1. Almog B, Al-Shalaty J, Sheizaf B. Difference between serum beta-human chorionic gonadotropin levels in pregnancies after in vitro maturation and in vitro fertilization treatments [J]. Fertil Steril. 2011;95(1):85–8.
2. Yuan Xuefei, Cao Yang, Zhang Tingting. Research status and prospects of traditional Chinese medicine in in vitro fertilization-embryo transfer [J]. Hebei Tradit Chin Med. 2016;38(1):130–4.
3. Zegers-Hochschild F, Mansour R, Ishihara O, et al. International committee for monitoring assisted reproductive technology: world report on assisted reproductive technology 2005 [J]. Fertil Steril. 2014;101(2):366–78.
4. Cao H, Han M, Ng EH, et al. Can Chinese herbal medicine improve outcomes of in vitro fertilization? A systematic review and meta - analysis of randomized controlled trials [J]. PLoS One. 2013;8(12):e81650.
5. Ried K, Stuart K. Efficacy of traditional Chinese herbal medicine in the management of female infertility: a systematic review [J]. Complement Ther Med. 2011;19(6):319.
6. Ge Mingxiao, Zhang Jinyu, Deng Weimin, et al. Clinical study on prevention and treatment of ovarian hyperstimulation syndrome by invigorating kidney and strengthening spleen and dampness Chinese medicine in in vitro fertilization-embryo transfer cycle [J]. J Guangzhou Univ Tradit Chin Med. 2012;29(3):257–60.
7. Zhang Rong, Deng Weimin. Effect of traditional Chinese medicine menstrual cycle therapy on ovarian hyporesponsiveness [J]. Guangdong Med J. 2013;34(18):2873–5.
8. Lian Fang, Teng Yili, Zhang Jianwei, et al. Effects of granules on leukemia inhibitory factor and egg cell quality in human follicular fluid during in vitro fertilization-embryo transfer [J]. Chin J Integr Tradit West Med. 2007;27(11):976–9.
9. Xu Xiaofeng. Study on the effect mechanism and clinical evidence of the intervention of Bushen Huoxue method on ovarian reserve dysfunction [D]. Nanjing: Nanjing University of Traditional Chinese Medicine; 2010.
10. Deng Weimin, Zhao Yanpeng, Ge Mingxiao, et al. Effects of Yiqi Xuebu Ganshen Chinese medicine on clinical outcome of in vitro fertilization-embryo transfer [J]. J Liaoning Univ Tradit Chin Med. 2011;13(6):5–7.
11. Zhang Xubin, Sun Jingruo. Anlu two days of soup plus flavor treatment of 36 cases of spleen and kidney deficiency type threatened abortion after in vitro fertilization-embryo transfer [J]. Henan Tradit Chin Med. 2012;32(7):918–9.
12. Liu Ying, Wu Jingzhi. Clinical study on 126 cases of pregnancy induced abortion in vitro fertilization-embryo transfer [J]. J Tradit Chin Med. 2006;47(4):272–3.
13. Liu Xiaofeng, Lian Fang, Wang Ruixia. Professor Lian Fang's experience in treating 40cases of threatened abortion after in vitro fertilization-embryo transfer[J]. J Liaoning Univ Tradit Chin Med. 2011;13(5):169–70.

14. Lian Fang, Xin Mingwei. The essence of kidney deficiency after in vitro fertilization and embryo transfer [J]. J Shandong Univ Tradit Chin Med. 2008;32(2):109–10.
15. Ceyle M, Smith C. A survey comparing TCM diagnosis, health status and medical diagnosis in won°Cn undergoing assisted reproduction [J]. Acupunct Med. 2005;23(2):62–9.
16. Li Dong. Clinical study of Wenshen Antai decoction combined with assisted reproductive technology to improve pregnancy rate of patients with embryo transplant failure [J]. J Beijing Univ Chin Med. 2009;32(2):139–41.
17. Feng Donglan, Li Gaifei. 30 cases of sterility due to hydrosalpinx treated by combination of Chinese and Western medicine and laparoscopy [J]. Chin J Basic Med Tradit Chin Med. 2013;19(5):591–2.
18. Cai Jing, Wu Keming. Treatment of follicular dysplasia by invigorating kidney and activating blood [J]. J Changchun Univ Tradit Chin Med. 2012;28(6):1050.
19. Zhang Ning. Effect of tonifying kidney and activating blood circulation on follicular blood flow in patients with PCOS during IVF cycle [J]. J Mod Integr Tradit Chi West Med. 2011;20(29):3641–3.
20. Sun Danjie, Zhang Xiaoqing. Progress in the application of traditional Chinese medicine in assisted reproductive technology [J]. Zhejiang J Integr Tradit Chin West Med. 2016;26(9):873–6.
21. Niu Yu, Lin Yingxun. Clinical observation of Tonifying kidney and activating blood medicine instead of HCG to prevent OHSS [J]. Clin Study Tradit Chin Med. 2013;5(16):29.
22. Rong Z, Yanpeng Z, Dewei L, et al. Therapeutic effect of luteinizing granule on mild to moderate ovarian hyperstimulation syndrome [J]. J Emerg in Tradit Chin Med. 2011;20(8):1213.
23. Wu Jiani, Chen Ruixue, Liu Zhishun. Efficacy of electroacupuncture in regulating female hormone levels in patients with premature ovarian failure [J]. New Chin Med. 2012;44(12):108–11.
24. Mi Hui, Gong Ai-ling, Sun Wei, et al. Therapeutic effect of percutaneous acupoint electrical stimulation on 30 cases of ovarian hyporesponsiveness [J]. J Shandong Univ Tradit Chin Med. 2013;37(6):495–6.
25. Xu Yin, Zhang Miao. Efficacy observation on 40 cases of anovulatory infertility treated by acupuncture and moxibustion [J]. World J Acupunct Moxibustion. 2013;23(1):40–3.
26. Zhou Li, Xia Youbing, Lu Jing, et al. Clinical study of sequential acupuncture and moxibustion for treatment of ovarian reserve function in IVF-ET30 cases [J]. Jiangsu J Tradit Chin Med. 2015;47(8):58–60.
27. Cui Wei, Li Jing, Sun Wei, et al. Effects of electroacupuncture on egg cell quality and pregnancy in in vitro fertilization-embryo transfer in patients with polycystic ovary syndrome [J]. Chin J Acupunct Moxibustion. 2011;31(8):686–91.
28. Lian Fang, Chen Wei, Xiang Shan. Study on the improvement of egg cell quality in patients with kidney deficiency type infertility [J]. Chin Acupunct. 2015;35(2):109–13.
29. Yin Dehui, Zhu Ye, Pei Kongjin, et al. Clinical study on 40 cases of ovulatory infertility treated by electroacupuncture [J]. Hainan Med J. 2011;22(11):20–2.
30. Zhang Dan. Clinical observation on the treatment of ovulatory infertility by acupuncture at the ovary axillary stalk [J]. Asia-Pacific Tradit Med. 2015;11(19):95–6.
31. Sheng Yonghui, Liu Haizhen, Jiang Chunyu, et al. Therapeutic effect of acupuncture combined with medicine on ovulatory infertility in 59 cases [J]. Hebei Tradit Chin Med. 2015;37(8):1216–7.
32. Xu Mei, Yang Jing, Zhao Meng. Effects of percutaneous acupoint electrical stimulation on patients with repeated implantation and freeze-thaw embryo transfer [J]. J Reprod Med. 2014;23(8):624–7.
33. Li Yu, Feng Xiaojun, Sun Wei, Feng Xue. Clinical study of percutaneous acupoint electrical stimulation to improve endometrial receptivity in patients undergoing freeze-thaw embryo transfer [J]. Modern Chinese Medicine. 2012;32(3):12–5.
34. Yan Honglian, He Shuzhen, Xing Yanjun, et al. Clinical application of acupuncture treatment in in vitro fertilization-embryo transfer technology [J]. Guangzhou Pharm. 2015;46(1):13–6.

35. Zhai Zhijian, Li Lifei, Li Na, et al. Evaluation of different anesthesia methods in transvaginal puncture and oocyte retrieval [J]. International Journal of Reproductive Health/Family Planning. 2014;33(3):103–6.
36. Chen Huan, Wang Yinping, Xing Jianqiu, et al. Application of electroacupuncture at auricular acupoints in in vitro fertilization-embryo transfer [J]. Jiangsu Med. 2015;41(23):2863–5.
37. He Xiaoxia, Zhang Xuehong, Wei Qinglin. Preliminary study on the effect of acupuncture on ovarian hyperstimulation syndrome (OHSS) [J]. Reprod Contracept. 2011;31(12):817–21.
38. Yang Ting. Study on the mechanism of acupuncture treatment in reducing [D]. Gansu: Lanzhou University; 2013.
39. Cong Dejun, Hu Jinfeng, Wang Yufeng. Effects of massage techniques on basal body temperature and progesterone in functional infertile women [J]. J Changchun Univ Tradit Chin Med. 2012;28(4):620–1.
40. Zheng Huiying, Yang Xinjiang. Treatment of 50 cases of infertility with integrated Chinese and Western medicine [J]. J Anhui Univ Tradit Chin Med. 2006;25(5):13–5.
41. Zhang Shunhe. Treatment of 20 cases of infertility by massage [J]. Chin Folk Ther. 2000;8(12):19.
42. Zhang Zongsheng, Li Aimei. Observation on the efficacy of Bushen recipe in the treatment of ovulatory infertility [J]. J Pract Tradit Chin Med. 2013;(8):631–2.
43. Wang Heming. Source and development of chiropractic therapy [J]. J Rehabil. 2007;17(5):37–9.
44. Liu Yun, Zhang Lifang. Acupuncture and chiropractic therapy for infertility [C]. International Traditional Medicine Conference Abstracts. 2000.
45. Feng Tianyou. Diagnosis and treatment of lumbar disc herniation [J]. Chin J Integr Tradit West Med. 1991;(4):237–8.
46. Feng Tianyou. Discussion on the diagnosis and treatment of lumbar disc herniation [J]. Air Force Med J. 1990;(3):127–31.
47. Wang Lei. Comparative study of localization and diagnosis procedures in two auricular acupuncture systems in China and Europe [D]. Beijing University of Chinese Medicine, 2016.
48. Zhang Mingmin, Huang Guangying, Lu Fuer, et al. Effect of acupuncture on pregnancy rate of embryo transfer and its mechanism: a randomized placebo study [J]. Chin Acupunct. 2003;23(1):3–5.
49. Wu Hongye. Observation of 33 cases of endometriosis infertility treated with traditional Chinese medicine enema [J]. Mod Chin Doct. 2009;47(13):77.
50. Lu Rongqing, Lu Ronghua. Treatment of 90 cases of tubal obstruction infertility with Chinese medicine enema [J]. J External Med Chin Med. 2010;19(5):29.
51. Zhang Jianchao, Chen Xiaoyan. Experience in laparoscopic surgery combined with traditional Chinese medicine enema for chronic pelvic inflammatory infertility [J]. Chin J Endosc. 2004;10(11):95–6.
52. Xiang Chunyan, Guo Quan, Liao Juan, et al. Effect of Chinese medicine five elements of music combined with music electroacupuncture on depression in patients with malignant tumors [J]. Chin J Nurs. 2006;41(11):969–72.
53. Johnson RC, Slade P. Obstetric complications and anxiety during pregnancy: is there a relationship? [J]. J Psychosom Obstet Gynecol. 2003;24(1):1–14.

Chapter 7
Controlled Ovarian Stimulation Protocols for IVF: From First IVF Baby in the United States and Beyond

Hakan E. Duran

7.1 What Is Controlled Ovarian Stimulation?

Ovarian stimulation is a means to stimulate follicular growth beyond recruitable stage, also known as class 5 follicles [1]. This is usually achieved by an increase in follicle-stimulating hormone (FSH) concentration in serum, since ovarian follicles are sensitive to and dependent on this hormone at this developmental stage and beyond. In the absence of adequate gonadotropin levels, follicular growth typically arrests at this stage. Abundance of FSH, on the other hand, will help recruit several to all ovarian follicles that are at this stage of development and enable their simultaneous growth. Ovarian stimulation has been suggested to differ from ovulation induction: the goal of the former is to induce ongoing development of multiple preovulatory follicles, whereas monofollicular development is the objective of the latter term [2].

Folliculogenesis is generally defined as the process of ovarian follicle growth from primordial stage to ovulation. Primordial, also known as resting follicles, is composed of an oocyte surrounded by a single layer of flat granulosa cells and comprises the ovarian reserve in women. A certain number of them are initiated regularly, as the first step in folliculogenesis, whereas some others constantly undergo atresia. How they are initiated is largely unknown in primates, as is the case for atresia. The general consensus is that the number of resting follicles initiated for growth or atresia can be modulated either by the size of the pool or by endocrine or environmental factors, and multiple paracrine/autocrine factors determine these events, which are difficult to identify with the current technology. The initiation process and atresia of resting follicles continue until ovarian follicle reserve is completely depleted; it is not interrupted by any biological or pharmaceutical

H. E. Duran (✉)
Department of Obstetrics and Gynecology, REI Division, University of Iowa,
Iowa City, IA, USA
e-mail: hakan-duran@uiowa.edu

© Springer Nature Switzerland AG 2020
O. Bukulmez (ed.), *Diminished Ovarian Reserve and Assisted Reproductive Technologies*, https://doi.org/10.1007/978-3-030-23235-1_7

Fig. 7.1 Brief schematic representation of folliculogenesis. Ovarian follicles undergo atresia at every stage of development and differentiation throughout the reproductive life span. They become sensitive to gonadotropins at recruitable stage (class 5) and remain that way afterward. RFP: resting follicle pool, also known as primordial follicles

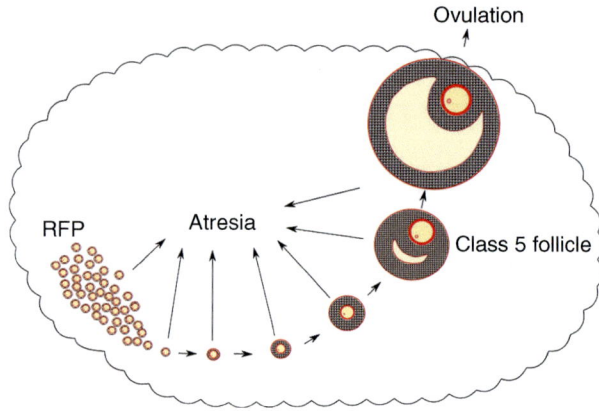

phenomena, including pregnancy, oral contraceptive use, or any other means of disruption in folliculogenesis (Fig. 7.1) [3]. Overall, it takes about 85 days for a resting follicle that was initiated for growth to reach to recruitable stage, thereby gaining FSH responsiveness [4].

There are two stages in a reproductive-aged woman's natural menstrual cycle when serum FSH is in abundance: early follicular phase and mid-cycle. Serum FSH level starts to rise by late luteal phase as a result of disinhibition from declining progesterone and inhibin A production by failing corpus luteum, which leads to a high-normal serum FSH level in the early follicular phase. The ovarian follicles that reach to the recruitable stage by completing their 85-day growth at this time of the cycle will therefore be successfully recruited for further growth. The endocrine environment, however, may not be favorable at mid-cycle for such recruitment despite the presence of FSH. During the first 5–6 days of this FSH abundance at early follicular phase, recruited follicles will simultaneously grow and compete for dominant follicle selection. Multiple factors may influence the number of dominant, preovulatory follicles, although it is typically one during a natural cycle. These factors include but may not be limited to the age of the woman, ovarian reserve, extent and duration of FSH abundance, existence of underlying ovulation dysfunction, and type of it. As the woman's ovarian reserve diminishes, the number of follicles in the recruitable pool decreases, and recruitment process typically occurs sooner in the cycle [5]. Controlled ovarian stimulation allows for follicular recruitment in women with ovulation dysfunction, who are unable to produce or maintain an adequate serum FSH level to regularly and consistently initiate this process on their own. This can be achieved by either inducing intrinsic FSH secretion or using extrinsic FSH. In the next several sections, we will review the history of ovarian stimulation in a more or less chronological fashion, but let us first define ovulatory dysfunction, which constitutes the main indication for this intervention.

7.1.1 Ovulatory Dysfunction and Use of Clomiphene Citrate for Ovulation Induction

Ovulatory dysfunction is the cause of infertility in 20–40% of women presenting for treatment [6]. It is typically characterized by the loss of regular menstrual cycles, which is an indicator of regular follicular recruitment in the ovaries that eventually lead to ovulation. Anovulation, and less commonly used oligoovulation, are terms used interchangeably with ovulatory dysfunction. There are essentially three types of anovulation based on serum gonadotropin levels as defined by the World Health Organization (WHO) [7]:

  I. Hypogonadotropic anovulation
 II. Eugonadotropic anovulation
III. Hypergonadotropic anovulation

Hypogonadotropic anovulation typically refers to a central problem, either hypothalamic or pituitary in origin, causing decreased secretion of gonadotropins into circulation. Suppression of the pacemaker cells of the reproductive clock, also known as gonadotropin-releasing hormone (GnRH) neurons in the arcuate nucleus of the hypothalamus, by neighboring autonomic centers, physical destruction of hypothalamus, or congenital defects that interfere with the migration of GnRH neurons to the arcuate nucleus, may lead to this type of ovulatory dysfunction. The secretion of both FSH and luteinizing hormone (LH) is affected, and their serum levels are typically low (<3 IU/L). The GnRH neurons gain sensitivity to serum estradiol levels with puberty, and their pulse frequency and amplitude decrease with estrogen negative feedback, which may be elucidated by either as a direct action on GnRH neurons or indirectly through other neurons or nuclei [8, 9]. Activin and inhibin, both products of the granulosa cells of the ovarian follicle, contribute to this feedback mechanism, which is typically interrupted with this type of anovulation, either by functional suppression of the GnRH neurons, their absence, or physical destruction. Therefore, hypoestrogenic state does not increase GnRH pulse frequency and amplitude in women with hypogonadotropic anovulation, like it normally would do. With this lack of change in the pacemaker activity, downstream FSH and LH secretion by the pituitary gland remains unchanged and low despite the hypoestrogenic state.

Eugonadotropic anovulation typically refers to an ovulatory dysfunction in the setting of normal serum gonadotropin levels. There are various pathophysiologic mechanisms that may lead to this type of anovulation; polycystic ovarian syndrome (PCOS) and obesity are the most common examples. These women typically require high-normal FSH levels in serum to "jump-start" folliculogenesis by recruiting available follicles as indicated above.

Hypergonadotropic anovulation refers to either severely diminished or depleted ovarian reserve, since this would typically lead to high serum gonadotropin levels.

Ovarian stimulation in women with this type of ovulatory dysfunction is usually disappointing and associated with a high risk of cancellation due to the lack of ovarian response. Strategies to optimize outcome in this type of ovulatory dysfunction will be reviewed in detail in Part I of this book.

7.1.2 Clomiphene Citrate

Clomiphene citrate was first synthesized in 1956, used in clinical trials in 1960, and approved for clinical use in 1967 [10, 11]. It is a nonsteroidal triphenylethylene derivative that acts as a selective estrogen receptor modulator (SERM) with both estrogen agonist and mostly antagonist properties. It is a racemic mixture of two stereoisomers, enclomiphene and zuclomiphene [12, 13]. The former is the more potent isomer with a shorter half-life, whereas the latter stays in circulation for several weeks after a single dose [14]. Clomiphene competitively binds to nuclear estrogen receptors for an extended duration of time, interferes with their recycling, and depletes them causing perceived hypoestrogenemia at the GnRH neuron level [12]. This would effectively increase the frequency (in ovulatory women) [15], or amplitude (in women with PCOS) [16] of GnRH pulses, leading to increased FSH and LH release by pituitary gland downstream, assisting or inducing follicle recruitment as reviewed above. The exact nature of the mechanism of action of clomiphene is still uncertain [17], which may involve changes in the insulin-like growth factor (IGF) system [18].

Clomiphene is typically more effective in type II, eugonadotropic anovulation. In the case of an already suppressed or compromised GnRH neuron population, as may be the case for type I anovulation, clomiphene would typically not elucidate an increase in the gonadotropin secretion by the pituitary gland, and folliculogenesis would fail to resume in the ovary. However, due to its low cost and the presence of occasional patients with type I anovulation responding to clomiphene, it is relatively common to try this medication for such cases.

The use of clomiphene on patients with diminished ovarian reserve (DOR) has gained popularity in recent years, which is discussed extensively in the section of minimal stimulation for IVF in women with DOR. This is both due to its low cost and reports of IVF outcome with low-dose clomiphene containing stimulation protocols being comparable to traditional stimulation protocols. Again, these protocols and their effectiveness are reviewed in detail in Part II.

7.1.3 Use of Pituitary Gonadotropins for Ovulation Induction

Initial evidence of an endocrine pituitary-gonadal axis appeared by the observation of genital atrophy following lesions of the anterior pituitary gland [19]. Fevold et al. first confirmed the existence of two separate gonadotropins in 1931, formerly named as prolans A and B, by isolating, purifying, and renaming them as FSH and LH [20]. Even prior to this discovery, the capacity of urine from pregnant women was known to stimulate gonadal function [21], as well as the capacity of daily fresh implants of anterior pituitary gland tissue from various species of animals to stimulate precocious sexual maturity, marked enlargement of ovaries, and superovulation in immature female mice [22]. By 1930, swine pituitary extracts were started to be used clinically to treat patients. This was followed by the use of gonadotropins extracted from various species for the same purpose in the United States and Europe until the early 1960s, when a new phenomenon was discovered, the "antihormones" [23].

Several investigators reported that during chronic treatment with gonadotropins from animal origin, the ovary maintained its response only for a limited period of time; then the response became increasingly weaker and finally disappeared. Antihormones, formation of which was evoked by chronic gonadotropin treatment, were capable of inactivating gonadotropin hormone both in vivo and in vitro. This was effectively the very early description of antibody formation a few decades before the nature of immunological phenomena was fully recognized [24].

Carl Gemzell extracted gonadotropins from human pituitary gland in 1958 and reported clinical results [25]. These preparations remained in clinical use until 1988 throughout the world. However, the reservoir of human pituitaries was too small to meet the growing demand for gonadotropin preparations. Moreover, their use was linked to cases with iatrogenic Creutzfeldt-Jakob disease, which were identified in Australia, France, and the United Kingdom [26, 27]. Thus, these preparations were subsequently withdrawn from the market.

7.1.4 The Discovery of hCG

Blood and urine of pregnant women were discovered to contain a gonad-stimulating substance, as stated above; when immature female mice were injected by either of these fluids, their ovaries showed follicular maturation, luteinization, and bleeding into the ovarian stroma [21]. Initially, this gonadotropic substance was believed to be produced by the anterior pituitary gland; however, Seeger-Jones et al. showed that this gonadotropin was produced in vitro in placental tissue culture, reaching to the conclusion that the placenta was the source [28]. It was then named as human chorionic gonadotropin (hCG). Purified urinary preparations became available in 1940, from the urine obtained during the first half of pregnancy [29]. It was soon discovered that when hCG was administered during follicular phase of the cycle, no visual evidence of follicle stimulation, ovulation, or corpus luteum formation was present in the ovaries [30].

7.1.5 Use of Urinary hMG for Ovulation Induction

Gonadotropins are also readily available in the urine of postmenopausal women, which is a less expensive and more abundant resource than human pituitary glands. Methods were developed to obtain gonadotropins from this resource for clinical use in the early 1950s [31, 32]. Just like pituitary extracts, gonadotropins obtained from urinary source were a mixture of FSH and LH; the preparations were appropriately named as human menopausal gonadotropins (hMG). Despite the purity of available preparations being around 5%, hMG was in clinical use by 1960 [33], and successful ovulation was reported in type 1 (hypogonadotropic) anovulatory women with the use of hMG [34]. The Steelman and Pohley assay, a bioassay on hCG-primed immature rats, became the gold standard for FSH estimation in the hMG preparations [35]. Another problem with both hMG and human pituitary gonadotropin preparations was that the FSH/LH ratio varied from batch to batch. Variations within the range of 0.1 to 10 were deemed acceptable for clinic use in the 1970s. This opened the new challenge in the manufacturing of hMG: purification of FSH from LH and other urinary proteins. With the advancement in immunology, passive and active immunofiltration methods were developed to produce highly purified FSH preparations, which now contained <0.1 IU of LH activity and <5% of unidentified urinary proteins. The purity was also now 95%, raised from the original range of 1–2%. This enhanced purity also allowed subcutaneous administration instead of the traditional intramuscular one. The so-called highly purified FSH virtually eliminated the batch-to-batch variability and enabled the analysis of the end product by physicochemical methods in addition to the classical bioassay [23].

Although urine from postmenopausal women provided a more abundant resource than human pituitary glands as a resource for hMG, it also had its own shortcomings:

- Cross-contamination of communicable diseases cannot be avoided
- No regulatory control available
- Poor quality control
- Impossible-to-trace donor source
- Still limited source

The whole endeavor started with 600 postmenopausal women in 4 urine collection centers, mostly in Europe. Each and every urine donor was well-known by the collectors, and if any of them suffered a sickness or needed to use medications, including antibiotics, their urine samples were rejected. As the worldwide demand increased in time, the donor number grew to 600,000, and their meticulous monitoring became impossible, contributing to the shortcomings as listed above. Identification of protease-resistant prion proteins in humans with possible prion disease helped raise concerns for the use of urinary hMG [36].

7.1.6 Advent of Recombinant Gonadotropins

The amino acid sequences of FSH α- and β-subunits were described by Rathnam and Saxena [37], and Saxena and Rathnam [38], respectively, and the FSH gene was cloned by Howles [39]. However, producing recombinant FSH proved to be still difficult, mainly due to the posttranslational modification of the protein, including folding and glycosylation, which could not be accomplished by prokaryotes, a common host for recombinant gene technology. Eventually, vectors containing α- and β-subunits of FSH, along with transcription promoters, were used to transfect Chinese hamster ovary (CHO) cell line, which successfully produced the recombinant versions of this hormone [39, 40]. This was followed by the production of recombinant LH and hCG; however, recombinant LH is no longer available for clinical use in the United States. Recombinant FSH and hCG can be quantified reliably by protein content (mass in micrograms), rather than biological activity, allowing optimal risk reduction, superior quality, and batch-to-batch consistency due to its purity. Unfortunately, mass production of these hormones based on recombinant technology did not result in a significant change in their market prices, as expected.

Recombinant gonadotropins are now the first-line option for cases where gonadotropin treatment is needed, and the cost of treatment is not a greater concern. They provide comparable treatment results to urinary gonadotropins, which have been the gold standard for decades. They have a very low adverse effect profile, and their use is even simpler with the advent of subcutaneous injection pens with dose-adjustment dials.

7.2 Brief History of IVF

7.2.1 The Adventure Until Louise Brown

Stimulating ovaries for multi-follicular development for IVF was a natural thought due to several advantages, most importantly being able to work on several oocytes but also having a better control on the menstrual cycle and the timing of oocyte retrieval. The latter advantage can be better appreciated when one considers the need for laparoscopy for oocyte retrieval in the early days of IVF. Therefore, ovarian stimulation with the only available gonadotropin preparation that was safe to use during that time, urinary hMG, was undertaken in about 100 cases by the pioneers of IVF in England and the world, Robert Edwards and Patrick Steptoe. After achieving no pregnancy in those attempts, and starting to run out of options, they suspected that the progesterone production was the problem in such cycles and decided to switch to attempting IVF in natural cycles, despite its disadvantages mentioned above. Consequently, the first IVF baby was conceived and born during a natural cycle.

7.2.2 An International Race of ART

Natural cycle IVF was accepted as common norm following the first live birth and eventually led to the delivery of the second and third IVF babies born in Britain and Australia, respectively. Many flourishing IVF centers in the world, which were trying to replicate these successful results, chose the same strategy, including the Norfolk Group in the United States. There were several limitations of IVF practice at that time as compared to today, some of which may be listed as follows:

- No available medical means of pituitary desensitization during ovarian stimulation – GnRH agonist or antagonists were simply not available
- Transvaginal ultrasound was not available. Monitoring the follicular phase was accomplished by estradiol levels and transabdominal ultrasound imaging
- Detection of ovulation was difficult and usually late. There was no ELISA assay for LH, and urinary LH detection kits were unavailable
- Basal body temperature charting, vaginal smears, and cervical mucus testing were the only methods relied on for detection of ovulation, even though they were all known to be confirmatory only after ovulation

Given these limitations, managing a natural cycle IVF was extremely difficult, where there was minimal, if any, control over a patient's menstrual cycle. The Norfolk group initially treated 41 patients to retrieve 19 oocytes from them, 13 of which fertilized with no clinical pregnancy achieved. Based on these discouraging results, and Georgeanna Seeger-Jones' extensive clinical experience on hMG use, Norfolk Group made an executive decision to go against current common wisdom and started doing IVF in hMG-stimulated cycles. With this change in practice, it became possible to schedule oocyte retrievals, timing them 36 hours after hCG injection once the leading follicles were decided to reach maturity based on transabdominal ultrasound findings. Shortly after this change, specifically 13 patients and 6 embryo transfers later, the first clinical pregnancy was achieved in the United States, which eventually became the first live birth [41]. This paradigm shift allowed controlled ovarian stimulation to become the norm for most IVF cycles in the world shortly afterward due to its obvious advantages and cost-effectiveness and has remained to be the standard way of doing IVF ever since.

7.3   Controlled Ovarian Stimulation for IVF

True control over ovarian stimulation for IVF requires hypothalamic and pituitary desensitization to rising serum estradiol level, which would lead to the mid-cycle LH surge and ovulation. This became possible with the availability of GnRH analogs for clinical use. First, the decapeptide was isolated from porcine hypothalamus [42], and then GnRH analogs were created by substituting the amino acids in certain positions of the decapeptide with others [43]. While pulsatile administration of GnRH was established as an effective and safe means of type I anovulation [44], continuous administration was discovered to initially cause an increase in gonadotropin secretion by the pituitary gland (the flare effect), followed by a decrease in both gonadotropin levels and downstream gonadal function [45]. This is due to desensitization by clustering and internalization of pituitary GnRH receptor [46].

Immediate suppression and recovery of pituitary function favored GnRH antagonists particularly appropriate for short-term use in IVF. However, it has taken almost three decades to develop these compounds with acceptable safety and pharmacokinetic characteristics. Eventually, third-generation GnRH antagonists, ganirelix, and Cetrotide were registered in 2001 for use in IVF [47].

7.3.1 Agonist-Based Protocols

GnRH agonist-based controlled ovarian stimulation protocols take advantage of both initial, short-term agonistic (flare) effect of these medications and pituitary desensitization obtained by continuous, long-term administration (Fig. 7.2). For the former effect, they are used in very low doses to mimic and augment GnRH pulsatility from arcuate nucleus preceding follicular recruitment. This is the micro-dose flare protocol for ovarian stimulation. It is one of the classical poor responder protocols and will be reviewed in Chap. 8 in detail. The long agonist protocol, on the other hand, would rely on continuous and longer-term administration of GnRH agonists in a higher dose range to achieve complete pituitary desensitization. While intrinsic FSH release would be expected to contribute to the follicular recruitment and growth in micro-dose flare protocol, this process would completely rely on extrinsic gonadotropin administration in long agonist protocol. Both of these protocols are

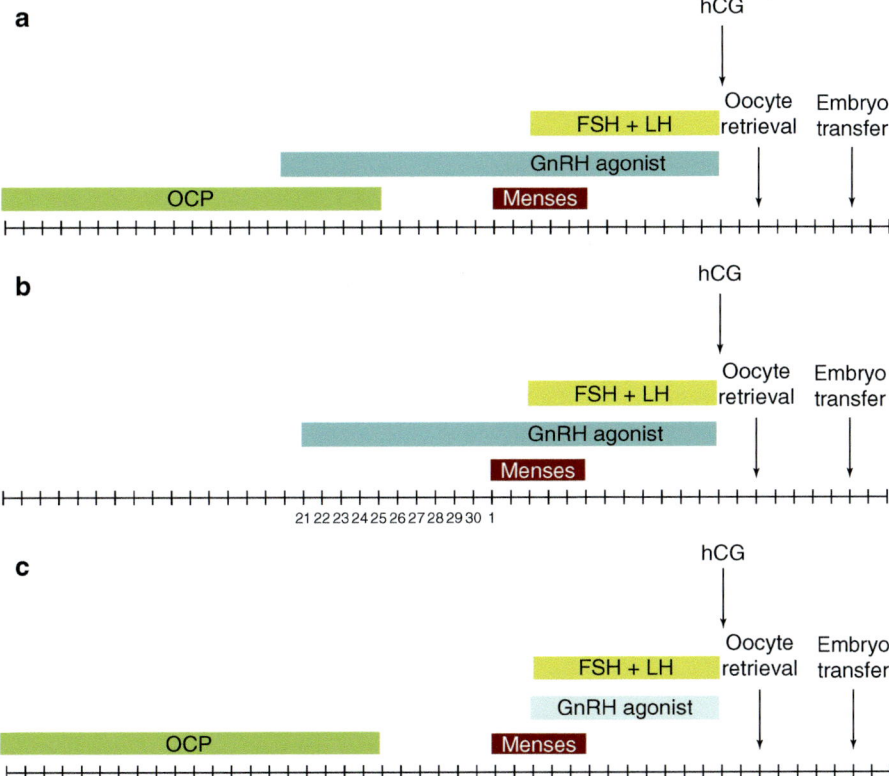

Fig. 7.2 Schematic representation of GnRH agonist protocols. Each tick mark on the line represents a day in the menstrual cycle; numbers represent cycle days, if present. The lighter tone of cyan indicates micro dose of GnRH agonist, as opposed to darker tone, which represents regular dose. OCP: oral contraceptive pills. (**a**) OCP-long agonist protocol, (**b**) non-OCP long-agonist protocol, (**c**) OCP-micro-dose flare protocol

usually combined with and preceded by oral contraceptive use for better cycle timing, predictability, and improved follicular synchrony. Long agonist protocol has long been the most commonly used method of ovarian stimulation for IVF in normal responders with optimal follicular synchrony. However, due to several advantages provided by GnRH antagonists, including immediate pituitary desensitization, shorter duration of use, and better prevention of ovarian hyperstimulation syndrome (OHSS), it is not as commonly used now as before.

7.3.2 Antagonist-Based Protocols

GnRH antagonist-based protocols have the advantage of immediate pituitary desensitization when needed. Unlike the flare effect caused by GnRH agonists resulting in depletion of pituitary FSH and LH reserves, GnRH antagonist use maintains FSH and LH vesicles in gonadotrophs, which allows immediate reversal of their actions. This feature allows the use of a GnRH agonist triggering LH release from pituitary reserves, mimicking the natural preovulatory surge. This strategy has been very effective in prevention of OHSS, since half-life of LH is significantly shorter than that of hCG (20 minutes versus 24 hours, respectively). Due to this effectiveness, ovulation trigger by GnRH agonist has become the most preferred strategy for patients with anticipated high response, such as younger patients or those with PCOS, as well as oocyte donors.

The timing of initiation of GnRH antagonists to prevent preovulatory LH surge during the ovarian stimulation is critical, and this is classically determined by fixed and flexible protocols (Fig. 7.3). GnRH antagonists are also used in patients with diminished ovarian reserve, to prevent early follicular recruitment, which is a common occurrence in such patients, by suppressing the luteal phase FSH rise preceding the ovarian stimulation cycle along with estradiol administration. All of these protocols are reviewed in detail in Chap. 8.

Another application of GnRH antagonists is as an attempt to limit OHSS development following oocyte retrieval in high-risk patients, although the efficacy of such use has not been proven [48].

Advances in oncofertility have allowed fertility preservation to become available for more and more women with cancer diagnosis. Some of these women choose oocyte cryopreservation as the preferred option and do not have the luxury to wait until the right time in their cycle to initiate ovarian stimulation with GnRH agonist-based protocols. GnRH antagonists allow the use of so-called crash ovarian stimulation for fertility preservation in these patients; who need to proceed with cancer treatment immediately following their oocyte cryopreservation cycle. Ovarian stimulation can be initiated at any time during the menstrual cycle along with GnRH antagonist use for such situations.

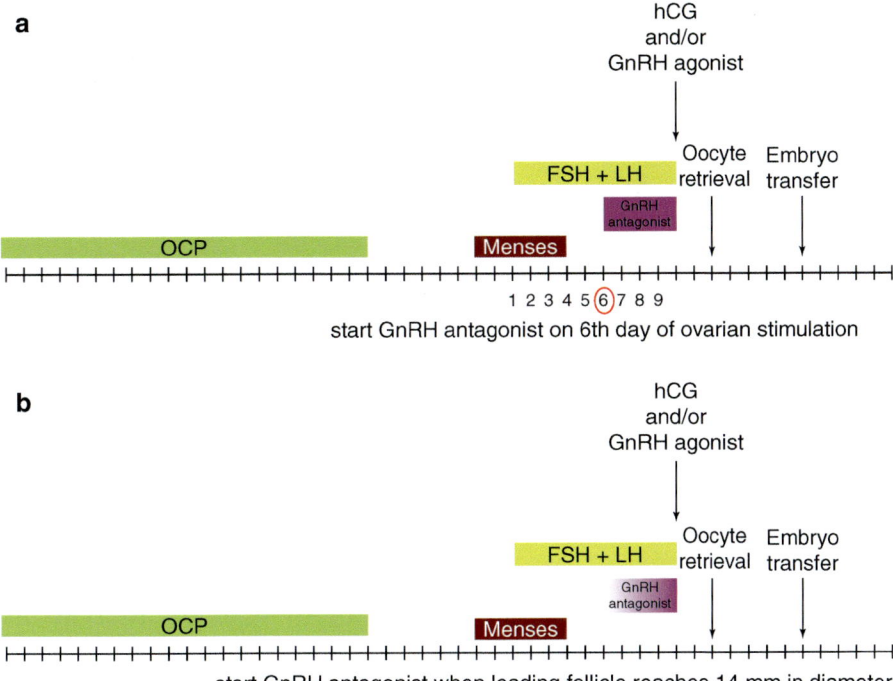

Fig. 7.3 Schematic representation of GnRH antagonist protocols. Each tick mark on the line represents a day in the menstrual cycle; numbers represent cycle days, if present. The gradient in the tone of GnRH antagonist box represents the contingency of this agent's initiation on the leading follicle diameter. Please note that the ovulation may be triggered by hCG, GnRH agonist or, both in these protocols. OCP: oral contraceptive pills. (**a**) Fixed GnRH antagonist protocol, (**b**) flexible GnRH antagonist protocol

References

1. Gougeon A. Dynamics of follicular growth in the human: a model from preliminary results. Hum Reprod. 1986;1:81–7.
2. Fauser BC, Van Heusden AM. Manipulation of human ovarian function: physiological concepts and clinical consequences. Endocr Rev. 1997;18:71–106.
3. Gougeon A. Regulation of ovarian follicular development in primates: facts and hypotheses. Endocr Rev. 1996;17:121–55.
4. Oktay K, Newton H, Mullan J, Gosden RG. Development of human primordial follicles to antral stages in SCID/hpg mice stimulated with follicle stimulating hormone. Hum Reprod. 1998;13:1133–8.
5. Treloar AE, Boynton RE, Behn BG, Brown BW. Variation of the human menstrual cycle through reproductive life. Int J Fertil. 1967;12:77–126.

6. Fritz M, Speroff L. Clinical gynecologic endocrinology and infertility. Philadelphia: Lipincott Williams & Wilkins, Wolters Kluwer Health; 2011. p. 1137–90.
7. Group WHOS. Agents stimulating gonadal function in the human. 1976.
8. Plant TM, Dubey AK. Evidence from the rhesus monkey (Macaca mulatta) for the view that negative feedback control of luteinizing hormone secretion by the testis is mediated by a deceleration of hypothalamic gonadotropin-releasing hormone pulse frequency. Endocrinology. 1984;115:2145–53.
9. Smith JT, Shahab M, Pereira A, Pau KYF, Clarke IJ. Hypothalamic expression of KISS1 and gonadotropin inhibitory hormone genes during the menstrual cycle of a non-human primate. Biol Reprod. 2010;83:568–77.
10. Greenblatt RB, Barfield WE, Jungck EC, Ray AW. Induction of ovulation with MRL/41. Preliminary report. JAMA. 1961;178:101–4.
11. Dickey RP, Holtkamp DE. Development, pharmacology and clinical experience with clomiphene citrate. Hum Reprod Update. 1996;2:483–506.
12. Clark JH, Markaverich BM. The agonistic-antagonistic properties of clomiphene: a review. Pharmacol Ther. 1981;15:467–519.
13. Ernst S, Hite G, Cantrell JS, Richardson A, Benson HD. Stereochemistry of geometric isomers of clomiphene: a correction of the literature and a reexamination of structure-activity relationships. J Pharm Sci. 1976;65:148–50.
14. Mikkelson TJ, Kroboth PD, Cameron WJ, Dittert LW, Chungi V, Manberg PJ. Single-dose pharmacokinetics of clomiphene citrate in normal volunteers. Fertil Steril. 1986;46:392–6.
15. Kerin JF, Liu JH, Phillipou G, Yen SS. Evidence for a hypothalamic site of action of clomiphene citrate in women. J Clin Endocrinol Metab. 1985;61:265–8.
16. Kettel LM, Roseff SJ, Berga SL, Mortola JF, Yen SS. Hypothalamic-pituitary-ovarian response to clomiphene citrate in women with polycystic ovary syndrome. Fertil Steril. 1993;59:532–8.
17. Adashi EY. Clomiphene citrate-initiated ovulation: a clinical update. Semin Reprod Endocrinol. 1986;4:255–75.
18. Bützow TL, Kettel LM, Yen SS. Clomiphene citrate reduces serum insulin-like growth factor I and increases sex hormone-binding globulin levels in women with polycystic ovary syndrome. Fertil Steril. 1995;63:1200–3.
19. Crowe SJ, Cushing H, Homans J. Experimental hypophysectomy. Bull Johns Hopkins Hosp. 1910;21:127–67.
20. Fevold SL, Hisaw FL, Leonard SL. The gonad-stimulating and the luteinizing hormones of the anterior lobe of the hypophysis. Am J Physiol. 1931;97:291–301.
21. Ascheim S, Zondek B. Hypophysenvorderlappen hormone und ovarialhormone in Harn von Schangeren. Klin Wochenschr. 1927;6:13–21.
22. Smith PE. Hastening of development of female genital system by daily hemoplastic pituitary transplants. Proc Soc Exp Biol Med. 1926;24:1311–33.
23. Lunenfeld B. Historical perspectives in gonadotrophin therapy. Hum Reprod Update. 2004;10:453–67.
24. Zondek B, Sulman F. The Antigonadotropic factor. Baltimore: Williams and Wilkins; 1942.
25. Gemzell CA, Diczfalusy E, Tillinger G. Clinical effect of human pituitary follicle-stimulating hormone (FSH). J Clin Endocrinol Metab. 1958;18:1333–48.
26. Cochius JI, Burns RJ, Blumbergs PC, Mack K, Alderman CP. Creutzfeldt-Jakob disease in a recipient of human pituitary-derived gonadotrophin. Aust N Z J Med. 1990;20:592–3.
27. Dumble LJ, Klein RD. Creutzfeldt-Jakob legacy for Australian women treated with human pituitary gonadotropins. Lancet. 1992;340:847–8.
28. Seeger-Jones GE, Gey GO, Ghisletta M. Hormone production by placental cells maintained in continuous culture. Bull Johns Hopkins Hosp. 1943;72:26–38.
29. Gurin S, Bachman G, Wilson DW. The gonadotropic hormone of urine of pregnancy. ii) Chemical studies of preparations having high biological activity. J Biol Chem. 1940;133:467–76.

30. Hamblen EC, Davis CD, Durham NC. Treatment of hypo-ovarianism by the sequential and cyclic administration of equine and chorionic gonadotropins – so-called one-two cyclic gonadotropic therapy. Summary of 5 years' results. Am J Obstet Gynecol. 1945;50:137–46.
31. Bradbury JT, Brown ES, Brown WE. Adsorption of urinary gonadotrophins on kaolin. Proc Soc Exp Biol Med. 1949;71:228–32.
32. Albert A. Procedure for routine clinical determination of urinary gonadotropin. Proc Staff Meet Mayo Clin. 1955;30:552–6.
33. Lunenfeld B, Menzi A, Volet B. Clinical effects of a human postmenopausal gonadotropin. Rass Clin Ter. 1960;59:213–6.
34. Rosemberg E, Coleman J, Demany M, Garcia CR. Clinical effect of human urinary postmenopausal gonado-tropin. J Clin Endocrinol Metab. 1963;23:181–90.
35. Steelman SL, Pohley FM. Assay of the follicle stimulating hormone based on the augmentation with human chorionic gonadotropin. Endocrinology. 1953;53:604–16.
36. Shaked GM, Shaked Y, Kariv-Inbal Z, Halimi M, Avraham I, Gabizon R. A protease-resistant prion protein isoform is present in urine of animals and humans affected with prion diseases. J Biol Chem. 2001;276:31479–82.
37. Rathnam P, Saxena BB. Primary amino acid sequence of follicle-stimulating hormone from human pituitary glands. I. alpha subunit. J Biol Chem. 1975;250:6735–46.
38. Saxena BB, Rathnam P. Amino acid sequence of the beta subunit of follicle-stimulating hormone from human pituitary glands. J Biol Chem. 1976;251:993–1005.
39. Howles CM. Genetic engineering of human FSH (Gonal-F). Hum Reprod Update. 1996;2:172–91.
40. Olijve W, de Boer W, Mulders JW, van Wezenbeek PM. Molecular biology and biochemistry of human recombinant follicle stimulating hormone (Puregon). Mol Hum Reprod. 1996;2:371–82.
41. Jones HW Jr. In vitro fertilization comes to America, memoir of a medical breakthrough. Williamsburg: Jamestowne Bookworks; 2014.
42. Schally AV, Baba Y, Nair RM, Bennett CD. The amino acid sequence of a peptide with growth hormone-releasing activity isolated from porcine hypothalamus. J Biol Chem. 1971;246:6647–50.
43. Schally AV. Luteinizing hormone-releasing hormone analogs: their impact on the control of tumorigenesis. Peptides. 1999;20:1247–62.
44. Leyendecker G, Wildt L, Hansmann M. Pregnancies following chronic intermittent (pulsatile) administration of Gn-RH by means of a portable pump ("Zyklomat") – a new approach to the treatment of infertility in hypothalamic amenorrhea. J Clin Endocrinol Metab. 1980;51:1214–6.
45. Labrie F, Auclair C, Cusan L, Lemay A, Bélanger A, Kelly PA, et al. Inhibitory effects of treatment with LHRH or its agonists on ovarian receptor levels and function. Adv Exp Med Biol. 1979;112:687–93.
46. Conn PM, Crowley WF. Gonadotropin-releasing hormone and its analogs. Annu Rev Med. 1994;45:391–405.
47. Fauser BCJM, Devroey P. Why is the clinical acceptance of gonadotropin-releasing hormone antagonist cotreatment during ovarian hyperstimulation for in vitro fertilization so slow? Fertil Steril. 2005;83:1607–11.
48. Lee D, Kim SJ, Hong YH, Kim SK, Jee BC. Gonadotropin releasing hormone antagonist administration for treatment of early type severe ovarian hyperstimulation syndrome: a case series. Obstet Gynecol Sci. 2017;60:449–54.

Chapter 8
Conventional Controlled Ovarian Stimulation Protocols for Diminished Ovarian Reserve Patients and Poor Responders

Bala Bhagavath

8.1 Introduction

A substantial number of women (10–24%) undergoing controlled ovarian stimulation (COS) for in vitro fertilization (IVF) do not respond well and may have very few oocytes retrieved or have the cycle cancelled [1]. These women have been collectively called "poor responders," and considerable energy has been devoted to finding a suitable way to stimulate their ovaries to achieve the ultimate goal of live birth.

At least 75 randomized controlled trials have been published on poor responders to COS leading up to IVF cycles. Despite this, no clear consensus has materialized on the appropriate stimulation protocol to achieve success in these women [2]. Numerous problems have been identified with these trials including lack of uniform definition of poor responders and lack of blinding of patients and/or staff. ESHRE came up with the Bologna criteria to define poor ovarian response (POR) to alleviate this problem as discussed in Chaps. 1 and 4 of this book. These criteria have been shown to predict poor ovarian response in women aged <40. Regardless of the prediction, women over the age of 40 had poor response uniformly [3].

Historically, there were three protocols for COS leading to IVF: long agonist protocol, microdose agonist flare protocol, and the antagonist protocol. In the last decade, numerous other innovative protocols have been introduced in the hope of obtaining a better response in women with POR. As a result, the original three protocols have been called "conventional stimulation protocols." Conventional IVF is defined by the American Society for Reproductive Medicine as "COS with exogenous gonadotropins to induce multiple oocyte development for retrieval" [4]. The

B. Bhagavath (✉)
University of Rochester Medical Center, Rochester, NY, USA
e-mail: bala_bhagavath@urmc.rochester.edu

© Springer Nature Switzerland AG 2020
O. Bukulmez (ed.), *Diminished Ovarian Reserve and Assisted Reproductive Technologies*, https://doi.org/10.1007/978-3-030-23235-1_8

purpose of this chapter is to review the various strategies that have been examined to optimize the conventional protocols to elicit the best ovarian response in women with expected poor ovarian response or known poor responders.

8.2 Conventional Stimulation Protocols

As physicians taking care of women desiring to achieve a pregnancy, we are eternal optimists. We refuse to give up hope that our patients cannot have biological children of their own – the very existence of IVF today is testament to that hope and tireless struggle! It is therefore not surprising that faced with poor response to COS, we are constantly engaged in finding a better protocol which would achieve a live birth for our patients [5–7]. Despite our best intentions, we have come to realize that quality evidence is still lacking for robust recommendations of any of the described protocols to date [1, 8]. Lack of perfect evidence notwithstanding, it is clear that a good number of these POR women will ultimately achieve a successful pregnancy using one or many of the described protocols [9–16].

In a study of 1152 women, the live birth rate was 23.8% in women meeting the Bologna criteria for POR [9]. In the same study, the cumulative birth rate was 18.6% in women with <3 eggs retrieved compared with 44% if they had >3 eggs retrieved. Other studies have confirmed that although the success rate is as expected, low, it is not nonexistent and the live birth rates range from 9.9% to 20.5% [10, 11].

The three stimulation protocols that fall under the definition of "conventional IVF protocols" are well described and will be briefly reviewed here for the sake of completion. All three protocols may be preceded by a few weeks of oral contraceptive pills intake. This is usually for ease of starting the gonadotropin releasing hormone agonist (GnRHa, usually leuprolide) at a convenient time prior to commencing the stimulation cycle. The long agonist (LA) protocol consists of 10 to 14 days of pituitary downregulation using GnRHa followed by about 10 days of stimulation using gonadotropin with a combination of pelvic ultrasound and serum hormone monitoring ultimately culminating in release of oocytes using human chorionic gonadotropin (Fig. 8.1). The microdose flare (MDF) protocol consists of using microdose quantities of GnRHa to stimulate and at the same time downregulate the pituitary while exogenously stimulating the ovary with gonadotropins. The idea is to augment the stimulation of ovary using exogenous and endogenous follicle stimulating hormone (FSH) (Fig. 8.2). The antagonist (ANT) protocol differs in that the ovary is stimulated using exogenous gonadotropins without any downregulation of the pituitary. Approximately 5 days into the stimulation, the antagonist is started to prevent the LH surge while the ovary continues to be stimulated. The idea is to stimulate the ovary using endogenous and exogenous gonadotropins in the first half of the cycle before downregulating the pituitary in the latter half of the cycle (Fig. 8.3).

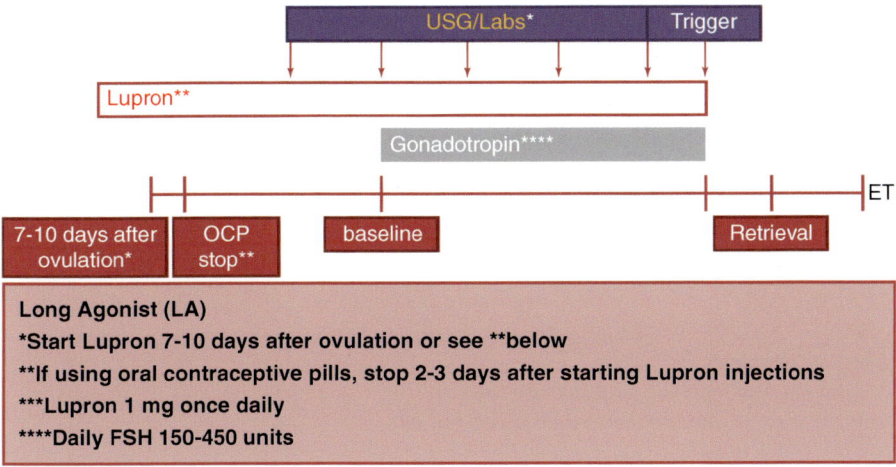

Fig. 8.1 Long Agonist protocol

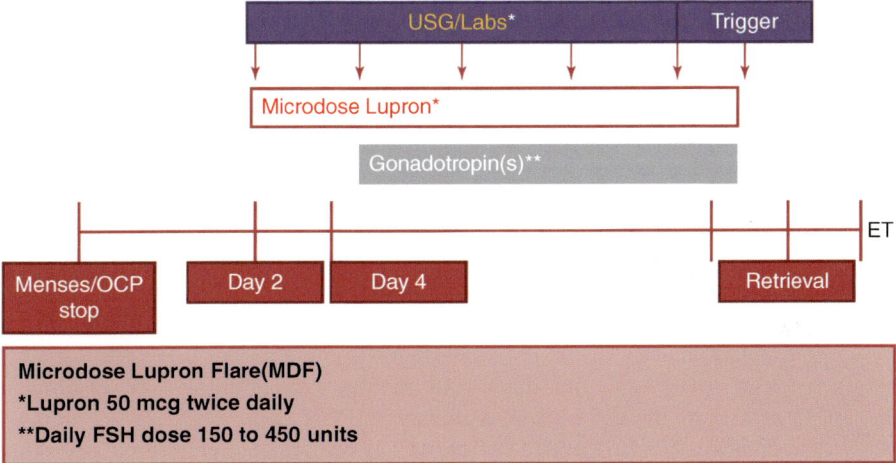

Fig. 8.2 Microdose lupron flare protocol (MDF)

In the following text, the various factors within an individual protocol that can affect cycle response in patients with POR will be reviewed such as FSH dose, use of augmentation agents growth hormone (GH), dehydroepiandrosterone (DHEA) and testosterone, dual trigger, follicular flushing, freezing all the embryos for later transfer, progesterone supplementation, conversion to IUI as a strategy, comparison of the conventional protocols against each other, followed finally by comparison of the conventional protocols with newer protocols.

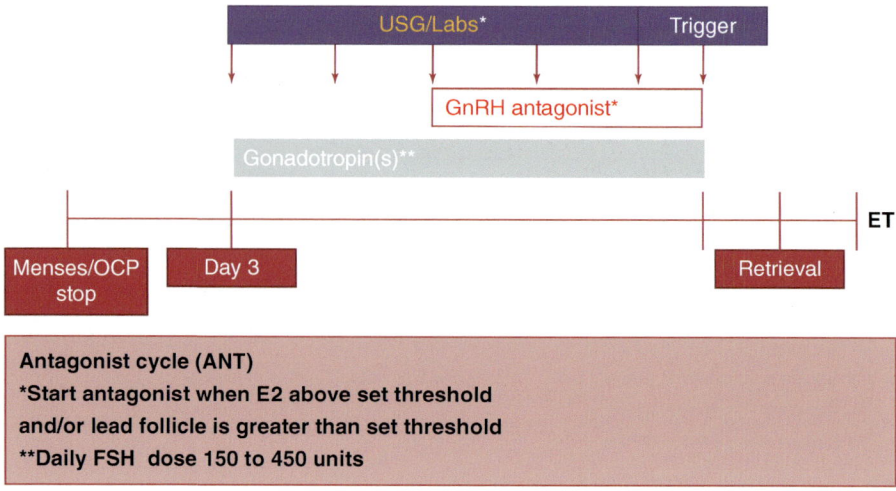

Fig. 8.3 Antagonist Cycle (ANT)

8.2.1 Dose of Gonadotropins

A randomized controlled trial (RCT) of 308 patients used AMH levels to individualize the FSH dosing for patients using the LA protocol. In fact, the study showed that cycles using AMH to dose were more likely to yield <5 oocytes compared to the other arm (25.7% vs 11%) [17].

A systematic review including seven RCTs concluded that more trials are needed to prove or disprove a benefit for individualized dosing of FSH in women with POR [18].

A recent Cochrane Review included 20 trials and concluded that lack of blinding, severe heterogeneity of the trials, and poor-to-moderate quality of the studies hampered firm conclusions, but dosing differences were unlikely to be of clinical benefit in increasing the live birth in women with POR [19].

On the contrary, a retrospective review of 1394 treatment cycles concluded that increasing the daily dose of FSH to >450 units is unlikely to be of benefit and is more likely to do harm [20]. A similar conclusion was arrived at by two other sets of investigators using MDF protocol and comparing 450 units with 600 units of FSH daily [21, 22].

8.2.2 Augmentation Agents

8.2.2.1 Growth Hormone

Many studies have been published regarding the use of GH to improve pregnancy rate in POR as also discussed extensively in Chap. 5. Almost all of them have study design problems including insufficient numbers and inconsistent definition of POR. A few studies are worth reviewing; however, and not surprisingly, they provide conflicting results. An open randomized trial using LA protocol included 240 women who fit the Bologna criteria. There was no difference in the live birth rate between the two groups [23]. In contrast, a meta-analysis of 16 eligible studies, including 663 patients, showed a significant difference in live birth rate (RR 1.73) with use of GH [24]. In direct contrast, a meta-analysis of 6 RCTs and 5 controlled clinical trials including 3788 patients concluded that there was no difference in pregnancy rates [25].

Another open-label, randomized trial included 287 patients and randomized them to 3 arms comparing the 3 conventional stimulation protocols with augmentation using GH. There was no statistically significant difference in pregnancy rates between the three groups [26].

8.2.2.2 Testosterone

Studies using testosterone as an adjuvant in POR patients are beset with the same problems as other studies in POR also echoed in Chap. 5. There are many studies proving a lack of efficacy as there are showing benefit [27–29]. A meta-analysis of 3 RCTs with 221 subjects showed a twofold increase in LBR (RR 2.01). The duration of treatment with testosterone may hold the key to success according to one study that compared different duration of exposure to testosterone ranging from 2 weeks to 4 weeks. The maximum benefit was seen in women who had used testosterone for at least 4 weeks [28].

8.2.2.3 DHEA

DHEA has probably been studied the most as an adjuvant agent for patients with POR and almost all studies are small with heterogeneity in the study population. As is the case with other adjuvants, many studies seem to show a benefit, and a similar number of studies don't show any benefit. Nevertheless, a 2015 Cochrane Review included 17 RCT with 1496 subjects and concluded that pretreatment with DHEA or testosterone may improve the live birth rates in poor responder patients [30].

8.2.2.4 Double Trigger

The idea behind the double trigger is to ensure ovulation by giving the injection at staggered times before the retrieval (GnRHa at 40 hours and hCG at 34 hours prior to retrieval) [31]. In a small pilot study, double trigger was compared with GnRHa alone or hCG alone. A higher number of top-quality embryos were noticed in the double-trigger arm compared with the other two arms. More studies are needed to confirm if this translated into more live births [32].

8.2.3 Follicular Flushing with Conventional Stimulation

Follicular flushing has been advocated as a strategy in normal responders and proven to be ineffective [33]. Each follicle is flushed three times with 2 mL of culture medium using a double lumen needle [34]. In the first RCT in POR patients, 50 women were randomized to have direct aspiration or follicular flushing. The average number of oocytes retrieved was four in the direct aspiration group and three in the follicular flushing group. Significantly, a lower pregnancy rate of 4 vs 36% was observed [33]. In another RCT, 80 patients were randomized, and similar live birth rates (25 vs 22.5%) were observed [34]. Similarly, another RCT recruited 80 patients and did not show any difference between the 2 groups for birth rate. Both the above trials showed a significant doubling of procedure time, however [35].

8.2.4 Freezing All Embryos After Conventional Stimulation

The optimal embryo transfer (ET) strategy was studied retrospectively in 2263 women undergoing IVF; 879 women fit the criteria for POR, and 645 had day 2 or cleavage stage transfer while remaining 234 had blastocyst transfer. Of the latter group, 59 had fresh transfer, and 87 had frozen embryo transfer. The cycle cancellation was lowest in the women who had day 2 or cleavage stage transfers, but the live birth rate per ET (LBR/ET) was also the lowest. Whereas the former group had an LBR/ET of 21.5%, the blastocyst transfer group had an LBR/ET of 41.1%. Among those, the LBR/ET was 30.5% and 40.2% for fresh transfer and frozen transfers (FET), respectively [36].

Another retrospective study reviewed 433 women with POR. Two hundred and seventy-seven women underwent fresh transfer, and 156 had FET. The clinical pregnancy rate was not different between the two groups (14.1 vs 13.7%) [37]. Another retrospective study included 559 patients with POR and failed to show a significant difference between the fresh transfer and FET groups [38].

8.2.5 Conversion to Intrauterine Insemination

A multicenter retrospective study looked into the strategy of cycle cancellation vs intrauterine insemination (IUI vs IVF) when two or less follicles were recruited during COS. Of the 461 cycles that met the criteria, 136 were cancelled, 141 were converted to IUI, and 184 completed IVF. LBR was significantly higher (11.6 vs 1.6%) in the IVF group regardless of the age of the patient and was even more significant in women aged <40 (13.1 vs 2%) [39]. More studies are needed to confirm that even in women with only one or two follicles, it is worthwhile to continue with IVF rather than cycle cancellation or converting to IUI.

8.3   Comparison of the Three Conventional Stimulation Protocols

The three conventional stimulation protocols were compared in an RCT involving 111 women with POR. The duration of stimulation and the total dose of gonadotropins used were significantly greater with the LA protocol compared to the other two protocols. The ongoing pregnancy rate was highest (16.2%) with the ANT protocol, and the other two protocols had an ongoing pregnancy rate of 8.1% [40].

In contrast, another RCT showed an entirely different outcome. The researchers allocated 330 women between ANT protocol (168 women) and LA protocol (162 women). The cycle cancellation rate was higher in the ANT group compared to the LA group but was not statistically significant (22.15 vs 15.2%). The clinical pregnancy rate per transfer was also not significant (42.3 vs 33.1%). However, when the cycle cancellation rates were considered, the clinical pregnancy rate per cycle initiated was significantly lower in the ANT group compared to the LA group (25.6 vs 35.8%) [41].

Interestingly, 2 years before the publication of the above trials, a meta-analysis of 14 studies involving 566 patients in ANT protocol and 561 patients in LA protocol was performed. This showed a shorter duration of stimulation in the ANT group as the only significant difference between the two groups. There was no difference in cycle cancellation rate or the clinical pregnancy rates [42]. Taken together, it is likely that there is no significant difference in pregnancy rates between the three protocols.

8.4   Comparison of the Conventional Protocols with Newer Protocols

8.4.1   Mild Stimulation

Multiple studies have been published on using mild stimulation of ovaries for IVF in POR patients compared to conventional protocols that traditionally use high or very high doses of gonadotropins. The common features of many of the protocols described under this category are use of clomiphene citrate, aromatase inhibitors, and low-dose gonadotropins, as discussed in the chapter in Part II. ASRM Practice Committee recently reviewed the available studies and recommended that mild-stimulation IVF protocols be considered as primary stimulation protocols in POR patients as the pregnancy rates are similar and the cost of stimulation is lower [4].

8.4.2 Luteal Phase Estrogen Priming with Flexible Antagonist Start

This protocol was first described by Dragisic in 2005 using luteal phase estrogen followed by GnRH antagonist and gonadotropin started at the same time. The underlying principle is suppression of luteal follicle recruitment and decreasing follicular heterogeneity. In a retrospective study, 117 patients underwent estrogen priming protocol, and 69 underwent MDF protocol. Although similar number of oocytes were retrieved in both groups, the ongoing pregnancy rate was 37% in the estrogen priming group vs 25% in the MDF group which was not statistically significant [43].

In another retrospective study, 86 patients had luteal estrogen with antagonist start midway through stimulation compared with 69 patients who had ANT protocol for COS. The ongoing pregnancy rates were 27.1 vs 20% which did not reach statistical significance [44].

8.4.3 Delayed Start

Delayed start with GnRH antagonist protocol for young POR patients was first described in 2014 [45]. The modification in delayed-start protocol compared to estrogen priming with flexible antagonist start protocol is that estrogen priming is followed by 7 days of GnRH antagonist treatment before starting ovarian stimulation with gonadotropins.

One hundred women were randomly assigned to receive the delayed-start protocol or the MDF protocol. There was no significant difference between clinical or ongoing pregnancy rate between the two groups [46]. Similarly, another smaller RCT with 54 patients did not show any difference in any of the measured outcomes including pregnancy rate [47].

8.5 Conclusion

Conventional IVF stimulation protocols are likely equally effective and better than IUI for patients with POR. There is no consensus on one specific conventional IVF stimulation protocol for patients with POR. However, mild-stimulation IVF may be more cost-effective and may at least result in similar outcome as using conventional IVF protocols with fresh embryo transfers. More detailed discussions on mild approaches for COS are extensively discussed in the upcoming chapters.

References

1. Patrizio P, Vaiarelli A, Levi Setti PE, Tobler KJ, Shoham G, Leong M, et al. How to define, diagnose and treat poor responders? Responses from a worldwide survey of IVF clinics. Reprod Biomed Online. 2015;30(6):581–92.
2. Papathanasiou A, Searle BJ, King NM, Bhattacharya S. Trends in 'poor responder' research: lessons learned from RCTs in assisted conception. Hum Reprod Update. 2016;22(3):306–19.
3. Yakin K, Oktem O, Balaban B, Urman B. Bologna criteria are predictive for ovarian response and live birth in subsequent ovarian stimulation cycles. Arch Gynecol Obstet. 2019;299(2):571–7.
4. Practice Committee of the American Society for Reproductive Medicine. Comparison of pregnancy rates for poor responders using IVF with mild ovarian stimulation versus conventional IVF: a guideline. Fertil Steril. 2018;109(6):993–9.
5. Check JH, Slovis B. Choosing the right stimulation protocol for in vitro fertilization-embryo transfer in poor, normal, and hyper-responders. Clin Exp Obstet Gynecol. 2011;38(4):313–7.
6. Busnelli A, Papaleo E, Del Prato D, La Vecchia I, Iachini E, Paffoni A, et al. A retrospective evaluation of prognosis and cost-effectiveness of IVF in poor responders according to the Bologna criteria. Hum Reprod. 2015;30(2):315–22.
7. Giovanale V, Pulcinelli FM, Ralli E, Primiero FM, Caserta D. Poor responders in IVF: an update in therapy. Gynecol Endocrinol. 2015;31(4):253–7.
8. Polat M, Bozdag G, Yarali H. Best protocol for controlled ovarian hyperstimulation in assisted reproductive technologies: fact or opinion? Semin Reprod Med. 2014;32(4):262–71.
9. Chai J, Lee VC, Yeung TW, Li HW, Ho PC, Ng EH. Live birth and cumulative live birth rates in expected poor ovarian responders defined by the Bologna criteria following IVF/ICSI treatment. PLoS One. 2015;10(3):e0119149.
10. Polyzos NP, Nwoye M, Corona R, Blockeel C, Stoop D, Haentjens P, et al. Live birth rates in Bologna poor responders treated with ovarian stimulation for IVF/ICSI. Reprod Biomed Online. 2014;28(4):469–74.
11. Ke H, Chen X, Liu YD, Ye DS, He YX, Chen SL. Cumulative live birth rate after three ovarian stimulation IVF cycles for poor ovarian responders according to the bologna criteria. J Huazhong Univ Sci Technolog Med Sci. 2013;33(3):418–22.
12. Sefrioui O, Madkour A, Aboulmaouahib S, Kaarouch I, Louanjli N. Women with extreme low AMH values could have in vitro fertilization success. Gynecol Endocrinol. 2019;35(2):170–3.
13. Xu B, Chen Y, Geerts D, Yue J, Li Z, Zhu G, et al. Cumulative live birth rates in more than 3,000 patients with poor ovarian response: a 15-year survey of final in vitro fertilization outcome. Fertil Steril. 2018;109(6):1051–9.
14. Gonda KJ, Domar AD, Gleicher N, Marrs RP. Insights from clinical experience in treating IVF poor responders. Reprod Biomed Online. 2018;36(1):12–9.
15. Busnelli A, Somigliana E. Prognosis and cost-effectiveness of IVF in poor responders according to the Bologna criteria. Minerva Ginecol. 2018;70(1):89–98.
16. Bozdag G, Polat M, Yarali I, Yarali H. Live birth rates in various subgroups of poor ovarian responders fulfilling the Bologna criteria. Reprod Biomed Online. 2017;34(6):639–44.
17. Magnusson Å, Nilsson L, Oleröd G, Thurin-Kjellberg A, Bergh C. The addition of anti-Müllerian hormone in an algorithm for individualized hormone dosage did not improve the prediction of ovarian response-a randomized, controlled trial. Hum Reprod. 2017;32(4):811–9.
18. van Tilborg TC, Broekmans FJ, Dólleman M, Eijkemans MJ, Mol BW, Laven JS, et al. Individualized follicle-stimulating hormone dosing and in vitro fertilization outcome in agonist downregulated cycles: a systematic review. Acta Obstet Gynecol Scand. 2016;95(12):1333–44.

19. Lensen SF, Wilkinson J, Leijdekkers JA, La Marca A, Mol BWJ, Marjoribanks J, et al. Individualised gonadotropin dose selection using markers of ovarian reserve for women undergoing in vitro fertilisation plus intracytoplasmic sperm injection (IVF/ICSI). Cochrane Database Syst Rev. 2018;2:CD012693.
20. Friedler S, Meltzer S, Saar-Ryss B, Rabinson J, Lazer T, Liberty G. An upper limit of gonadotropin dose in patients undergoing ART should be advocated. Gynecol Endocrinol. 2016;32(12):965–9.
21. Lefebvre J, Antaki R, Kadoch IJ, Dean NL, Sylvestre C, Bissonnette F, et al. 450 IU versus 600 IU gonadotropin for controlled ovarian stimulation in poor responders: a randomized controlled trial. Fertil Steril. 2015;104(6):1419–25.
22. Haas J, Zilberberg E, Machtinger R, Kedem A, Hourvitz A, Orvieto R. Do poor-responder patients benefit from increasing the daily gonadotropin dose during controlled ovarian hyperstimulation for IVF? Gynecol Endocrinol. 2015;31(1):79–82.
23. Dakhly DMR, Bassiouny YA, Bayoumi YA, Hassan MA, Gouda HM, Hassan AA. The addition of growth hormone adjuvant therapy to the long down regulation protocol in poor responders undergoing in vitro fertilization: randomized control trial. Eur J Obstet Gynecol Reprod Biol. 2018;228:161–5.
24. Li XL, Wang L, Lv F, Huang XM, Wang LP, Pan Y, et al. The influence of different growth hormone addition protocols to poor ovarian responders on clinical outcomes in controlled ovary stimulation cycles: a systematic review and meta-analysis. Medicine (Baltimore). 2017;96(12):e6443.
25. Yu X, Ruan J, He LP, Hu W, Xu Q, Tang J, et al. Efficacy of growth hormone supplementation with gonadotrophins in vitro fertilization for poor ovarian responders: an updated meta-analysis. Int J Clin Exp Med. 2015;8(4):4954–67.
26. Dakhly DM, Bayoumi YA, Gad Allah SH. Which is the best IVF/ICSI protocol to be used in poor responders receiving growth hormone as an adjuvant treatment? A prospective randomized trial. Gynecol Endocrinol. 2016;32(2):116–9.
27. Doan HT, Quan LH, Nguyen TT. The effectiveness of transdermal testosterone gel 1% (androgel) for poor responders undergoing in vitro fertilization. Gynecol Endocrinol. 2017;33(12):977–9.
28. Bosdou JK, Venetis CA, Dafopoulos K, Zepiridis L, Chatzimeletiou K, Anifandis G, et al. Transdermal testosterone pretreatment in poor responders undergoing ICSI: a randomized clinical trial. Hum Reprod. 2016;31(5):977–85.
29. Kim CH, Ahn JW, Moon JW, Kim SH, Chae HD, Kang BM. Ovarian features after 2 weeks, 3 weeks and 4 weeks transdermal testosterone gel treatment and their associated effect on IVF outcomes in poor responders. Dev Reprod. 2014;18(3):145–52.
30. Nagels HE, Rishworth JR, Siristatidis CS, Kroon B. Androgens (dehydroepiandrosterone or testosterone) for women undergoing assisted reproduction. Cochrane Database Syst Rev. 2015;(11):CD009749.
31. Kasum M, Kurdija K, Orešković S, Čehić E, Pavičić-Baldani D, Škrgatić L. Combined ovulation triggering with GnRH agonist and hCG in IVF patients. Gynecol Endocrinol. 2016;32(11):861–5.
32. Haas J, Zilberberg E, Nahum R, Mor Sason A, Hourvitz A, Gat I, et al. Does double trigger (GnRH-agonist + hCG) improve outcome in poor responders undergoing IVF-ET cycle? A pilot study. Gynecol Endocrinol. 2019;35(7):628–30.
33. Mok-Lin E, Brauer AA, Schattman G, Zaninovic N, Rosenwaks Z, Spandorfer S. Follicular flushing and in vitro fertilization outcomes in the poorest responders: a randomized controlled trial. Hum Reprod. 2013;28(11):2990–5.
34. Haydardedeoglu B, Gjemalaj F, Aytac PC, Kilicdag EB. Direct aspiration versus follicular flushing in poor responders undergoing intracytoplasmic sperm injection: a randomised controlled trial. BJOG. 2017;124(8):1190–6.

35. von Horn K, Depenbusch M, Schultze-Mosgau A, Griesinger G. Randomized, open trial comparing a modified double-lumen needle follicular flushing system with a single-lumen aspiration needle in IVF patients with poor ovarian response. Hum Reprod. 2017;32(4):832–5.
36. Berkkanoglu M, Coetzee K, Bulut H, Ozgur K. Optimal embryo transfer strategy in poor response may include freeze-all. J Assist Reprod Genet. 2017;34(1):79–87.
37. Roque M, Valle M, Sampaio M, Geber S. Does freeze-all policy affect IVF outcome in poor ovarian responders? Ultrasound Obstet Gynecol. 2018;52(4):530–4.
38. Xue Y, Tong X, Zhu H, Li K, Zhang S. Freeze-all embryo strategy in poor ovarian responders undergoing ovarian stimulation for in vitro fertilization. Gynecol Endocrinol. 2018;34(8):680–3.
39. Quinquin M, Mialon O, Isnard V, Massin N, Parinaud J, Delotte J, et al. In vitro fertilization versus conversion to intrauterine insemination in Bologna-criteria poor responders: how to decide which option? Fertil Steril. 2014;102(6):1596–601.
40. Sunkara SK, Coomarasamy A, Faris R, Braude P, Khalaf Y. Long gonadotropin-releasing hormone agonist versus short agonist versus antagonist regimens in poor responders undergoing in vitro fertilization: a randomized controlled trial. Fertil Steril. 2014;101(1):147–53.
41. Prapas Y, Petousis S, Dagklis T, Panagiotidis Y, Papatheodorou A, Assunta I, et al. GnRH antagonist versus long GnRH agonist protocol in poor IVF responders: a randomized clinical trial. Eur J Obstet Gynecol Reprod Biol. 2013;166(1):43–6.
42. Pu D, Wu J, Liu J. Comparisons of GnRH antagonist versus GnRH agonist protocol in poor ovarian responders undergoing IVF. Hum Reprod. 2011;26(10):2742–9.
43. Shastri SM, Barbieri E, Kligman I, Schoyer KD, Davis OK, Rosenwaks Z. Stimulation of the young poor responder: comparison of the luteal estradiol/gonadotropin-releasing hormone antagonist priming protocol versus oral contraceptive microdose leuprolide. Fertil Steril. 2011;95(2):592–5.
44. Chang EM, Han JE, Won HJ, Kim YS, Yoon TK, Lee WS. Effect of estrogen priming through luteal phase and stimulation phase in poor responders in in-vitro fertilization. J Assist Reprod Genet. 2012;29(3):225–30.
45. Cakmak H, Tran ND, Zamah AM, Cedars MI, Rosen MP. A novel "delayed start" protocol with gonadotropin-releasing hormone antagonist improves outcomes in poor responders. Fertil Steril. 2014;101(5):1308–14.
46. Davar R, Neghab N, Naghshineh E. Pregnancy outcome in delayed start antagonist versus microdose flare GnRH agonist protocol in poor responders undergoing IVF/ICSI: an RCT. Int J Reprod Biomed (Yazd). 2018;16(4):255–60.
47. DiLuigi AJ, Engmann L, Schmidt DW, Benadiva CA, Nulsen JC. A randomized trial of microdose leuprolide acetate protocol versus luteal phase ganirelix protocol in predicted poor responders. Fertil Steril. 2011;95(8):2531–3.

Chapter 9
Natural Cycle Approaches for ART

Jennifer Shannon

9.1 Introduction

The first neonate created through in vitro fertilization (IVF) was the result of an oocyte retrieved during a natural cycle in a young woman with tubal disease [1]. By definition, natural cycle means "oocytes are collected … from a spontaneous menstrual cycle without administration of any medication at any time during the cycle [2]." Natural cycle IVF as a strategy in most patients is limited by premature ovulation and low live birth rates per cycle due to low oocyte yield. The development of GnRH agonists and the isolation of urinary gonadotropins made it possible to hyperstimulate the ovaries and retrieve multiple oocytes, resulting in increased pregnancy and live birth rates. This strategy became referred to as conventional IVF. Since it is a more effective strategy for most couples, conventional IVF quickly replaced natural cycle IVF as the most effective means for achieving live birth.

Natural cycle IVF was further improved through the development of gonadotropin-releasing hormone (GnRH) antagonists and improved methods for freezing and long-term storage of embryos. GnRH antagonists effectively resolved the problem of premature ovulation and resultant cycle cancellation. However, with their use, the practice is to supplement follicular growth with low doses of human gonadotropins, referred to as modified natural cycle IVF. Furthermore, the advent of embryo cryopreservation allowed the accumulation of embryos for transfer, with subsequent improved live birth rates as discussed in the outcomes section.

Considering natural cycle IVF as an option for patients involves a paradigm shift in the thought process regarding cycle dynamics. With conventional IVF, the thought process is to retrieve a goal number of oocytes with one cycle to optimize

J. Shannon (✉)
Division of Reproductive Endocrinology & Infertility, Department of Obstetrics
and Gynecology, University of Texas Southwestern Medical Center, Dallas, TX, USA
e-mail: jennifer.shannon@utsouthwestern.edu

© Springer Nature Switzerland AG 2020   131
O. Bukulmez (ed.), *Diminished Ovarian Reserve and Assisted Reproductive
Technologies*, https://doi.org/10.1007/978-3-030-23235-1_9

live birth rates. With natural cycle IVF, live birth rates will not be optimized until a cohort of embryos has been obtained. This is particularly useful in the patients who showed poor ovarian response (POR) to conventional stimulation protocols.

According to the SART database in 2011, women who can be classified as poor ovarian response make up about 30% of the patient population seeking reproductive assistance [3]. Data from the CDC suggest that while the total population's mean age at first birth has not increased from around 23 years old, about one-third of women with college education and women living well above the poverty line have their first child at 30 years or older [4]. Data from the National Center for Education Statistics would suggest that the percentage of females seeking higher education is going to increase [5]. Thus, one could project that the proportion of females with advanced reproductive age (ARA), with the associated risk of diminished ovarian response (DOR) and POR, will be expected to increase. Some women with advanced reproductive age (ARA) and diminished ovarian reserve (DOR) may benefit from natural cycle approaches.

9.2 Natural Cycle Protocols for IVF

Traditional natural cycle IVF does not involve the use of any exogenous medication. The risk of premature LH surge and premature ovulation can make this approach impractical for many clinics, so alternative protocols have been created to help manage this. We would like to summarize these protocols in individual figures below (modified from Datta 2017) [6]. *Figure 9.1 describes a typical natural cycle protocol for IVF. Natural cycle IVF is defined as the natural selection of the dominant follicle without addition of exogenous medication. Traditional natural cycle may be troubled by premature LH surges and cycle cancellations. It requires a 24/7 high-functioning lab, both due to cycle demands and low oocyte yield at retrieval.

Figures 9.2 and 9.3 summarize modified natural cycle protocols for timely oocyte retrieval and/or prevention of the LH surge. In Fig. 9.2, a natural cycle is modified with an human chorionic gonadotropin (hCG) trigger to induce oocyte maturation. Modified natural cycle with an hCG trigger allows more flexibility in the timing of

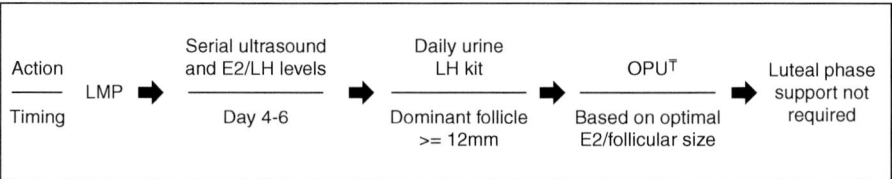

ᵀIf at risk of premature ovulation, use indomethacin. If premature ovulation occurs, OPU within 24 hours.

Fig. 9.1 Traditional Natural Cycle IVF*. ᵀIf at risk of premature ovulation, use indomethacin. If premature ovulation occurs, OPU within 24 hours. E2 estradiol, LH luteinizing hormone, OPU oocyte pickup

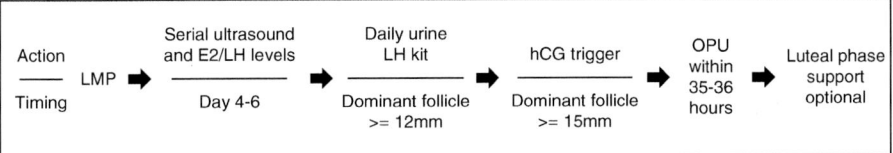

Fig. 9.2 Modified Natural Cycle IVF with hCG Trigger*

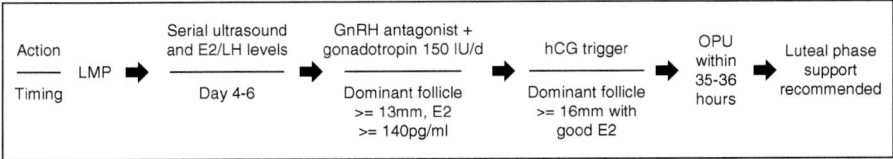

*Abbreviations: LH luteinizing hormone. E2 estradiol. OPU Oocyte pick up. hCG human chorionic gonadotropin. GnRH gonadotropin-releasing hormone. FSH Follicle stimulating hormone. HMG human menopausal gonadotropin.

Fig. 9.3 Modified Natural Cycle IVF with a GnRH Antagonist*. *Abbreviations: LH luteinizing hormone, E2 estradiol, OPU Oocyte pick up, hCG human chorionic gonadotropin, GnRH gonadotropin-releasing hormone, FSH Follicle stimulating hormone, HMG human menopausal gonadotropin

oocyte retrieval; however, this protocol can still be plagued by premature ovulation. In Fig. 9.3, the addition of a GnRH antagonist all but eliminates premature ovulation; however, it dramatically increases cost for the patient as add-back therapy is needed. Some practitioners also add low-dose gonadotropins for few days. As with traditional natural cycle, a high-functioning lab is a requirement with low oocyte yields.

9.3   Natural Cycle IVF Outcomes

In the early days of IVF, Edwards reported an ongoing pregnancy rate of 14.7% per oocyte retrieval and 19% per embryo transfer with natural cycles, which leads to a rate of 1 clinical pregnancy per 6.8 embryos [7]. More recently, a randomized controlled trial showed a clinical pregnancy rate of 14.9% per embryo transfer with natural cycle IVF, but the rate did not improve after three cycles [8]. In 2016, Sunkara found that it would take 4.8 natural cycles with fresh embryo transfer to achieve the pregnancy rates observed in one conventional cycle [9]. A prospective cohort study that looked at 844 natural cycles found that the ongoing pregnancy rate after 3 modified natural cycles was 20.8% with a cancellation rate of 17.7% [10]. The author comments that the occurrence of cancellation of oocyte retrieval, unsuccessful oocyte retrieval, and fertilization failure are recurrent events, and patients should receive counseling in such cases. When the patients were pushed toward nine cycles [11], the ongoing pregnancy rates approached 35.8%, but the dropout rate was significant at 47.8%. The dropout rate was noted to increase sharply after three cycles.

Given that women with POR, by definition, do not respond well to conventional stimulation, natural cycle IVF has been studied as a less expensive and more patient-friendly approach for reproductive assistance in this specific subpopulation. A randomized controlled trial comparing natural cycle to microdose flare high-dose FSH protocol in women with POR, defined as three or fewer follicles recruited or cycle cancelled because of no follicular activation, did not show a significant difference in pregnancy per cycle (6.1 vs 6.9%, respectively). However, implantation rate was significantly higher with natural cycle [7]. In 2009, Schimberni showed a similar pregnancy rate of 9.8% per cycle and 16.7% per embryo transfer in women with POR, defined as patients ≤ 44 years old with a previous cycle that was cancelled due to no follicular activation or only one follicle recruited [12]. In a general poor responder population, defined as ≤ 4 oocytes retrieved and/or E2 level <1000 pg/mL on day of hCG administration, Elizur reported a pregnancy rate of 9% [13]. In poor responders defined by an increased baseline FSH >10mIU/mL and possibly <7AFC, Papaleo found a pregnancy rate of 11.5% per cycle and 20% per embryo transfer [14].

In 2011, the ESHRE created a definition of poor ovarian response in an attempt to standardize the literature. In order to be diagnosed with poor ovarian response, women must meet two of the following three criteria: (1) advanced maternal age or any other risk factor for poor ovarian response, (2) a previous poor ovarian response, and (3) an abnormal ovarian reserve test [15]. When applying this definition, the outcomes appear to worsen. Kedem compared modified natural cycle to conventional IVF and, in poor responders per ESHRE definition, found that the live birth rate was less than 1%, meeting ASRM criteria for futility [16]. Lainas also found very low chances of live birth with modified natural cycle (MNC) but makes the comment that MNC may be more patient-friendly and cost-effective when anticipated live birth rates are low [17]. While Polyzos does not endorse natural cycle in Bologna-criteria poor responders, he does note that pregnancy rates approach 10% after four cycles. Interestingly, Shaulov showed divergent clinical pregnancy rates (CPR) with regard to age in poor responders. In 1503 MNC cycles, the CPR in those ≥36 years old with normal ovarian response was 26.26% per embryo transfer and with poor ovarian response was 6.25% per embryo transfer. However, the CPRs were not divergent between normal and poor ovarian responders ≤35 years old [18].

Lastly, more recent data question the relationship of gonadotropin dosing with both aneuploidy rates and oocyte quality. Baart showed that the proportion of abnormal embryos per patient significantly reduced after mild, versus high, dose stimulation protocols. She also noted that the percentage of mosaic embryos was increased in conventional cycle, and hypothesizes that this is due to an increased incidence of mitotic errors with high doses of gonadotropins [19]. She interestingly comments that the long GnRH agonist protocol shuts down the mechanisms of early follicular recruitment, while milder protocols maintain this mechanism. Sekhon looked at 1122 cycles and noted that patients who required a prolonged stimulation had an elevated risk of aneuploidy with an increasing gonadotropin dosage [20]. Finally, Wu looked at 1088 cycles and found no association with total gonadotropin dosage and aneuploidy rates [21]. With regard to potential oocyte quality, Baker found that as total gonadotropin dose increases, pregnancy rates decrease [22].

To conclude and well stated by Inge, it still only takes one oocyte/embryo to produce a baby, irrespective of level of stimulation. Then the goal is still to find and identify the right oocyte/embryo [7].

9.4   Patient Population

Classically, natural cycle IVF has been thought of either as the historical initial approach to IVF or as a similarly effective, cheaper, and more patient-friendly approach than conventional stimulation for women with POR due to either poor ovarian response, DOR, or ARA. As more data are gathered on this method in different patient populations, clarity has been gained on populations that would benefit the most from its use.

Natural cycle IVF may be an appealing option for those patients who wish to avoid the use of medications for ovarian stimulation. It can also be an option for those opposed to the creation of excess embryos. Natural cycle IVF may also be the safest option in those who are at very high risk of ovarian hyperstimulation syndrome.

With regard to poor ovarian response, both Gordon and Ho suggest that natural cycle is best suited for ovulatory women with normal ovarian reserve testing and normal ovarian response to stimulation [23, 24]. Ho further comments that natural cycle may be a better second-line option in poor ovarian responders after they have failed conventional ovarian stimulation [24]. Datta comments that conventional IVF does not appear to be superior to natural cycle IVF in women with poor ovarian response [6]. Shaulov draws a line at older women with POR, who show very poor outcomes with modified natural cycle IVF, and rather states that MNC-IVF is a reasonable option for both normal and poor ovarian responders ≤ 35 years old and normal ovarian responders ≥36 years old [18]. Kadoch suggests that natural cycle can be considered as a first-line therapy in young poor ovarian responders [25]. Meanwhile, Papathanasiou does not believe there are enough data to make a final conclusion on the place of natural cycle in women with poor ovarian response [26], and Lainas rejects its use in women with POR [17].

Finally, women with poor ovarian response may have elevated basal levels of follicle-stimulating hormone. Chapters in this book will discuss the relationship of elevated basal FSH and IVF cycle outcome. In these cases, alternative protocols, such as luteal phase mild stimulation or long GnRH agonist suppression with estrogen priming and mild stimulation protocols, may be of benefit.

9.5   Conclusion

Natural cycle IVF involves various approaches. Natural cycle IVF may be an option for those patients who wish to avoid the use of medications for ovarian stimulation, those opposing to the creation of excess embryos, and, lastly, in those who are at very high risk of ovarian hyperstimulation syndrome. The women with expected POR or those with DOR may also show some benefits as compared to conventional IVF especially in women younger than 36 years of age with reliable menstrual cycles. Some women with ARA may also benefit. These approaches may require multiple oocyte retrieval cycles. More data are needed to compare its efficacy as compared to other stimulation protocols suggested for women with expected POR such as those with DOR and ARA.

References

1. Steptoe PC, Edwards RG. Birth after the reimplantation of a human embryo. Lancet. 1978;2(8085):366.
2. Nargund G, Fauser BC, Macklon NS, Ombelet W, Nygren K, Frydman R, Rotterdam ISMAAR Consensus Group on Terminology for Ovarian Stimulation for IVF. The ISMAAR proposal on terminology for ovarian stimulation for IVF. Hum Reprod. 2007;22(11):2801–4.
3. Devine K, Mumford SL, Wu M, DeCherney AH, Hill MJ, Propst A. Diminished ovarian reserve in the United States assisted reproductive technology population: diagnostic trends among 181,536 cycles from the Society for Assisted Reproductive Technology Clinic Outcomes Reporting System. Fertil Steril. 2015;104(3):612–19.e3.
4. Martinez GM, Daniels K, Febo-Vazquez I. Fertility of men and women aged 15–44 in the United States: National Survey of Family Growth, 2011–2015. Nat Health Stat Rep. 2018;113:1–17.
5. https://nces.ed.gov/fastfacts/display.asp?id=372. Accessed 10/28/2018.
6. Datta AK, Deval B, Campbell S, Nargund G. Chapter 8: which women are suitable for natural and modified natural cycle IVF? In: Development of in vitro maturation for human oocytes. London: Springer International Publishing; 2017.
7. Inge GB, Brinsden PR, Elder KT. Oocyte number per live birth in IVF: were Steptoe and Edwards less wasteful? Hum Reprod. 2005;20(3):588–92.
8. Morgia F, Sbracia M, Schimberni M, Giallonardo A, Piscitelli C, Giannini P, Aragona C. A controlled trial of natural cycle versus microdose gonadotropin-releasing hormone analog flare cycles in poor responders undergoing in vitro fertilization. Fertil Steril. 2004;81(6):1542–7.
9. Sunkara SK, LaMarca A, Polyzos NP, Seed PT, Khalaf Y. Live birth and perinatal outcomes following stimulated and unstimulated IVF: analysis of over two decades of a nationwide data. Hum Reprod. 2016;31(10):2261–7.
10. Pelinck MJ, Vogel NE, Hoek A, Simons AH, Arts EG, Mochtar MH, Beemsterboer S, Hondelink MN, Heineman MJ. Cumulative pregnancy rates after three cycles of minimal stimulation IVF and results according to subfertility diagnosis: a multicentre cohort study. Hum Reprod. 2006;21(9):2375–83.
11. Pelinck MJ, Vogel NE, Arts EG, Simons AH, Heineman MJ, Hoek A. Cumulative pregnancy rates after a maximum of nine cycles of modified natural cycle IVF and analysis of patient drop-out: a cohort study. Hum Reprod. 2007;22(9):2463–70.

12. Schimberni M, Morgia F, Colabianchi J, Giallonardo A, Piscitelli C, Giannini P, Montigiani M, Sbracia M. Natural-cycle in vitro fertilization in poor responder patients: a survey of 500 consecutive cycles. Fertil Steril. 2009;92(4):1297–301.
13. Elizur SE, Aslan D, Shulman A, Weisz B, Bider D, Dor J. Modified natural cycle using GnRH antagonist can be an optional treatment in poor responders undergoing IVF. J Assist Reprod Genet. 2005;22(2):75–9.
14. Papaleo E, De Santis L, Fusi F, Doldi N, Brigante C, Marelli G, Persico P, Cino I, Ferrari A. Natural cycle as first approach in aged patients with elevated follicle-stimulating hormone undergoing intracytoplasmic sperm injection: a pilot study. Gynecol Endocrinol. 2006;22(7):351–4.
15. Ferraretti AP, La Marca A, Fauser BC, Tarlatzis B, Nargund G, Gianaroli L, ESHRE working group on Poor Ovarian Response Definition. ESHRE consensus on the definition of 'poor response' to ovarian stimulation for in vitro fertilization: the Bologna criteria. Hum Reprod. 2011;26(7):1616–24.
16. Kedem A, Tsur A, Haas J, Yerushalmi GM, Hourvitz A, Machtinger R, Orvieto R. Is the modified natural in vitro fertilization cycle justified in patients with "genuine" poor response to controlled ovarian hyperstimulation? Fertil Steril. 2014;101(6):1624–8.
17. Lainas TG, Sfontouris IA, Venetis CA, Lainas GT, Zorzovilis IZ, Tarlatzis BC, Kolibianakis EM. Live birth rates after modified natural cycle compared with high-dose FSH stimulation using GnRH antagonists in poor responders. Hum Reprod. 2015;30(10):2321–30.
18. Shaulov T, Vélez MP, Buzaglo K, Phillips SJ, Kadoch IJ. Outcomes of 1503 cycles of modified natural cycle in vitro fertilization: a single-institution experience. J Assist Reprod Genet. 2015;32(7):1043–8.
19. Baart EB, Martini E, Eijkemans MJ, Van Opstal D, Beckers NG, Verhoeff A, Macklon NS, Fauser BC. Milder ovarian stimulation for in-vitro fertilization reduces aneuploidy in the human preimplantation embryo: a randomized controlled trial. Hum Reprod. 2007;22(4):980–8.
20. Sekhon L, Shaia K, Santistevan A, Cohn KH, Lee JA, Beim PY, Copperman AB. The cumulative dose of gonadotropins used for controlled ovarian stimulation does not influence the odds of embryonic aneuploidy in patients with normal ovarian response. J Assist Reprod Genet. 2017;34(6):749–58.
21. Wu Q, Li H, Zhu Y, Jiang W, Lu J, Wei D, Yan J, Chen ZJ. Dosage of exogenous gonadotropins is not associated with blastocyst aneuploidy or live-birth rates in PGS cycles in Chinese women. Hum Reprod. 2018;33(10):1875–82.
22. Baker VL, Brown MB, Luke B, Smith GW, Ireland JJ. Gonadotropin dose is negatively correlated with live birth rate: analysis of more than 650,000 assisted reproductive technology cycles. Fertil Steril. 2015;104(5):1145–52.
23. Gordon JD, DiMattina M, Reh A, Botes A, Celia G, Payson M. Utilization and success rates of unstimulated in vitro fertilization in the United States: an analysis of the Society for Assisted Reproductive Technology database. Fertil Steril. 2013;100(2):392–5.
24. Ho JR, Paulson RJ. Modified natural cycle in in vitro fertilization. Fertil Steril. 2017;108(4):572–6.
25. Kadoch IJ, Phillips SJ, Bissonnette F. Modified natural-cycle in vitro fertilization should be considered as the first approach in young poor responders. Fertil Steril. 2011;96(5):1066–8.
26. Papathanasiou A, Searle BJ, King NM, Bhattacharya S. Trends in 'poor responder' research: lessons learned from RCTs in assisted conception. Hum Reprod Update. 2016;22(3):306–19.

Part II
Minimal and Mild Stimulation Protocols

Chapter 10
The International Society for Mild Approaches in Assisted Reproduction (ISMAAR) Definitions for Mild Stimulation and Their Rationale for Assisted Reproductive Technologies

Orhan Bukulmez

10.1 Introduction: Earlier Concerns for Ovarian Stimulation for In Vitro Fertilization

The first test-tube baby was delivered in 1978 in the United Kingdom. In vitro fertilization was performed during a natural cycle with laparoscopic oocyte retrieval [1]. This group lead by Drs. Edwards and Steptoe also studied granulosa cell steroid hormone production collected from follicles during a natural cycle or with human menopausal gonadotropin (HMG) stimulation followed by human chorionic gonadotropin (HCG) administration. They reported concerns about multiple asynchronous follicle development with HMG/HCG. The granulosa cells collected from follicles of various sizes in fact showed different progesterone and estradiol production. The authors discussed the potential adverse effects of multiple but asynchronous follicle development on oocyte maturation [2, 3].

The same pioneering British group tested gonadotropin treatment for ovarian stimulation in 100 cases. Mostly due to progesterone elevation before oocyte retrieval, they were never successful. In the United States, Howard W. and Georgeanna S. Jones started using gonadotropins to stimulate the ovaries despite Dr. Bob Edwards' warning. Per Dr. Howard W. Jones memoir, "the trick might be to administer a smaller dose than Bob (Edwards) had used…. Two ampoules (pergonal) a day from 4th day of menstrual cycle continuing until day 6th or 7….we allowed the follicles to coast until oocyte retrieval…we often harvested 2,3, or even 4 follicles most with mature oocytes." [4]. We have to consider that each

O. Bukulmez (✉)
Division of Reproductive Endocrinology and Infertility, Fertility and Advanced Reproductive Medicine Assisted Reproductive Technologies Program, Department of Obstetrics and Gynecology, University of Texas Southwestern Medical Center, Dallas, TX, USA
e-mail: Orhan.Bukulmez@UTSouthwestern.edu

© Springer Nature Switzerland AG 2020
O. Bukulmez (ed.), *Diminished Ovarian Reserve and Assisted Reproductive Technologies*, https://doi.org/10.1007/978-3-030-23235-1_10

ampoule of pergonal was 75 international units (IU). They did not use HCG for trigger first, but then they calculated from natural cycles that laparoscopic oocyte retrieval should be performed at 36 hours after HCG trigger, which was used as the luteinizing hormone (LH) surrogate. Eventually in December 1981, the same group delivered the first test-tube baby in the United States. Then in 1981, by using HMG, 55 women were stimulated; 31 of them had the transfer, and 7-term healthy live births resulted [4, 5].

10.2 Controlled Ovarian Stimulation Protocols for In Vitro Fertilization

Since the efficiency of the process seemed to improve with ovarian stimulation using gonadotropins, very fast innovation in ovarian stimulation drugs and the protocols followed. The terms controlled ovarian hyperstimulation (COH) and controlled ovarian stimulation (COS) were introduced with direct relevance to IVF although it has become highly debatable if these protocols deserve the term "controlled." The doses of gonadotropins used in the stimulation protocols increased with a rationale that more oocytes would lead to better IVF outcomes. Thereafter, the concerns about complications like ovarian hyperstimulation syndrome, multiple pregnancies due to the transfer of high number of embryos, and high levels steroids and endometrial receptivity issues were associated with various prenatal complications. In addition, there were worries about the financial cost and the emotional burden of IVF with such high-dose protocols. Then some countries imposed strict embryo transfer policies to minimize multiple gestations.

10.2.1 Concerns with Conventional Controlled Ovarian Stimulation Protocols for In Vitro Fertilization

There are concerns that COS protocols for IVF may be associated with increased rates of embryonic aneuploidy and inferior IVF outcomes [6, 7]. High doses of FSH use which is associated with high estradiol levels may be associated with problems in chromosome segregation during meiosis [8]. In an earlier prospective randomized study, the chromosome abnormality rates for embryos developed from mild and conventional stimulation were 55% and 73%, respectively. Hence even some additional oocytes may be obtained with conventional stimulation, the euploid embryo outcome may be higher with mild stimulation, largely minimizing the importance of retrieving more oocytes with conventional stimulation [6].

It was also demonstrated that high concentrations of FSH added to the in vitro maturation medium increased the first meiotic division errors, with increased number of aneuploidy in in vitro matured human oocytes when the polar bodies and the oocytes were assessed with fluorescent in situ hybridization, although there were no differences between the low-dose FSH and very high-dose FSH treated group when the spindle morphology was assessed. Euploid and aneuploid oocytes showed comparable meiotic spindle visualization rates under PolScope as well [9].

A randomized controlled study conducted in women younger than 38 years of age compared eight-cell stage blastomere biopsy results testing for ten chromosomes with fluorescent in situ hybridization (FISH) in patients randomized to either mild stimulation antagonist (recombinant FSH 150 IU daily, started on day 5 of the menstrual cycle) or conventional FSH luteal agonist protocols (recombinant FSH dose 225 IU/daily, starting with withdrawal bleeding). The authors had to terminate the study early after interim analysis revealed a lower embryo aneuploidy rate with mild stimulation IVF. Actually, the number of euploid embryos with conventional stimulation was not higher than the mild stimulation group even with twice the number of embryos obtained with conventional stimulation. In addition, increased mosaic embryos with conventional stimulation was observed with concerns about higher doses of FSH that may also lead to mitotic segregation errors [6].

In another randomized dose-response trial for a new recombinant human FSH preparation, it was shown that increasing FSH dose for stimulation correlated with decreased fertilization rate and decreased blastocyst development per oocyte-recovered ratio [10].

Conventional stimulation protocols for IVF may affect ovarian follicular hormonal milieu. A cross-sectional study of leading follicular fluid samples has revealed that a conventional HMG (150–300 IU daily initiated day 3–5 of the menstrual cycle) stimulation with antagonist protocol resulted in lower AMH, testosterone, androstenedione, dehydroepiandrosterone, estradiol, and LH levels as compared to leading follicular fluid samples collected from women who underwent natural cycle IVF. Both treatment cycles were triggered by HCG (10,000 IU with conventional stimulation and 5000 IU with >18 mm follicle with natural cycle) [11]. Then recently the same researchers again studied the follicular fluid samples collected from first dominant follicle of patients who underwent natural cycle IVF or conventional stimulation IVF with HMG and GnRH antagonist. Follicular fluid obtained from conventional stimulation group contained more CD45+ leucocytes but fewer CD8+ cytotoxic T cells than those obtained from natural cycle IVF group. There were also differences between the levels of IL-8 and vascular endothelial growth factor (VEGF), former being lower and the latter being higher in conventional stimulation IVF group as compared to natural cycle IVF [12]. Therefore, the use of gonadotropins per se is associated with intrafollicular changes.

10.2.2 Clinical Data on Gonadotropin Doses and In Vitro Fertilization Outcomes in Women with Advanced Reproductive Age and/or Expected Poor Ovarian Response

Increasing the dose of gonadotropins to enhance oocyte yield in women with advanced reproductive age (ARA) may not work as rationalized. An earlier prospective double-blind multicenter study conducted in women between 30 and 39 years of age compared the fixed daily dose use of a recombinant (rec-) FSH preparation at either 150 IU or 250 IU for COS for IVF. The number of oocytes collected between the low- and high-dose groups was comparable. In younger women between the age of 30 and 33 years, high-dose regimen resulted in higher mean number of oocytes (14.8 versus 10.6) than the low-dose regimen. However, in advanced reproductive age group between 37 and 39 years of age, the mean number of oocytes was comparable between high- and low-dose protocols (8.1 versus 7.4, respectively). Advancing female age was associated with decreased oocyte yield regardless of the rec-FSH dose used. Average FSH concentrations on the day of hCG administration for triggering for final oocyte maturation was 13 IU/L in 250 IU group but only 9.3 IU in the 150 IU group. Again higher FSH levels did not help with the oocyte yield. When the secondary outcomes were assessed, it was obvious that the pregnancy rates were comparable between 150 IU and 250 IU groups. However, in the general patient population, those stimulated with 150 IU daily dose resulted in somewhat higher clinical pregnancy rates per started cycle or per embryo transfer than the 250 IU arm. The implantation rates seemed to be higher in the lower-dose group as well although none of these differences reached statistical significance. Therefore, increasing the daily dose of recombinant FSH did not compensate for age-related decrease in retrievable oocytes [13].

A recent Cochrane review analyzed whether individualized gonadotropin dosing based on ovarian reserve tests (AMH, basal FSH, antral follicle count) effects IVF outcome. The authors included 20 such clinical trials, but meta-analysis was limited due to heterogeneity. Lack of blinding also influenced the quality of the evidence. The authors concluded that modifying FSH dose for IVF according to low, normal, or high ovarian reserve patients did not affect live birth or ongoing pregnancy rates. Consequently, the current evidence did not justify increasing the standard daily dose of 150 IU in poor or normal responders [14].

Multicenter prospective cohort study and two embedded randomized controlled trials assessed the IVF/intracytoplasmic sperm injection (ICSI) outcomes of the women with antral follicle counts (AFC) < 11 who were randomized to individualized dosing with 450 IU (women with AFC ≤ 7) or 225 IU (women with AFC 8–10) of daily gonadotropins and standard daily 150 IU dose of gonadotropins. IVF/ICSI live birth outcomes were comparable between the general high-dose individualized dose group and the standard daily 150 IU dose group, while the cost was much higher for the high-dose group. The authors recommended starting 150 IU daily dose of gonadotropins to all women with regular cycles for IVF including those with predicted poor ovarian response (POR) per AFC [15, 16]. In addition, in women at ≤ 39 years of age, receiving standard fixed daily dose of 150 IU of recombinant FSH, the serum FSH levels on the day of trigger were not different between poor and normal responders. The authors concluded that POR is not due to low serum FSH levels achieved on the day of trigger. Therefore, increasing the dose of recombinant FSH above 150 IU daily dose may not be justified to improve outcomes in women with POR [17].

10.3   International Society for Mild Approaches in Assisted Reproduction (ISMAAR): Mild Stimulation Versus Minimal Stimulation

A large national registry study from the United States of autologous cycles performed between 2004 and 2012 suggested that with increasing FSH dose, regardless of the number of oocytes retrieved, the live birth rates declined. This was also true for the good prognosis patients as well. The authors suggested that perhaps the providers may avoid using high-dose FSH but noted that this study's results does not support the use of minimal stimulation or natural cycle approaches for IVF [18]. Interestingly the lead author of this paper commented earlier that since its cost effectiveness was not established, the acceptability of mild stimulation protocols for IVF might not be acceptable for patients in the United States [19].

The European group though recently suggested that with the recent research evidence, the mild stimulation approaches for IVF should lead to their widespread acceptance [20]. This was entailing using more gentle approaches for ovarian stimulation for IVF and elective single embryo transfer. Then some societies and organizations started promoting low cost and safe IVF stimulation protocols. One of these organizations is the International Society for Mild Approaches in Assisted Reproduction (ISMAAR) [21].

The ISMAAR defines mild stimulation IVF when FSH or HMG is administered at a lower dose and/or shorter duration in a gonadotropin-releasing hormone (GnRH) antagonist co-treated cycle or when oral compounds, oral antiestrogens, or aromatase inhibitors are used either alone or in combination with gonadotropins with the aim of collecting fewer oocytes.

Mild stimulation IVF definition may be considered somewhat vague. Mild stimulation includes the stimulation protocols with reduced gonadotropin dose and/or duration leading to low cumulative doses of gonadotropins and perhaps aiming to develop 3–5 follicles per IVF cycle. The ISMAAR defines that the daily maximum dose of FSH or HMG should be 150 IU as the described threshold to differentiate between conventional controlled ovarian stimulation protocols for IVF. We agree with the daily dose threshold, but we also consider that the cycles including oral agents like clomiphene citrate or aromatase inhibitor letrozole may even require less cumulative FSH doses per treatment cycle. We chose to call such approaches as minimal stimulation for IVF as some others suggested [22].

10.3.1 Natural Cycle Paradigm for IVF

Natural cycle protocols have been revisited and implemented especially taking advantage of the advances in embryo freezing and the availability of GnRH antagonists. These protocols were especially gaining acceptance in patients with POR and/or diminished ovarian reserve (DOR).

In a small study involving DOR and ARA patients between the ages of 37 and 43 years, natural cycle IVF with ICSI resulted in comparable pregnancy rates as compared to those rates achieved with conventional stimulation in historical controls [23]. In a randomized controlled study, natural cycle IVF in women with history of POR (59 patients 114 cycles) has been shown to result in better implantation rates (14.9% vs 5.5%) than those achieved by GnRH agonist microdose flare protocol (70 women, 101 cycles). Otherwise, the patients treated with natural cycle IVF and those treated with GnRH agonist microdose flare showed similar pregnancy rates per cycle and per transfer. Especially those patients ≤35 years of age benefited better than older patients from natural cycle IVF in terms of pregnancy rates [24]. A small within-patient study has suggested that natural cycles may result in higher oocyte retrieval rates with higher clinical pregnancy rate per started cycle in patients with history POR with conventional IVF stimulation [25]. Considering the overall reduced adverse impact of such approaches in terms of decreased cost per cycle and possibly better endometrial receptivity and oocyte quality and possibility of doing multiple cycles at reduced cost as compared to conventional high-dose stimulation protocols, natural cycle approaches have been favored especially for DOR and ARA patients.

10.3.2 Mild Stimulation for IVF

In regard to mild stimulation, a prospective randomized study compared GnRH agonist long protocol to two flexible-start GnRH antagonist protocols, one commencing rec-FSH on day 2 of the cycle and the other one was commencing on day 5 of the cycle. Daily rec-FSH dose for GnRH antagonist protocols was kept at 150 IU. Although with day 5 rec-FSH start more cycles were canceled before oocyte retrieval, overall, the quality of the embryos were reported to be higher in day 5 start group. The transfer rate per oocyte retrieval as a result became higher with higher pregnancy rates in women with ≤4 oocytes retrieved in the group with day 5 rec-FSH start. This group showed the least median cumulative dose of rec-FSH use (1200 IU, while with GnRH agonist and GnRH antagonist, day 2 rec-FSH start used median of 1650 IU and 1350 IU, respectively). All treatment groups showed comparable pregnancy rates per started cycle suggesting that mild stimulation regimens are as effective as higher dose regimens in COS for IVF. This may be related to better oocyte and embryo quality with lower doses of FSH [26].

At least in normal to high responders, there are randomized trials demonstrating comparable or a trend of higher rate of good-quality embryos or blastocysts via mild stimulation approaches [26, 27].

In terms of elective single embryo transfer applications with mild stimulation, which entails cycle day 5 start of 150 IU/day rec-FSH and late follicular phase GnRH antagonist co-treatment in women younger than 38 years of age, the ongoing pregnancy rates of 28% per single embryo transfer were reported [28].

Recently the American Society for Reproductive Medicine (ASRM) recommended, "in patients who are classified as poor responders and pursuing IVF, strong consideration should be given to mild ovarian stimulation protocol...." This practice committee of ASRM recommendation is based on the findings that mild stimulation has low cost and comparable low pregnancy rates with conventional stimulation protocols [29]. This last suggestion may also be challenged since such protocols can be optimized if combined with the sole use of frozen embryo transfers as we discussed in this book.

10.4 Conclusion

Ovarian stimulation to increase oocyte yield was commenced in the early 1980s albeit starting with low gonadotropin doses. In a short time, controlled ovarian stimulation protocols evolved to include high daily doses of FSH. Shortly, many concerns about using high-dose FSH lead to revisiting the dose of gonadotropins to assure optimum outcomes. The efforts to increase oocyte yield in women with DOR and ARA by using high-dose conventional COS protocol did not result in the expected improvement in IVF outcomes. The ISMAAR proposed mild stimulation definition, and since then many studies supported their use especially in women with predicted POR, i.e., DOR and/or ARA. Natural cycle approaches to IVF found ground for DOR population. Mild and minimal stimulation approaches are beginning to have some acceptance from the assisted reproductive technology establishment as well.

References

1. Steptoe PC, Edwards RG. Birth after the reimplantation of a human embryo. Lancet. 1978;2(8085):366.
2. Fowler RE, Edwards RG, Walters DE, Chan ST, Steptoe PC. Steroidogenesis in preovulatory follicles of patients given human menopausal and chorionic gonadotrophins as judged by the radioimmunoassay of steroids in follicular fluid. J Endocrinol. 1978;77(2):161–9.
3. Fowler RE, Fox NL, Edwards RG, Walters DE, Steptoe PC. Steroidogenesis by cultured granulosa cells aspirated from human follicles using pregnenolone and androgens as precursors. J Endocrinol. 1978;77(2):171–83.

4. Jones HW Jr. In vitro fertilization comes to America. Memoir of a medical breakthrough. Williamsburg: Jamestown Bookworks; 2014. p. 234.

5. Jones HW Jr, Jones GS, Andrews MC, Acosta A, Bundren C, Garcia J, et al. The program for in vitro fertilization at Norfolk. Fertil Steril. 1982;38(1):14–21.

6. Baart EB, Martini E, Eijkemans MJ, Van Opstal D, Beckers NG, Verhoeff A, et al. Milder ovarian stimulation for in-vitro fertilization reduces aneuploidy in the human preimplantation embryo: a randomized controlled trial. Hum Reprod. 2007;22(4):980–8.

7. Kovacs P, Sajgo A, Kaali SG, Pal L. Detrimental effects of high-dose gonadotropin on outcome of IVF: making a case for gentle ovarian stimulation strategies. Reprod Sci. 2012;19(7):718–24.

8. Edwards RG. IVF, IVM, natural cycle IVF, minimal stimulation IVF – time for a rethink. Reprod Biomed Online. 2007;15(1):106–19.

9. Xu YW, Peng YT, Wang B, Zeng YH, Zhuang GL, Zhou CQ. High follicle-stimulating hormone increases aneuploidy in human oocytes matured in vitro. Fertil Steril. 2011;95(1):99–104.

10. Arce JC, Andersen AN, Fernandez-Sanchez M, Visnova H, Bosch E, Garcia-Velasco JA, et al. Ovarian response to recombinant human follicle-stimulating hormone: a randomized, antimullerian hormone-stratified, dose-response trial in women undergoing in vitro fertilization/intracytoplasmic sperm injection. Fertil Steril. 2014;102(6):1633–40 e5.

11. von Wolff M, Kollmann Z, Fluck CE, Stute P, Marti U, Weiss B, et al. Gonadotrophin stimulation for in vitro fertilization significantly alters the hormone milieu in follicular fluid: a comparative study between natural cycle IVF and conventional IVF. Hum Reprod. 2014;29(5):1049–57.

12. Kollmann Z, Schneider S, Fux M, Bersinger NA, von Wolff M. Gonadotrophin stimulation in IVF alters the immune cell profile in follicular fluid and the cytokine concentrations in follicular fluid and serum. Hum Reprod. 2017;32(4):820–31.

13. Out HJ, Braat DD, Lintsen BM, Gurgan T, Bukulmez O, Gokmen O, et al. Increasing the daily dose of recombinant follicle stimulating hormone (Puregon) does not compensate for the age-related decline in retrievable oocytes after ovarian stimulation. Hum Reprod. 2000;15(1):29–35.

14. Lensen SF, Wilkinson J, Leijdekkers JA, La Marca A, Mol BWJ, Marjoribanks J, et al. Individualised gonadotropin dose selection using markers of ovarian reserve for women undergoing in vitro fertilisation plus intracytoplasmic sperm injection (IVF/ICSI). Cochrane Database Syst Rev. 2018;(2):CD012693.

15. van Tilborg TC, Oudshoorn SC, Eijkemans MJC, Mochtar MH, van Golde RJT, Hoek A, et al. Individualized FSH dosing based on ovarian reserve testing in women starting IVF/ICSI: a multicentre trial and cost-effectiveness analysis. Hum Reprod. 2017;32(12):2485–95.

16. van Tilborg TC, Torrance HL, Oudshoorn SC, Eijkemans MJC, Koks CAM, Verhoeve HR, et al. Individualized versus standard FSH dosing in women starting IVF/ICSI: an RCT. Part 1: the predicted poor responder. Hum Reprod. 2017;32(12):2496–505.

17. Oudshoorn SC, van Tilborg TC, Hamdine O, Torrance HL, Eijkemans MJC, Lentjes E, et al. Ovarian response to controlled ovarian hyperstimulation: what does serum FSH say? Hum Reprod. 2017;32(8):1701–9.

18. Baker VL, Brown MB, Luke B, Smith GW, Ireland JJ. Gonadotropin dose is negatively correlated with live birth rate: analysis of more than 650,000 assisted reproductive technology cycles. Fertil Steril. 2015;104(5):1145–52 e1-5.

19. Baker VL. Mild ovarian stimulation for in vitro fertilization: one perspective from the USA. J Assist Reprod Genet. 2013;30(2):197–202.

20. Nargund G, Datta AK, Fauser B. Mild stimulation for in vitro fertilization. Fertil Steril. 2017;108(4):558–67.

21. Nargund G, Fauser BC, Macklon NS, Ombelet W, Nygren K, Frydman R, et al. The ISMAAR proposal on terminology for ovarian stimulation for IVF. Hum Reprod. 2007;22(11):2801–4.

22. Teramoto S, Kato O. Minimal ovarian stimulation with clomiphene citrate: a large-scale retrospective study. Reprod Biomed Online. 2007;15(2):134–48.

23. Papaleo E, De Santis L, Fusi F, Doldi N, Brigante C, Marelli G, et al. Natural cycle as first approach in aged patients with elevated follicle-stimulating hormone undergoing intracytoplasmic sperm injection: a pilot study. Gynecol Endocrinol. 2006;22(7):351–4.
24. Morgia F, Sbracia M, Schimberni M, Giallonardo A, Piscitelli C, Giannini P, et al. A controlled trial of natural cycle versus microdose gonadotropin-releasing hormone analog flare cycles in poor responders undergoing in vitro fertilization. Fertil Steril. 2004;81(6):1542–7.
25. Bassil S, Godin PA, Donnez J. Outcome of in-vitro fertilization through natural cycles in poor responders. Hum Reprod. 1999;14(5):1262–5.
26. Hohmann FP, Macklon NS, Fauser BC. A randomized comparison of two ovarian stimulation protocols with gonadotropin-releasing hormone (GnRH) antagonist cotreatment for in vitro fertilization commencing recombinant follicle-stimulating hormone on cycle day 2 or 5 with the standard long GnRH agonist protocol. J Clin Endocrinol Metab. 2003;88(1):166–73.
27. Casano S, Guidetti D, Patriarca A, Pittatore G, Gennarelli G, Revelli A. MILD ovarian stimulation with GnRH-antagonist vs. long protocol with low dose FSH for non-PCO high responders undergoing IVF: a prospective, randomized study including thawing cycles. J Assist Reprod Genet. 2012;29(12):1343–51.
28. Verberg MF, Eijkemans MJ, Macklon NS, Heijnen EM, Fauser BC, Broekmans FJ. Predictors of ongoing pregnancy after single-embryo transfer following mild ovarian stimulation for IVF. Fertil Steril. 2008;89(5):1159–65.
29. Practice Committee of the American Society for Reproductive Medicine. Electronic address, ASRM@asrm.org. Comparison of pregnancy rates for poor responders using IVF with mild ovarian stimulation versus conventional IVF: a guideline. Fertil Steril. 2018;109(6):993–9.

Chapter 11
Current Outlook of Minimal and Mild Stimulation Protocols for Assisted Reproductive Technologies in Women with Diminished Ovarian Reserve and/or Advanced Reproductive Age

Orhan Bukulmez

11.1 Relevant Studies in Milder Approaches in Ovarian Stimulation in Women with Advanced Reproductive and/or Diminished Ovarian Reserve

Mild and minimal stimulation protocols have been favored more for women with expected poor ovarian response (POR) due to diminished ovarian reserve (DOR) and/or advanced reproductive age (ARA). A review from 2017 identified five randomized studies in poor responders comparing conventional high-dose FSH protocols to mild stimulation IVF protocols [1]. One of these was with gonadotropin-releasing hormone (GnRH) antagonist high-dose (500 international units (IU)/day of total FSH) protocol (n:33) versus letrozole plus FSH (150 IU/day) (n:31). This study showed comparable clinical pregnancy rates with much less gonadotropin use [2]. Another trial randomized patients with history of one or more failed cycles to mild stimulation with letrozole 5 mg/day for 5 days between cycle days 2–6 and human menopausal gonadotropin (HMG) 150 IU daily from cycle day 7 with flexible GnRH antagonist protocol (n:30) and conventional high-dose (purified HMG 300 IU daily) GnRH agonist short flare protocol (n:30). This study showed comparable clinical pregnancy rates per cycle with no differences in mean number of oocytes/embryos ratio [3].

Then there were three larger studies. In one of these prospective randomized studies, the authors treated women with DOR and POR (between ages of 18 and 42) with either clomiphene citrate 150 mg daily for 5 days between cycle days 3

O. Bukulmez (✉)
Division of Reproductive Endocrinology and Infertility, Fertility and Advanced Reproductive Medicine Assisted Reproductive Technologies Program, Department of Obstetrics and Gynecology, University of Texas Southwestern Medical Center, Dallas, TX, USA
e-mail: Orhan.Bukulmez@UTSouthwestern.edu

© Springer Nature Switzerland AG 2020
O. Bukulmez (ed.), *Diminished Ovarian Reserve and Assisted Reproductive Technologies*, https://doi.org/10.1007/978-3-030-23235-1_11

and 7 (n:148) or GnRH agonist short flare protocol with daily use of recombinant FSH at 450 IU (n:156). Live birth rate per cycle (3% versus 5%, respectively) and live birth rate per embryo transfer (9% versus 9%, respectively) were comparable among groups [4] .

In one other trial, women with ARA (age $\geq$ 35 years) or DOR or history of POR were randomized to one cycle of a mild stimulation protocol with a fixed dose of FSH at 150 IU daily started on cycle day 5 after oral contraceptive pre-treatment, which was combined with fixed dose antagonist start on day 6 of stimulation (n:195). The authors had a set cancellation criteria. If the patients showed less than 2 follicles 15 mm or above after day 7, the cycles were canceled. Other group was randomized to one cycle of GnRH agonist long protocol with daily use of HMG at 450 IU (n:199). The clinical (15.3% versus 15.5%, respectively) and ongoing pregnancy (12.8% versus 13.6%, respectively) rates per patient were comparable. There were no data concerning the cryopreservation of surplus embryos, and therefore cumulative pregnancy rates could not be calculated [5].

Lastly, patients <43 years of age with DOR were randomized to mild stimulation with clomiphene citrate 100 mg daily for 5 days between cycle days 2 and 6 and recombinant follitropin alfa 150 IU/lutropin alfa 75 IU (Pergoveris) started daily on day 5. GnRH antagonist was started on day 8 (n:309). Other randomized groups received long GnRH agonist protocol with HMG with starting dose of 300 IU daily and with a maximum dose of 450 IU daily (n:331). Cycle cancellation rate was significantly higher in the mild stimulation arm (13% versus 2.7%). However, clinical pregnancy rate per cycle (13.2% versus 15.3%, respectively) and ongoing pregnancy rate per embryo transfer (17.8% versus 16.8%, respectively) were comparable among groups even if significantly more metaphase II oocytes were retrieved in conventional high-dose stimulation group as compared to the mild stimulation arm. There were no differences in top-grade embryos [6].

A meta-analysis published in 2016 investigated the efficiency of mild stimulation protocols with clomiphene citrate in women with POR [7]. There were only four studies, two of which were by Ragni et al. and Revelli et al. as described above. Other two studies were from 2004 and 2011, and the earlier study was quasi-randomized since protocols were assigned per weekday of the stimulation start [8, 9]. In these two studies, the description of the mild stimulation protocols with clomiphene citrate actually included high gonadotropin doses. D'Amato et al. described the stimulation protocol as recombinant FSH 300 IU twice daily with clomiphene citrate 100 mg for 5 days, and Karimzadeh et al. gave recombinant FSH or HMG at 225–300 IU daily doses along with 100 mg daily and 5-day regimen of clomiphene citrate. Therefore, relevance of this meta-analysis to the defined mild stimulation protocols may not be relevant. Still the authors did not show any difference between the protocols with and without clomiphene citrate in terms of live birth rate and clinical pregnancy rate [7].

Recently the American Society for Reproductive Medicine (ASRM) came up with a practice committee opinion on mild stimulation as compared to conventional stimulation for IVF in women POR [10]. After reviewing two publications

[5, 11], it was concluded that although live birth rates cannot be estimated, in women with POR, there is fair evidence that clinical pregnancy rates after IVF are not substantially different when mild stimulation protocols using low-dose gonadotropins (defined as ≤150 IU/day) are compared to conventional stimulation protocols. A similar conclusion was reached in terms of similar clinical pregnancy rates with mild stimulation protocols with oral superovulating agents like clomiphene citrate and letrozole when these mild stimulation protocols are compared to conventional stimulation protocols for IVF in poor responders [2, 3, 6, 12, 13]. However, the evidence was found insufficient to recommend for or against for using oral agents alone for IVF versus using conventional IVF stimulation protocols for poor responders while assessing one trial [4], but that trial also suggested that mild ovarian stimulation with clomiphene citrate alone may be cost effective.

The summary conclusion of ASRM was in POR patients for IVF; strong consideration should be given for mild ovarian stimulation protocols due to lower cost and comparable pregnancy rates to conventional IVF stimulation protocols [10].

11.2   Issues with Prospective Randomized Controlled Trials and Their Interpretation

Certainly, the practice of IVF is a more outcome-based field more than any other field in medicine. The short-term accepted outcomes for IVF are clinical pregnancy rates and ongoing pregnancy rates. These are readily available from prospective randomized controlled trials within a short time period. The midterm outcome and the desired outcome include live birth rates, which may be accounted as live births anywhere between 24th and 40th weeks of pregnancy. Perhaps, even more important outcomes are take-home baby rates and general developmental outcomes of the offspring conceived with IVF. These outcomes are least reported in the literature for any specific IVF approach for POR and DOR patients.

One other point to consider is how the success is defined in IVF. Per cycle pregnancy rate paradigm was created by government agencies when the mandatory IVF data registries were set up in Europe and in the United States. This rate has been typically used for marketing while ignoring the impact of frozen-thawed embryo transfers on IVF treatment outcomes. Therefore, per fresh cycle pregnancy rates are not reflecting the true outcome. Currently the paradigm is shifting toward pregnancy rate per patient. This definition opens venues for more widespread acceptance of mild stimulation approaches for patients with DOR and/or ARA. Such protocols cannot be properly implemented without the presence of a highly successful embryo-freezing program, because especially in protocols involving minimal stimulation or luteal phase mild stimulation, fresh embryo transfers are not considered as explained in subsequent sections.

The studies reviewed above are set protocols without patient-tailored modifications during the protocol implementation although we are living in the era of personalized medicine or precision medicine. The patient-specific approaches may be expected to achieve better outcomes rather than firmly set and "cookie-cutter" protocols.

It is difficult to tailor many parameters at once within the context of a prospective randomized controlled trial. On the other hand, it is observed that DOR and POR patients are profoundly heterogeneous groups. We and others noted that DOR patients present with different basal FSH and estradiol levels and different antral follicle counts with each menstrual cycle. Hence, their oocyte and embryo yield may change over repetitive cycles. In that respect, treatment cycle preparation and choosing the right cycle to start the stimulation are the important aspects of treatment regimens for women with DOR and/or ARA or with history of POR. Some protocols for DOR patients may be associated with a sub-receptive endometrium as well. Considering these and many other factors, achieving conformity in management of DOR patients can easily be deemed impossible. Therefore, customization of the approaches for each such patient should be the norm rather than the exception.

11.3   Conclusion

Milder approaches of ovarian stimulation for IVF in women with DOR and/or ARA are finally met with some acceptance. In the upcoming sections on minimal and mild stimulation protocols for women with DOR and/or ARA and those with predicted POR, we will cover the customization aspects of such protocols. We will go-over stimulation cycle preparation, which minimal or mild stimulation protocol to use, endogenous or exogenous LH activity support while preventing premature LH surge and others. Most importantly, like many others, in order to reach higher pregnancy and live birth rates than those reported in prospective randomized trials, such protocols cannot be performed properly without having an excellent embryo freezing and successful frozen-thawed embryo transfer program as we also discuss in subsequent sections.

References

1. Nargund G, Datta AK, Fauser B. Mild stimulation for in vitro fertilization. Fertil Steril. 2017;108(4):558–67.
2. Bastu E, Buyru F, Ozsurmeli M, Demiral I, Dogan M, Yeh J. A randomized, single-blind, prospective trial comparing three different gonadotropin doses with or without addition of letrozole during ovulation stimulation in patients with poor ovarian response. Eur J Obstet Gynecol Reprod Biol. 2016;203:30–4.
3. Mohsen IA, El Din RE. Minimal stimulation protocol using letrozole versus microdose flare up GnRH agonist protocol in women with poor ovarian response undergoing ICSI. Gynecol Endocrinol. 2013;29(2):105–8.

  4. Ragni G, Levi-Setti PE, Fadini R, Brigante C, Scarduelli C, Alagna F, et al. Clomiphene citrate versus high doses of gonadotropins for in vitro fertilisation in women with compromised ovarian reserve: a randomised controlled non-inferiority trial. Reprod Biol Endocrinol. 2012;10:114.
  5. Youssef MA, van Wely M, Al-Inany H, Madani T, Jahangiri N, Khodabakhshi S, et al. A mild ovarian stimulation strategy in women with poor ovarian reserve undergoing IVF: a multi-center randomized non-inferiority trial. Hum Reprod. 2017;32(1):112–8.
  6. Revelli A, Chiado A, Dalmasso P, Stabile V, Evangelista F, Basso G, et al. "Mild" vs. "long" protocol for controlled ovarian hyperstimulation in patients with expected poor ovarian responsiveness undergoing in vitro fertilization (IVF): a large prospective randomized trial. J Assist Reprod Genet. 2014;31(7):809–15.
  7. Song D, Shi Y, Zhong Y, Meng Q, Hou S, Li H. Efficiency of mild ovarian stimulation with clomiphene on poor ovarian responders during IVF\ICSI procedures: a meta-analysis. Eur J Obstet Gynecol Reprod Biol. 2016;204:36–43.
  8. D'Amato G, Caroppo E, Pasquadibisceglie A, Carone D, Vitti A, Vizziello GM. A novel protocol of ovulation induction with delayed gonadotropin-releasing hormone antagonist administration combined with high-dose recombinant follicle-stimulating hormone and clomiphene citrate for poor responders and women over 35 years. Fertil Steril. 2004;81(6):1572–7.
  9. Karimzadeh MA, Mashayekhy M, Mohammadian F, Moghaddam FM. Comparison of mild and microdose GnRH agonist flare protocols on IVF outcome in poor responders. Arch Gynecol Obstet. 2011;283(5):1159–64.
 10. Practice Committee of the American Society for Reproductive Medicine. Electronic address, ASRM@asrm.org. Comparison of pregnancy rates for poor responders using IVF with mild ovarian stimulation versus conventional IVF: a guideline. Fertil Steril. 2018;109(6):993–9.
 11. Klinkert ER, Broekmans FJ, Looman CW, Habbema JD, te Velde ER. Expected poor responders on the basis of an antral follicle count do not benefit from a higher starting dose of gonadotrophins in IVF treatment: a randomized controlled trial. Hum Reprod. 2005;20(3):611–5.
 12. Goswami SK, Das T, Chattopadhyay R, Sawhney V, Kumar J, Chaudhury K, et al. A randomized single-blind controlled trial of letrozole as a low-cost IVF protocol in women with poor ovarian response: a preliminary report. Hum Reprod. 2004;19(9):2031–5.
 13. Pilehvari S, Shahrokh Tehraninejad E, Hosseinrashidi B, Keikhah F, Haghollahi F, Aziminekoo E. Comparison pregnancy outcomes between minimal stimulation protocol and conventional GnRH antagonist protocols in poor ovarian responders. J Family Reprod Health. 2016;10(1):35–42.

Chapter 12
Minimal Stimulation Protocol for Assisted Reproductive Technologies in Women with Diminished Ovarian Reserve and/or Advanced Reproductive Age

Orhan Bukulmez

12.1 Conditions for Minimal Stimulation IVF

In order to implement the minimal and mild stimulation approaches for in vitro fertilization (IVF) in women with diminished ovarian reserve (DOR) and/or advanced reproductive age (ARA), building an appropriate team of professionals is essential. Apart from physician providers, IVF laboratory professionals, nursing, front desk, and financial counseling teams understanding the essentials of this process are important components to run an efficient and smooth minimal or mild stimulation cycles for IVF. Minimal stimulation protocol at a glance seems to be very easy on the paper, but it requires extremely close monitoring, more frequently than the conventional IVF stimulation protocols, which necessitates profound understanding of reproductive endocrinology, and complex decision-making daily, from the physicians. Many fertility physicians may need additional training for the implementation of such protocols in women with DOR and/or ARA. Application of minimal/mild stimulation protocols for women with poor ovarian response (POR) or with DOR and/ARA should be considered as a typical example of personalized medicine. Each age and ovarian reserve matched patient will show different responses during each of their repetitive cycles, which requires extreme plasticity from the physician providers while the patients should be prepared to meet the daily demands of these protocols.

Physician providers, nursing team, and laboratory professionals should acknowledge that these patients will stay in treatment cycles for a while due to the proposed plans for multiple ovarian stimulation cycles with the aim of accumulating mul-

O. Bukulmez (✉)
Division of Reproductive Endocrinology and Infertility, Fertility and Advanced Reproductive Medicine Assisted Reproductive Technologies Program, Department of Obstetrics and Gynecology, University of Texas Southwestern Medical Center, Dallas, TX, USA
e-mail: Orhan.Bukulmez@UTSouthwestern.edu

© Springer Nature Switzerland AG 2020
O. Bukulmez (ed.), *Diminished Ovarian Reserve and Assisted Reproductive Technologies*, https://doi.org/10.1007/978-3-030-23235-1_12

tiple frozen embryos. Therefore, everyone in the care team should be familiar with each patients'/couples' needs for proper scheduling and should set expectations. For example, although a sample treatment calendar is provided for patients to explain the daily medication and time estimates for a given cycle, the team should assure that the patients will primarily follow the recommendations of the fertility clinic after the first 3 days of stimulation, following the approval of starting the treatment cycle after baseline ultrasound and serum testing for estradiol (E2), luteinizing hormone (LH), and progesterone (P4). Medication teaching sessions are important to understand the proper drug administration by the patients in the evening or when needed. Patients should be trained, for example, how to administer half-dose gonadotropin-releasing hormone (GnRH) antagonist when required. Sometimes we may ask the patients to keep their GnRH antagonist preparation handy since its administration may be required as soon as the E2 and LH levels are available in the late morning or early afternoon rather than typical nighttime administration of such medications.

Multiple cycles of minimal stimulation IVF with close monitoring will require weekend and holiday work for the team of physicians and laboratory and nursing staff. Therefore, proper staffing for such days should be assured.

We cannot emphasize the importance of human embryology laboratory enough. Environmental control, assuring air quality and being on top of quality control and quality assurance parameters and close observation of fertilization, embryo progression, pregnancy, and biochemical pregnancy rates to be able to make fast interventions is essential. In addition, many embryologists were trained to process multiple oocytes from each patient undergoing IVF. Hence, many laboratory professionals want to be provided with more "head room" to work with when it comes to the number of oocytes. The protocols that we discuss in upcoming sections usually result in "0"–"4" oocytes. Some patients only have one oocyte retrieved each time. Therefore, embryologists' mental readiness and motivation to work with such patients' oocytes and embryos should not be underestimated. Our team is always cheerful once we find "an egg." Our team treats each oocyte of such patients as their only oocyte.

Minimal and mild stimulation protocols require accumulation of frozen embryos for a future elective frozen-thawed embryo transfer (FET). This approach, rather than planning to transfer embryos during the stimulation cycle, makes all the difference in outcomes. We cannot be assured about proper endometrial receptivity due to how we manage minimal and mild stimulation cycles for patients with DOR and/or ARA. Therefore, implementing such stimulation approaches in DOR and/or ARA patients without having a successful embryo freezing and FET program is unconceivable.

12.2 Pretreatment Cycle Considerations

As we discussed in prior sections, we consider minimal stimulation when it is combined with an oral agent like an aromatase inhibitor or clomiphene citrate while starting the 150 IU of gonadotropin on day 5 of stimulation while dosing it as an every other day regimen. All other low-dose alternatives with 150 IU daily gonado-tropins are considered as mild stimulation.

Patients with DOR require a customized approach even with minimal stimula-tion. The aims in this population is to assure a follicle synchronization as much as possible before starting the stimulation. This type of cycle programming may not be reliably done with oral contraceptive pills (OCPs) which primarily suppress luteinizing hormone (LH), and the LH suppression may be profound, and at times long lasting as the treatment with OCPs is extended. It is already known that, in conventional GnRH antagonist IVF protocols, OCP pretreatment is associated with longer duration of stimulation and higher dose requirements for gonadotropins [1, 2]. Prolonged use of OCPs more than 5 weeks also decreases AMH levels, which is a reflection of arrest in follicle development [3]. Likewise, minimal stimulation protocols may not work well in the presence of hypothalamic dysfunction since the gonadotropin response to clomiphene citrate or aromatase inhibitor will be blunted.

Estradiol use especially during the luteal phase prior to starting stimulation has been found beneficial in POR patients [4–8]. Diminished ovarian reserve is associ-ated with early follicle selection with follicle asynchrony and short follicular phase with early ovulation. Luteal phase use of estradiol can decrease the inter-cycle increase of follicle-stimulating hormone (FSH), which in turn leads to follicle syn-chronization. Estradiol also increases the follicle granulosa cell FSH sensitivity. In return, luteal phase estradiol use results in lower FSH level in the beginning of the following cycle and avoids early and multiple follicle selections and assures a slower and more synchronous follicle growth during the stimulation [9–11]. Decreased pace of follicle growth with follicle synchronization may result in more competent oocytes for fertilization and follicle development.

Therefore, we use 17β-estradiol in the form of oral micronized estradiol at 4 mg daily dose during the luteal phase of prior cycle before starting minimal stimulation. In DOR patients, it is difficult to limit the start day of micronized estradiol strictly to cycle day 20 as reported by Fanchin et al. [11]. Especially, those with profound DOR and ARA at or over 40 years of age, the follicular phase may be very short, and in return, corpus luteum may not function as long as it is expected from a regu-lar natural cycle. Therefore, in such patients we start checking serum progesterone (P4) level on day 10–11 of a natural cycle. According to the first result, we deter-mine the day of the next serum P4 level. Eventually when serum P4 is at or above 3 ng/mL, patients are placed on oral micronized estradiol 4 mg daily. Patients call with the first day of their next menstrual period. Then the patients are scheduled to have a baseline ultrasound and at least one time blood work is recommended dur-ing the patient's first minimal stimulation cycle on the day of baseline ultrasound to have some understanding about how that particular patient responded to luteal phase estradiol treatment. Typically, serum E2, LH, and P4 levels are assessed. In general, follicle synchronization is mostly assured if the serum E2 level is at around 150 pg/mL. When E2 levels are below 100 pg/mL, early follicle selection and fol-licle asynchrony may still be a problem. Therefore, for the planning of another treat-ment cycle, oral micronized estradiol dose can be adjusted for each patient to reach the desired serum E2 level on the day of baseline sonogram. Variation of serum E2 levels among patients are due to the batch-to-batch variation of the generic medication used, the degree of liver metabolism of the micronized estradiol, and some differences may be associated with body mass index. Per patient customization of luteal phase priming is an essential element for preparation of a patient for a minimal stimulation.

A similar observation regarding the relationship between the serum E2 and FSH levels was also made by the group from Japan [12]. Their findings from the natural cycles suggested that the mean FSH level on day 3 of a natural cycle was 10.5 ± 2.1 IU/L, while the mean serum E2 was 69 ± 14 pg/mL. Then when the E2 level increased above 140 pg/mL, the mean FSH levels dropped below 8 IU/L, and FSH further reduced to 6 IU/L just before the LH surge. It was observed that the follicle growth from antral follicles for eventual dominant follicle growth might require FSH levels at or above 8 IU/L, and below that level either other growing follicles undergo apoptosis or no more new follicle growth could be noted. Our observation is almost similar that if serum E2 levels are maintained at around 150 pg/mL, antral follicle synchrony can often be assured.

With luteal phase estradiol priming, it is very rare to see suppressed LH levels below 2 IU/L. It is even possible to see little higher LH levels on baseline tests of >5 IU/L when the tests are performed on day 2 or 3 of the menstrual cycle, while the patients are still on micronized estradiol. This should not be surprising acknowledging the effects of chronic tonic elevation of estradiol on the hypothalamus and pituitary, which may be instrumental in enhancing LH synthesis and secretion [13–17]. Avoiding LH suppression in the beginning of the cycle is essential to assure appropriate response from hypothalamus acting agents like clomiphene citrate or aromatase inhibitor, letrozole.

Since minimal stimulation is recommended for multiple cycles for frozen embryo accumulation, in women who desire starting another minimal stimulation cycle right after their retrievals, oral micronized estradiol can be started about 3–4 days after the oocyte retrieval to prime the follicles for the next minimal stimulation IVF cycle.

12.2.1 Considerations if Treatment Cycle Scheduling Is Required

At times, readily proceeding with a minimal stimulation after luteal phase estradiol priming may not be feasible for the patient or for the practice. Many patients may have some work- or family-related events and travel but may still want to avoid postponing the treatment cycle. IVF laboratory may need a day or two of maintenance, or laboratory staff vacations may require short-term lab closures. In addition, some practices prefer to batch the IVF cycles throughout the certain weeks of the month for various reasons. In such cases, either prolongation of estrogen priming for few days or for a week or, if longer time is needed, then in patients without strict contraindications to OCPs, estradiol-OCP-estradiol conversion will provide the best results. OCPs suppress both FSH and LH levels. Short-term use of OCPs for about 2 weeks will not totally stall follicle development unlike the case when the OCPs are used more than 5 weeks, but again individual variation among women in terms of the OCPs' profound and sustained LH suppressive effects can still be observed even with short-term use. Therefore, micronized estradiol can be stopped with menses and OCPs can be started the same evening daily. Then after daily OCP use, while getting closer to stimulation cycle, OCPs are stopped and micronized estradiol at the patient specific dose is started. After at least 4 days of micronized estradiol use after stopping OCPs, a baseline transvaginal ultrasound and E2, LH levels can be checked to assure that LH is not suppressed below 2 IU/L and E2 levels are now about 150 pg/mL. If antral follicle count and follicle synchronicity are found satisfactory, then micronized estradiol is stopped, and the stimulation can be started as early as the day of discontinuing micronized estradiol or within 3 days of stopping the estradiol priming.

12.3   Starting Minimal Stimulation with Clomiphene Citrate

Clomiphene citrate (CC) was approved by the US Food and Drug Administration in 1967 with the indication of treatment of ovulatory dysfunction in women desiring pregnancy [18]. Clomiphene has become a very widely used fertility drug for many indications not only limited to chronic anovulation. The compound is a nonsteroidal triphenylethylene stilbene derivative (Fig. 12.1)

Clomiphene citrate is one of the selective estrogen receptor modulators (SERMs) with both agonistic and antagonistic activities for estrogen receptor. It is a racemic mixture of 62% enclomiphene (Cis-) and 38% zuclomiphene (trans-), the former considered to be the more potent isomere with much shorter half-life (about 24 hours) than zuclomiphene which is less potent, but its elimination from the body may take weeks after a single dose [19], although no clinical or ill effects from zuclomiphene accumulation over repetitive treatment cycles are anticipated [20–22].

Clomiphene use alone for ovulation induction was associated with delayed ovulation or luteinized unruptured follicle development. These issues have been associated with continued estrogen receptor antagonistic effects of enclomiphene

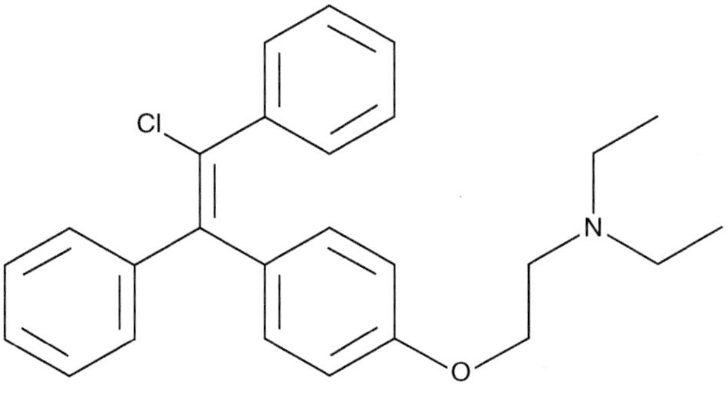

Fig. 12.1 (Creative common license tag by bing) clomiphene citrate

at the level of the hypothalamus, which can be mitigated by using human chorionic gonadotropin (HCG) or GnRH agonist to trigger ovulation or final oocyte maturation. If CC is used throughout the stimulation daily rather than limiting the duration solely to 5 days as the norm to induce ovulation in women with chronic anovulation due to polycystic ovary syndrome, then decreased estrogen sensitivity of the hypothalamus may lead to delay of LH surge while allowing for continued multiple follicle growths with continued endogenous FSH action on the ovary.

In one study, the prolonged use of CC at 100 mg daily dose for 15 days resulted in prolonged and continued increase in LH without any LH surge. With continued high levels of LH, some follicles may undergo luteinization without ovulation, which may become an issue. On the other hand, CC use at 100 mg daily dose for 5 days resulted in normal LH levels followed by LH surge [23]. This means that some washout period is required for enclomiphene for proper LH surge to occur. Actually, this effect of CC on LH can be exploited in minimal stimulation protocols for IVF in women with DOR and/or ARA [24].

The use of CC requires intact hypothalamic-pituitary function on the contrary to many conventional stimulation protocols for IVF, which largely rely on hypothalamic suppression with GnRH agonists or GnRH antagonists. Therefore, more physiological contributions of endogenous FSH and LH are ignored in conventional stimulation while relying on recombinant FSH, highly purified human menopausal gonadotropins (HMG) with more reliance on low-dose human chorionic gonadotropin (HCG) for LH activity support, especially in the United States where recombinant LH is not marketed currently. Therefore, conventional stimulation requires higher doses of gonadotropins. In that respect, the prolonged use of CC during a minimal stimulation protocol may result in more physiological stimulation of follicles with less reliance to commercial gonadotropin products. In terms of using gonadotropins, we also prefer alternate day dosing of highly purified HMG rather than the recombinant products.

The CC is started at 100 mg daily dose in minimal stimulation IVF for DOR and/or ARA, unlike using a lower-dose regimen in women with normal to high ovarian reserve who prefer minimal stimulation IVF. In such cases, typical daily dose of CC is 50 mg daily. Our reasoning of using higher doses in DOR and/or ARA patients is differential impact of LH between normal/high ovarian reserve cases and DOR and/or ARA cases. In general, higher LH levels during stimulation are not desirable in women with normal or high ovarian reserve. However, reverse is the case in women with DOR and/or ARA who are believed to be negatively affected from profound LH suppression. Hence, for normal responders, there is an impression that lower LH levels may be well tolerated or even can lead to better pregnancy outcomes [25, 26]. In women with expected POR, however, many conventional IVF stimulation protocols are based on the prevention of LH suppression with protocols like short agonist or micro-agonist dose flare protocols or focusing on appropriate LH activity support which seems to be beneficial in women with DOR and/or ARA [27–29].

12.4   Gonadotropin Co-treatment

Our gonadotropin of choice for minimal stimulation with CC is highly purified human menopausal gonadotropin (hp-HMG). Each vial of hp-HMG contains 75 IU of FSH and 75 IU of LH with some added HCG for additional LH activity support. Each 75 IU vial of hp-HMG contains about 10 IU of HCG [30]. After 4 days of daily CC, hp-HMG is added to CC on day 5 of stimulation and continued on every other day basis until the day of trigger for final oocyte maturation. This choice is based on some data showing beneficial effects of HCG addition to stimulation protocols to assure adequate LH activity support during the stimulation days that GnRH antagonist administration may be needed to prevent premature LH surge. Even with half dose of GnRH antagonist administration, profound LH suppression may be observed in some set of patients, which may result in plateauing E2 levels and slowing down of follicle growth. Theoretically, these unwanted effects may at least be partially mitigated by hp-HMG rather than recombinant FSH use. In conventional IVF stimulation protocols, the addition of HCG to recombinant FSH was found to be beneficial to achieve top-quality embryos [31].

12.5   Preventing Premature Luteinization

In DOR and/or ARA group, keeping the endogenous LH levels at an optimum level is of great importance. The upcoming section will review the control of LH in more detail. GnRH antagonists are mainly used to prevent LH surge during the minimal stimulation IVF cycles. GnRH antagonists promptly and reversibly suppress LH levels as can easily be detected shortly after GnRH antagonist administration due to the known short half-life of LH in the order of minutes [32]. Therefore, GnRH antagonist can be administered whenever it is needed if the serum LH levels are followed closely. The initial dose finding trials of one of the antagonists (ganirelix acetate) used in IVF stimulation protocols revealed that as the dose of daily antagonist increased, more profound suppression of LH was attained, while lower embryo implantation rates were observed. The optimal IVF outcomes were achieved by the 0.25 mg subcutaneous daily dose when it is used at a fixed dose starting on day 7 of stimulation as compared to the other higher dose regimens of 0.5 mg, 1 mg, and 2 mg [33]. As some studies have suggested, more intense dose regimens of GnRH antagonist may affect IVF outcomes at an adverse fashion, and GnRH antagonist may have some direct effects on the ovaries at granulosa cell level [34–36].

Considering the information as summarized above, we start monitoring E2 and LH levels as early as day 4 of stimulation in order to assess when GnRH antagonist would be required to prevent premature LH surge. Clomiphene citrate usually induces some LH flare in DOR and/or ARA patients, but again unless the level of LH is close to or above 10 IU/L while E2 levels are at or above 200 pg/mL, GnRH antagonist administration is not required. When needed, it is usually preferred at 1/2 of the suggested daily dose. Since the 0.25 mg cetrorelix acetate vial can be used in half doses without wasting the other half dose of the medication, we prefer cetrorelix acetate use. At least in the United States, ganirelix acetate is marketed in individual prefilled fixed needle syringes, and therefore with half dose use, the other half has to be wasted which will increase the cost of the treatment cycle for the patient.

12.6 Trigger for Final Oocyte Maturation

Once the E2 levels reach at or above 250 pg/mL, and the LH levels are maintained at less than 10 IU/L or more than 2 IU/L with appropriate administration of half dose cetrotide as needed, the E2 progression along with follicle growth rate is closely observed. The trigger agents are considered when the follicle sizes are between 16 and 20 mm in average diameters according to the patient factors and information obtained from the recent IVF cycles of some patients with such data available. Especially in profound DOR cases and DOR cases at or above 40 years of age, spontaneous follicle collapse shortly after trigger for final oocyte maturation can be a problem. In such cases if the leading follicle size is >18–19 mm, a nonsteroidal anti-inflammatory agent administration the day after trigger can be considered as we will discuss in another chapter.

Deciding on the leading size of the follicle to administer the trigger agent depends on many factors and highly customized for each patient. In women with ARA, at or above 43 years of age, it was recommended that the lead size of the follicles should be between 16 and 18 mm to minimize premature luteinization of granulosa cells in this population [37]. This was related to aging-induced aberration in proper proliferation of granulosa cells as they respond to high levels of FSH typically found in this patient population. Granulosa cell luteinization may be a reflection of the arrest in granulosa cell proliferation, one step away from apoptosis. This phenomenon may be associated with poor oocyte and embryo quality leading to lower pregnancy rates [38]. Although minimal stimulation is typically performed to avoid high levels of FSH and if the endogenous FSH is found high, resorting to other mild stimulation approaches is considered; with staggering E2 progression while noticing mildly elevated levels of progesterone with normal (<10 IU/L) LH levels, we do consider triggering between 16 and 18 mm size of the leading follicle if there are no other growing follicles below 16 mm. Otherwise, we can still proceed with trigger with a lead follicle size of 19–20 mm. We document the follicle sizes corresponding to oocyte yield in patients to assist with future trigger decisions for their subsequent minimal stimulation cycles.

For trigger agents, GnRH agonist and/or HCG can be considered. We typically consider GnRH agonist-only trigger as a single 2 mg subcutaneous dose of leuprolide acetate in cases when we plan a luteal phase mild stimulation shortly after oocyte retrieval following minimal stimulation. This is to avoid the lingering high

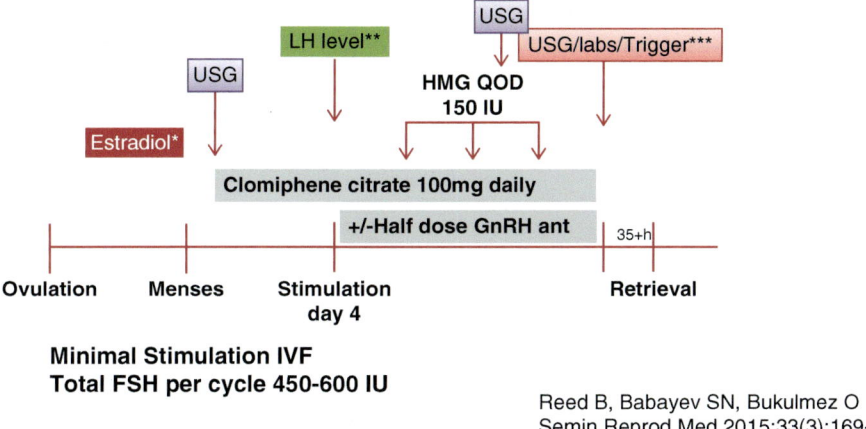

Fig. 12.2   Minimal stimulation protocol with clomiphene citrate

serum levels of HCG when it is administered at 10,000 IU due to concerns of premature luteinization of growing follicles exposed to HCG levels >10 IU/L. Otherwise, final oocyte maturation can be triggered with single s.c. dose of 10,000 IU of HCG. Oocyte retrieval is typically scheduled 35 or 35.5 hours after the trigger. Typical minimal stimulation IVF protocol with CC is depicted in Fig. 12.2.

12.7   Considerations for Oocyte Retrieval, Fertilization, and Embryo Freezing

Since still the number of oocytes is an important parameter for the number of embryos developed for future frozen embryo transfers, the method used for oocyte retrieval is important. All retrievals are performed under general anesthesia without intubation. We will have another section on oocyte retrieval in minimal and mild stimulation protocols for DOR and/or ARA patients. Briefly, we use 17G single lumen oocyte retrieval needle with the tubing extending toward the collection or sampling tube (K-OSN-1735-B-90-US, Cook Medical, Brisbane, Australia). We attach the tubing to the Rocket Craft R29655 suction pump (Rocket Medical plc, Washington, Tyne &Wear, NE38 9BZ, England). We keep the pressure at around 120 mm Hg never to exceed 180 mm Hg. The single lumen needle can also be used to flush the follicles by using the opening within the silicone rubber cork of the sampling tube by injecting warmed sterile media flush toward the needle with a 10 cc syringe while minimizing air within the tubing.

Follicle flush has been debated over several decades. The systematic review of five randomized controlled trials comparing follicular flushing to aspiration only in general IVF population suggested comparable number of oocytes and the clinical pregnancy and live birth rates (only one trial reported) between the groups. As expected, the duration of the oocyte retrieval is prolonged with flushing [39]. The quality of evidence was admitted to be moderate, and the results may show some imprecision per authors. Another recent Cochrane review also reported similar results from ten studies in general IVF population [40]. One study involving only minimal stimulation IVF cycles for women with POR demonstrated that, with only follicle aspiration alone, the oocyte recovery rate could be 46.8%, while with follicular flushing this rate may be increased to 84.6%. The same study even suggested that the oocytes retrieved with follicular flushing result in a better morphology and implantation rates than the oocytes readily recovered with first attempt of aspiration without flushing [41]. Consideration for follicular flushing is an essential element of minimal/mild stimulation and natural cycle approaches for DOR and/or ARA patients who typically present with limited number of follicles.

There will be a discussion in the upcoming chapters that the fertilization method for the oocytes, conventional insemination versus intracytoplasmic sperm injection (ICSI), should carefully be thought over. Although there is a tendency to use ICSI for the majority of ART cycles, conventional IVF may actually be considered in many women with DOR and/or ARA due to many physiological differences between these two fertilization methods [42].

Then the stage of the embryo considered for cryopreservation also depends on many factors. The information obtained from multiple minimal stimulation cycles, whether preimplantation testing for aneuploidy is desired or not, are important components of decision-making. Minimal stimulation approach for women with DOR requires accumulation of either day 3 or day 5/6 stage frozen embryos in appropriate grade for their stage to maximize success in their future frozen-thawed embryo transfer (FET) cycles. Frozen embryo transfer preparation should not be taken lightly as well. In patients with reliable menstrual cycles, natural cycle preparation can be considered especially if they show erratic response or compliance issues with oral or transdermal estradiol preparations that we will review in another chapter.

12.8   Aromatase Inhibitor Use for Minimal Stimulation

Letrozole is an oral aromatase inhibitor. Letrozole, by inhibiting conversion of androgens to estrogens by follicular granulosa cells and showing the same effects in the brain, will lead to increased gonadotropin release via a central mechanism somewhat similar to clomiphene citrate. Letrozole has a shorter half-life (about 45 hours) than CC, and it does not deplete estrogen receptors unlike CC. Letrozole may also have some proposed benefits in increasing FSH sensitivity while promoting early follicular growth due to increase in intraovarian androgens [43].

Letrozole use for ovulation induction and controlled ovarian stimulation had been impacted negatively by an abstract reporting increased risk of especially locomotor and cardiac defects in the babies conceived via letrozole or letrozole with gonadotropins [44]. Although various larger and better designed studies did not confirm any such findings, letrozole use in ovulation induction or other ovarian stimulation protocols stayed off-label. Recently, after critical analysis of studies based on letrozole use in ovulation induction for women with polycystic ovary syndrome (PCOS), the American College of Obstetricians and Gynecologists affirmed that letrozole, rather than CC, should be the first-line therapy for ovulation induction due to the increased live birth rate when compared to CC, also considering the recent safety data on letrozole [45].

Aromatase inhibitors like letrozole has been used in some conventional stimulation protocols for IVF to enhance cycle outcomes in women with expected poor ovarian response (POR). These studies involved using 5 days of letrozole in the beginning of stimulation for 5 days along with a high-dose gonadotropin protocols. These studies suggested some partial benefits of letrozole addition to gonadotropins as compared to those not using letrozole or those using GnRH agonist microdose flare protocol [46, 47]. A recent Cochrane review analyzed if letrozole or CC use with or without gonadotropins makes any difference in IVF outcome. Most of the studies included in this review actually included poor responders, and many were about letrozole co-treatment in this patient population. In general IVF patient population, live births or clinical pregnancy rates did not significantly change with letrozole or CC use with or without gonadotropins as compared to gonadotropin use with GnRH analogs. The addition of these oral agents though was associated with decreased risk of ovarian hyperstimulation syndrome. In poor responders, the conclusions on live births and clinical pregnancy rates did not change in terms of CC or letrozole use with or without gonadotropins versus gonadotropins with GnRH analogs. There was a moderate quality of evidence that co-treatment with CC or letrozole might decrease the mean gonadotropin dose. However, their use with gonadotropins may be associated with the increased cycle cancellation rate and decreased number of oocytes retrieved in both general IVF population and in women with POR [48].

The context of letrozole use is different from its use in conventional stimulation protocols where letrozole use is limited to 5 days with the daily doses ranging from 2.5 to 5 mg mostly with the intention of proceeding with fresh embryo transfer. It is known that further increase in daily dose of letrozole higher than 7.5 mg may result in thin endometrial lining as observed in CC [45, 49]. Also within the context of superovulation with intrauterine insemination for unexplained infertility, letrozole showed lower clinical pregnancy and live birth rates than CC and gonadotropins alone, although multiple gestation rates between letrozole and CC were comparable [50]. The authors suggested some potential mechanisms for such differences including the differential effects of letrozole on the endometrium, ovary, and central nervous system different from those with CC in unexplained infertility patients.

Letrozole use in minimal stimulation is similar to CC use. It is prescribed for everyday use at daily doses between 2.5 to 5 mg, while adding hMG 150 IU every other day on day 5 of stimulation. The use of letrozole daily until the day of triggering for final oocyte maturation during controlled ovarian stimulation is not a new concept and has been implemented in patients with estrogen receptor-positive breast cancer undergoing embryo or oocyte freezing cycles [51]. Using daily letrozole at 5 mg daily dose along with daily gonadotropin doses ranging from 150 to 300 IU resulted in much lower peak estradiol levels with decreased gonadotropin dose requirements as compared to historical controls with tubal factor infertility who underwent conventional IVF stimulation without daily letrozole, while keeping the fertilization and embryo development rates comparable if the letrozole arm is triggered with a leading follicle size of ≥ 20 mm rather than with the follicle size of ≥ 17–18 mm [52]. The reason for this increased diameter threshold for letrozole-treated cycles is the perception of decreased oocyte maturity rate. Even using this threshold, a compromised oocyte maturation with daily letrozole use was reported, and some authors demonstrated decreased fertilization rates and increased gonadotropin requirements with letrozole co-treatment in breast cancer patients as compared to age-matched infertile controls [53, 54]. One retrospective cohort multicenter study from Italy compared the oocyte cryopreservation outcomes between estrogen receptor-positive and estrogen receptor-negative breast cancer patients. Those with estrogen receptor-positive tumors received letrozole co-treatment with gonadotropins and demonstrated significantly decreased mean number of oocytes than the estrogen receptor-negative group treated only with gonadotropins. Letrozole co-treatment arm showed lower gonadotropin requirements to achieve the same number of developing follicles as the patients only treated with gonadotropins, while ending up with lower peak levels of estradiol. The authors argued whether scientific evidence was there to use letrozole co-treatment in estrogen receptor-positive breast cancer patients since mature oocyte yield may be 40% lower with letrozole co-treatment [55]. Certainly, there may be many biases in each of these retrospective reports, and the stimulation response may be different per estrogen receptor status and in breast cancer patients in general as compared to those with infertility [56].

Within the context of mild stimulation, most studies used letrozole in a classic 5-day course combined with daily gonadotropins at 150 IU daily. A retrospective study compared outcomes of mild stimulation protocol with 5-day courses of either letrozole 5 mg daily or CC 25 mg daily combined with HMG commenced at 75–150 IU daily dose started on day 3 of letrozole or CC treatment [57]. Pretreatment programming was made by using oral contraceptives. Patients with DOR were encouraged to try these protocols, and those with high ovarian reserve were excluded. Ovulation trigger was achieved with hCG 10,000 IU when the lead follicle was ≥ 17 mm, and the oocyte retrieval was performed 34 hours after. All follicles at or above 12 mm were accessed, and all follicles at or above 14 mm in size were flushed multiple times. Peak mean E2 level was significantly lower in the letrozole-treated group as compared to those treated with CC (516 versus 797 ng/mL). CC group produced significantly more mature oocytes (3.3 versus 2.4). All embryo transfers were performed on the third day after oocyte retrieval. CC co-treated group resulted in more mean number of embryos transferred than the letrozole arm (2.5 vs 1.5). Endometrial thicknesses between the groups were comparable. Live birth rates per embryo transfer were also comparable between letrozole (17.7%) and CC co-treated (21.4%) groups. Therefore, letrozole and CC co-treatment seemed to have comparable live birth outcomes with fresh transfers. Again the immature oocyte yield was higher in the letrozole arm [57].

With the daily use of letrozole, estradiol monitoring is less reliable, and at times due to low E2 levels, LH surge may not be observed, and low-dose GnRH antagonist may be required somewhat less frequently. However, continuous letrozole use may have less LH flare effects than CC, which may not work for some DOR and/or ARA patients. We prefer CC primarily for minimal stimulation for DOR and/or ARA patients. Letrozole is considered in women who cannot tolerate CC, who may have activation risk for an autoimmune or inflammatory condition with CC or those with history for estrogen receptor-positive breast cancer. In patients who did not have satisfactory outcomes with minimal stimulation using CC rather than switching to letrozole, we recommend other mild stimulation alternatives, like luteal phase mild stimulation. We still recommend freezing all the embryos for minimal stimulation with daily letrozole due to the frequent observation of thin and non-trilaminar endometrial stripe pattern with the letrozole protocol.

12.9   Costs of Minimal Stimulation Versus Conventional High-Dose FSH Protocols for Diminished Ovarian Reserve Patients

The typical minimal stimulation protocol was reviewed in detail above. If we attempt conventional high-dose FSH treatment, our protocol of choice is estradiol priming GnRH antagonist protocol as depicted in Fig. 12.3, which is also mentioned in Chap. 8. In this protocol, the stimulation is started with recombinant gonadotropin

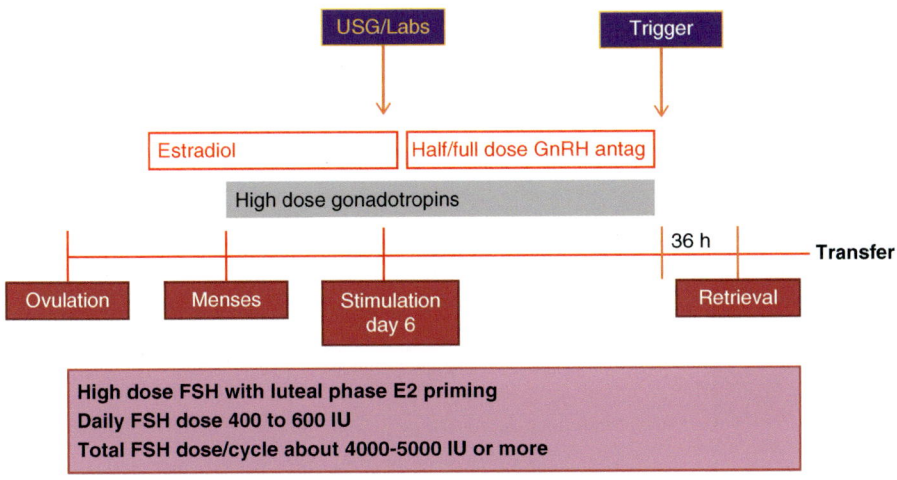

Fig. 12.3 Estradiol priming GnRH antagonist high-dose FSH protocol

at ≥300 IU daily, and this is combined with hp-HMG 150 IU or more with the commencing of daily GnRH antagonist.

Although many see the disadvantage of minimal stimulation for frozen embryo accumulation as being a longer process than the high-dose FSH protocols mostly with fresh embryo transfers, they also quote the impression of a higher cost for multiple cycles with an added cost of frozen-thawed embryo transfers. We will calculate the cost of one conventional high-dose stimulation IVF cycle with fresh embryo transfer and the combined costs of three minimal stimulation IVF cycles with one frozen-thawed embryo transfer (FET) cycle. The treatment cycle charges for our self-paying patients and the cost of the fertility medications as checked in July of 2018 were considered. The costs may be much lower in other practices or in other countries and may even be much lower in patients with insurance coverage. We summarized the cost calculation as given in Table 12.1.

Minimal stimulation IVF full 10 days of stimulation with purified HMG and HCG trigger costs:

- Drug cost: $30 + 509.94 + 263.98 + 99.9 = $903.82
- Per cycle cost including anesthesia for egg retrieval: $3800 ($600 for anesthesia)
- Total per cycle cost of minimal stimulation IVF: *$4703.82*
- High-dose FSH protocol with daily dose of 300 IU follitropin-α or follitropin-β with daily 150 IU purified HMG for full 10 days with 5-day course of antagonist with HCG trigger costs
- Drug cost: 1680 + 1699 + 649.35 + 99.9 = *$4128.25* (with follitropin-β: add ($2919–$1680=) *$1239*; becomes *$5367.25*)
- IVF with ICSI with embryo transfer and embryo freezing = $9030 ($600 for anesthesia)

Total per cycle cost of conventional high-dose FSH stimulation IVF:

- With follitropin-α = *$13,158.25*
- With follitropin-β = *$14,397.25*

Table 12.1 Approximate fertility medication costs as calculated in July 2018 in the United States

Medication	Price (USD)
Clomiphene citrate 50 mg tablet	1.5
Purified HMG 75 IU vial	84.99
Recombinant FSH 300 IU cartridge Follitropin-β	291.90
Recombinant FSH 300 IU cartridge Follitropin-α	168.00
Cetrorelix acetate 250 mcg	131.99
Ganirelix acetate 250 mcg prefilled syringe	129.87
HCG 10,000 IU vial	99.90
Progesterone in sesame oil 50 mg/mL vial	49.90
Micronized estradiol 2 mg 30 tablets	20.00

The total cost of 3 cycles of minimal stimulation plus 1 cycle of frozen-thawed embryo transfer:

- (3×$4703.82) + $2625 = <u>$16,736.46</u>

In summary there may be about $2000–$3000 higher cost for three consecutive minimal stimulation IVF cycles and one frozen embryo transfer cycle as compared to one cycle of high-dose FSH protocol with fresh embryo transfer. Good bulk of the cost difference is due to the charges for general anesthesia/deep sedation used during each oocyte retrieval. Some programs may also charge less for frozen embryo cycles. At least, by using local anesthesia and mild sedation, these costs can be decreased. However, the remaining cost difference, we believe, will be offset by higher pregnancy rates per embryo transfer in minimal stimulation IVF treatment as compared to high-dose FSH stimulation in patients with POR, DOR, and/or ARA.

12.10   Conclusion

Minimal stimulation protocol that we describe in this chapter is comprised of daily CC at 100 mg dose combined with hp-HMG 150 IU every other day added to CC on day 5 of stimulation. Half-dose antagonist cetrorelix acetate is administered only when decided by close monitoring of E2, LH, and P4 levels. Minimal stimulation is started after follicle synchronization is assured by using micronized estradiol orally at 4 mg daily dose during the luteal phase of the prior cycle. In some patients, letrozole can be used instead of CC; however, letrozole is not considered as an alternative to CC when the patients do not respond well to minimal stimulation with CC. Individualized decisions are required per each patient about when and how to trigger patients for final oocyte maturation. Minimal stimulation approach for women with DOR requires accumulation of either day 3 or day 5/6 stage frozen embryos in appropriate grade for their stage. The cost of three minimal stimulation IVF cycles plus one FET cycle can be close to one conventional high-dose FSH cycle with fresh embryos transfer.

References

1. Kolibianakis EM, Papanikolaou EG, Camus M, Tournaye H, Van Steirteghem AC, Devroey P. Effect of oral contraceptive pill pretreatment on ongoing pregnancy rates in patients stimulated with GnRH antagonists and recombinant FSH for IVF. A randomized controlled trial. Hum Reprod. 2006;21(2):352–7.
2. Pinkas H, Sapir O, Avrech OM, Ben-Haroush A, Ashkenzi J, Fisch B, et al. The effect of oral contraceptive pill for cycle scheduling prior to GnRH-antagonist protocol on IVF cycle parameters and pregnancy outcome. J Assist Reprod Genet. 2008;25(1):29–33.

3. Kallio S, Puurunen J, Ruokonen A, Vaskivuo T, Piltonen T, Tapanainen JS. Antimullerian hormone levels decrease in women using combined contraception independently of administration route. Fertil Steril. 2013;99(5):1305–10.
4. Chang EM, Han JE, Won HJ, Kim YS, Yoon TK, Lee WS. Effect of estrogen priming through luteal phase and stimulation phase in poor responders in in-vitro fertilization. J Assist Reprod Genet. 2012;29(3):225–30.
5. Fisch JD, Keskintepe L, Sher G. Gonadotropin-releasing hormone agonist/antagonist conversion with estrogen priming in low responders with prior in vitro fertilization failure. Fertil Steril. 2008;89(2):342–7.
6. Frattarelli JL, Hill MJ, McWilliams GD, Miller KA, Bergh PA, Scott RT Jr. A luteal estradiol protocol for expected poor-responders improves embryo number and quality. Fertil Steril. 2008;89(5):1118–22.
7. Hill MJ, McWilliams GD, Miller KA, Scott RT Jr, Frattarelli JL. A luteal estradiol protocol for anticipated poor-responder patients may improve delivery rates. Fertil Steril. 2009;91(3):739–43.
8. Lee H, Choi HJ, Yang KM, Kim MJ, Cha SH, Yi HJ. Efficacy of luteal estrogen administration and an early follicular Gonadotropin-releasing hormone antagonist priming protocol in poor responders undergoing in vitro fertilization. Obstet Gynecol Sci. 2018;61(1):102–10.
9. Fanchin R, Cunha-Filho JS, Schonauer LM, Kadoch IJ, Cohen-Bacri P, Frydman R. Coordination of early antral follicles by luteal estradiol administration provides a basis for alternative controlled ovarian hyperstimulation regimens. Fertil Steril. 2003;79(2):316–21.
10. Fanchin R, Cunha-Filho JS, Schonauer LM, Righini C, de Ziegler D, Frydman R. Luteal estradiol administration strengthens the relationship between day 3 follicle-stimulating hormone and inhibin B levels and ovarian follicular status. Fertil Steril. 2003;79(3):585–9.
11. Fanchin R, Salomon L, Castelo-Branco A, Olivennes F, Frydman N, Frydman R. Luteal estradiol pre-treatment coordinates follicular growth during controlled ovarian hyperstimulation with GnRH antagonists. Hum Reprod. 2003;18(12):2698–703.
12. Teramoto S. Clomiphene citrate for IVF. In: Chavez-Badiola A, Allahbadia GN, editors. Textbook of minimal stimulation IVF – milder, mildest or back to nature. 1st ed. New Delhi: Jaypee Brothers Medical Publishers; 2011. p. 37–43.
13. Marut EL, Williams RF, Cowan BD, Lynch A, Lerner SP, Hodgen GD. Pulsatile pituitary gonadotropin secretion during maturation of the dominant follicle in monkeys: estrogen positive feedback enhances the biological activity of LH. Endocrinology. 1981;109(6):2270–2.
14. Quyyumi SA, Pinkerton JV, Evans WS, Veldhuis JD. Estradiol amplifies the amount of luteinizing hormone (LH) secreted in response to increasing doses of gonadotropin-releasing hormone by specifically augmenting the duration of evoked LH secretory events and hence their mass. J Clin Endocrinol Metab. 1993;76(3):594–600.
15. Urban RJ, Veldhuis JD, Dufau ML. Estrogen regulates the gonadotropin-releasing hormone-stimulated secretion of biologically active luteinizing hormone. J Clin Endocrinol Metab. 1991;72(3):660–8.
16. Veldhuis JD, Beitins IZ, Johnson ML, Serabian MA, Dufau ML. Biologically active luteinizing hormone is secreted in episodic pulsations that vary in relation to stage of the menstrual cycle. J Clin Endocrinol Metab. 1984;58(6):1050–8.
17. Veldhuis JD, Rogol AD, Perez-Palacios G, Stumpf P, Kitchin JD, Dufau ML. Endogenous opiates participate in the regulation of pulsatile luteinizing hormone release in an unopposed estrogen milieu: studies in estrogen-replaced, gonadectomized patients with testicular feminization. J Clin Endocrinol Metab. 1985;61(4):790–3.
18. Dickey RP, Holtkamp DE. Development, pharmacology and clinical experience with clomiphene citrate. Hum Reprod Update. 1996;2(6):483–506.
19. Ghobadi C, Mirhosseini N, Shiran MR, Moghadamnia A, Lennard MS, Ledger WL, et al. Single-dose pharmacokinetic study of clomiphene citrate isomers in anovular patients with polycystic ovary disease. J Clin Pharmacol. 2009;49(2):147–54.

20. Ernst S, Hite G, Cantrell JS, Richardson A Jr, Benson HD. Stereochemistry of geometric isomers of clomiphene: a correction of the literature and a reexamination of structure-activity relationships. J Pharm Sci. 1976;65(1):148–50.
21. Mikkelson TJ, Kroboth PD, Cameron WJ, Dittert LW, Chungi V, Manberg PJ. Single-dose pharmacokinetics of clomiphene citrate in normal volunteers. Fertil Steril. 1986;46(3):392–6.
22. Young SL, Opsahl MS, Fritz MA. Serum concentrations of enclomiphene and zuclomiphene across consecutive cycles of clomiphene citrate therapy in anovulatory infertile women. Fertil Steril. 1999;71(4):639–44.
23. Messinis IE, Templeton A. Blockage of the positive feedback effect of oestradiol during prolonged administration of clomiphene citrate to normal women. Clin Endocrinol (Oxf). 1988;29(5):509–16.
24. Teramoto S, Kato O. Minimal ovarian stimulation with clomiphene citrate: a large-scale retrospective study. Reprod Biomed Online. 2007;15(2):134–48.
25. Kolibianakis EM, Zikopoulos K, Schiettecatte J, Smitz J, Tournaye H, Camus M, et al. Profound LH suppression after GnRH antagonist administration is associated with a significantly higher ongoing pregnancy rate in IVF. Hum Reprod. 2004;19(11):2490–6.
26. Orvieto R, Meltcer S, Liberty G, Rabinson J, Anteby EY, Nahum R. Does day-3 LH/FSH ratio influence in vitro fertilization outcome in PCOS patients undergoing controlled ovarian hyperstimulation with different GnRH-analogue? Gynecol Endocrinol. 2012;28(6):422–4.
27. Lehert P, Kolibianakis EM, Venetis CA, Schertz J, Saunders H, Arriagada P, et al. Recombinant human follicle-stimulating hormone (r-hFSH) plus recombinant luteinizing hormone versus r-hFSH alone for ovarian stimulation during assisted reproductive technology: systematic review and meta-analysis. Reprod Biol Endocrinol. 2014;12:17.
28. Hill MJ, Levens ED, Levy G, Ryan ME, Csokmay JM, DeCherney AH, et al. The use of recombinant luteinizing hormone in patients undergoing assisted reproductive techniques with advanced reproductive age: a systematic review and meta-analysis. Fertil Steril. 2012;97(5):1108–14.e1.
29. Mak SM, Wong WY, Chung HS, Chung PW, Kong GW, Li TC, et al. Effect of mid-follicular phase recombinant LH versus urinary HCG supplementation in poor ovarian responders undergoing IVF – a prospective double-blinded randomized study. Reprod Biomed Online. 2017;34(3):258–66.
30. Wolfenson C, Groisman J, Couto AS, Hedenfalk M, Cortvrindt RG, Smitz JE, et al. Batch-to-batch consistency of human-derived gonadotrophin preparations compared with recombinant preparations. Reprod Biomed Online. 2005;10(4):442–54.
31. Thuesen LL, Loft A, Egeberg AN, Smitz J, Petersen JH. Andersen AN. A randomized controlled dose-response pilot study of addition of hCG to recombinant FSH during controlled ovarian stimulation for in vitro fertilization. Hum Reprod. 2012;27(10):3074–84.
32. Choi J, Smitz J. Luteinizing hormone and human chorionic gonadotropin: origins of difference. Mol Cell Endocrinol. 2014;383(1–2):203–13.
33. A double-blind, randomized, dose-finding study to assess the efficacy of the gonadotrophin-releasing hormone antagonist ganirelix (Org 37462) to prevent premature luteinizing hormone surges in women undergoing ovarian stimulation with recombinant follicle stimulating hormone (Puregon). The ganirelix dose-finding study group. Hum Reprod 1998;13(11):3023–31.
34. Bukulmez O, Rehman KS, Langley M, Carr BR, Nackley AC, Doody KM, et al. Precycle administration of GnRH antagonist and microdose HCG decreases clinical pregnancy rates without affecting embryo quality and blastulation. Reprod Biomed Online. 2006;13(4):465–75.
35. Winkler N, Bukulmez O, Hardy DB, Carr BR. Gonadotropin releasing hormone antagonists suppress aromatase and anti-Mullerian hormone expression in human granulosa cells. Fertil Steril. 2010;94(5):1832–9.
36. Tan O, Carr BR, Beshay VE, Bukulmez O. The extrapituitary effects of GnRH antagonists and their potential clinical implications: a narrated review. Reprod Sci. 2013;20(1):16–25.

37. Wu YG, Barad DH, Kushnir VA, Wang Q, Zhang L, Darmon SK, et al. With low ovarian reserve, Highly Individualized Egg Retrieval (HIER) improves IVF results by avoiding premature luteinization. J Ovarian Res. 2018;11(1):23.
38. Wu YG, Barad DH, Kushnir VA, Lazzaroni E, Wang Q, Albertini DF, et al. Aging-related premature luteinization of granulosa cells is avoided by early oocyte retrieval. J Endocrinol. 2015;226(3):167–80.
39. Roque M, Sampaio M, Geber S. Follicular flushing during oocyte retrieval: a systematic review and meta-analysis. J Assist Reprod Genet. 2012;29(11):1249–54.
40. Georgiou EX, Melo P, Brown J, Granne IE. Follicular flushing during oocyte retrieval in assisted reproductive techniques. Cochrane Database Syst Rev. 2018;(4):CD004634.
41. Mendez Lozano DH, Brum Scheffer J, Frydman N, Fay S, Fanchin R, Frydman R. Optimal reproductive competence of oocytes retrieved through follicular flushing in minimal stimulation IVF. Reprod Biomed Online. 2008;16(1):119–23.
42. Babayev SN, Park CW, Bukulmez O. Intracytoplasmic sperm injection indications: how rigorous? Semin Reprod Med. 2014;32(4):283–90.
43. Mitwally MF, Casper RF. Aromatase inhibition improves ovarian response to follicle-stimulating hormone in poor responders. Fertil Steril. 2002;77(4):776–80.
44. Biljan MM, Hemmings R, Brassard N. The outcome of 150 babies following the treatment with letrozole or letrozole and gonadotropins. Fertil Steril. 2005;84(Suppl 1):S95.
45. ACOG Practice Bulletin No. 194: polycystic ovary syndrome. Obstet Gynecol 2018;131(6):e157–e171.
46. Ozmen B, Sonmezer M, Atabekoglu CS, Olmus H. Use of aromatase inhibitors in poor-responder patients receiving GnRH antagonist protocols. Reprod Biomed Online. 2009;19(4):478–85.
47. Yarali H, Esinler I, Polat M, Bozdag G, Tiras B. Antagonist/letrozole protocol in poor ovarian responders for intracytoplasmic sperm injection: a comparative study with the microdose flare-up protocol. Fertil Steril. 2009;92(1):231–5.
48. Kamath MS, Maheshwari A, Bhattacharya S, Lor KY, Gibreel A. Oral medications including clomiphene citrate or aromatase inhibitors with gonadotropins for controlled ovarian stimulation in women undergoing in vitro fertilisation. Cochrane Database Syst Rev. 2017;(11):CD008528.
49. Al-Fozan H, Al-Khadouri M, Tan SL, Tulandi T. A randomized trial of letrozole versus clomiphene citrate in women undergoing superovulation. Fertil Steril. 2004;82(6):1561–3.
50. Diamond MP, Legro RS, Coutifaris C, Alvero R, Robinson RD, Casson P, et al. Letrozole, gonadotropin, or clomiphene for unexplained infertility. N Engl J Med. 2015;373(13):1230–40.
51. Oktay K, Buyuk E, Libertella N, Akar M, Rosenwaks Z. Fertility preservation in breast cancer patients: a prospective controlled comparison of ovarian stimulation with tamoxifen and letrozole for embryo cryopreservation. J Clin Oncol. 2005;23(19):4347–53.
52. Oktay K, Hourvitz A, Sahin G, Oktem O, Safro B, Cil A, et al. Letrozole reduces estrogen and gonadotropin exposure in women with breast cancer undergoing ovarian stimulation before chemotherapy. J Clin Endocrinol Metab. 2006;91(10):3885–90.
53. Johnson LN, Dillon KE, Sammel MD, Efymow BL, Mainigi MA, Dokras A, et al. Response to ovarian stimulation in patients facing gonadotoxic therapy. Reprod Biomed Online. 2013;26(4):337–44.
54. Kim JH, Kim SK, Lee HJ, Lee JR, Jee BC, Suh CS, et al. Efficacy of random-start controlled ovarian stimulation in cancer patients. J Korean Med Sci. 2015;30(3):290–5.
55. Revelli A, Porcu E, Levi Setti PE, Delle Piane L, Merlo DF, Anserini P. Is letrozole needed for controlled ovarian stimulation in patients with estrogen receptor-positive breast cancer? Gynecol Endocrinol. 2013;29(11):993–6.
56. Shapira M, Raanani H, Meirow D. IVF for fertility preservation in breast cancer patients-efficacy and safety issues. J Assist Reprod Genet. 2015;32(8):1171–8.
57. Rose BI, Laky DC, Rose SD. A comparison of the use of clomiphene citrate and letrozole in patients undergoing IVF with the objective of producing only one or two embryos. Facts Views Vis Obgyn. 2015;7(2):119–26.

Chapter 13
Mild Stimulation Alternatives to Minimal Stimulation

Orhan Bukulmez

13.1 Luteal Phase Mild Stimulation to Mitigate High LH and FSH Levels

Although minimal stimulation has many advantages both financially and physiologically, some patients with diminished ovarian reserve (DOR) and/or advanced reproductive age (ARA) require other mild stimulation alternatives. The intention will still be to freeze all embryos for future frozen-thawed embryo transfer. During minimal stimulation, some patients may show high luteinizing hormone (LH) levels between 8 and 12 IU/L. If this occurs after first 3 days of clomiphene citrate use, while estradiol (E2) level is still less than100 pg/mL, we just watch E2 and LH progression over the next few days. Some patients may benefit from LH flare early in the stimulation phase. With continued stimulation, some of such patients may show sustained increase in their LH levels exceeding 10 IU/L although their E2 levels increase above 200 pg/mL while having follicles >12 mm in diameters, requiring gonadotropin-releasing hormone (GnRH) antagonist administration to prevent further LH increase or surge.

Per the classic knowledge, follicle-stimulating hormone (FSH) receptor is exclusively expressed on the granulosa cells, and LH receptor is constitutively expressed on theca and interstitial cells of the ovary [1]. During the follicular growth, however, granulosa cells start expressing LH receptors as well with various effects on cell proliferation and steroid hormone production [2, 3]. During controlled ovarian stimulation protocols, flexible GnRH antagonist protocol assumes that the rising LH would have more detrimental effects in terms of premature luteinization when the follicle

O. Bukulmez (✉)
Division of Reproductive Endocrinology and Infertility, Fertility and Advanced Reproductive Medicine Assisted Reproductive Technologies Program, Department of Obstetrics and Gynecology, University of Texas Southwestern Medical Center, Dallas, TX, USA
e-mail: Orhan.Bukulmez@UTSouthwestern.edu

© Springer Nature Switzerland AG 2020
O. Bukulmez (ed.), *Diminished Ovarian Reserve and Assisted Reproductive Technologies*, https://doi.org/10.1007/978-3-030-23235-1_13

size reaches >13 mm, and this should be the time that GnRH antagonist should be administered [4, 5]. Earlier data have suggested that a weak LH receptor expression in granulosa cells can be observed when the follicles are between 12 and 15 mm in diameter. Then the expression increases in preovulatory follicles between 18 and 22 mm to moderate levels with strong expression noted on corpus luteum [2]. A more recent study has reported that the highest LH expression is observed in follicles just before ovulation. However, low levels of LH receptor expression is still noted in antral follicles at or above the diameter of 5 mm [6]. In some women with DOR and ARA, we noted luteinization of follicles between 7 and 11 mm with the LH levels between 10 and 15 IU/L, which was marked by increased progesterone (P4) levels above 2 ng/mL with stalled and degenerating follicles. Using GnRH antagonist suppression frequently and at full doses, in such cases on the other hand, would counteract the desired effects of clomiphene citrate and may lead to undesirable direct effects of GnRH antagonists on follicle development [7]. It would also be difficult to maintain endogenous LH to the level that supports follicle growth with appropriate E2 progression. These women may rather benefit from one of the mild stimulation protocols.

During minimal stimulation, in some women, high LH levels above 10 IU/L is associated with low E2 levels below 75 pg/mL which may just be the reflection of high FSH levels >20 IU/L. In such profound DOR cases almost within the spectrum of premature ovarian insufficiency (POI), since the ovaries are already under the influence of FSH levels encountered in high-dose FSH stimulation protocols, it would be somewhat pointless to continue with the minimal stimulation. In such women, it would be best to stop the treatment and monitor the patient if in fact the patient has spontaneous ovulation on her own with P4 elevation. Such patients can be advised for luteal phase mild stimulation.

In DOR and/or ARA patients with suboptimal oocyte or frozen embryo outcome after minimal stimulation, we can also proceed with one of the mild stimulation protocols, which may again help control high LH combined with high endogenous FSH levels.

13.2   Luteal Phase Stimulation: Does It Lead to Competent Embryos?

Random start ovarian stimulation protocols in fertility preservation cycles before chemotherapy and/or radiation suggested that satisfactory number of oocytes and embryos can be obtained [8]. Due to multiple waves of follicle development on any day of natural cycle, ovarian stimulation can be started on any day of the menstrual cycle with comparable outcomes [9]. Even double stimulation, meaning, stimulation in both follicular and luteal phases of the same menstrual cycle, can be considered to maximize competent oocyte yield when oocyte or embryo cryopreservation is the main aim of the treatment [10].

In a prospective observational study, patients with DOR defined with AMH level of ≤1.5 ng/mL, antral follicle count of ≤6 and/or ≤ 5 oocytes retrieved in a previous cycle were subjected dual ovarian stimulation for preimplantation testing for aneuploidy. The age range of the 43 women who underwent oocyte retrieval was between 32 and 44 years. Fixed daily dose (high dose of recombinant FSH (300 IU) combined with recombinant LH (75 IU) with flexible antagonist protocol) was used in both follicular and luteal phases. Five days after the oocyte retrieval, the luteal phase stimulation was started. Gonadotropin-releasing hormone agonist (GnRHa) was used for both triggers. Both oocyte and blastocyst stage embryo yields were comparable between follicular and luteal phase stimulations. Euploid blastocyst rate calculated per biopsied blastocyst was also similar between the follicular and luteal phase stimulations [11]. The same team published another similar study including more patients and reporting the ongoing pregnancy rates. This study showed that less oocytes were obtained from follicular phase of the dual stimulation as compared to luteal phase, but euploid embryo rates and ongoing pregnancy rates were comparable from embryos obtained from follicular versus luteal phase [12]. Other authors also reported that the luteal phase stimulation results in competent oocytes [13, 14].

For women with poor ovarian response (POR), outcomes of dual or double – both in follicular phase and luteal phase –stimulation were reported with a minimal and then regular stimulation regimen. The authors excluded women with basal FSH level above 20 IU/L. The patients were subjected to a protocol with clomiphene citrate 25 mg/day continuously and letrozole 2.5 mg/day only for 4 days. Human menopausal gonadotropin (HMG) 150 IU every other day was added on cycle day 6. When the leading follicle size was at or above 18 mm, the final oocyte maturation was induced by GnRH agonist, and 600 mg sustained release ibuprofen daily for 2 days was used to prevent premature ovulation. Oocyte retrieval was performed in 32–36 hours. The authors left all follicles less than 10 mm for luteal phase stimulation. Just after oocyte retrieval if transvaginal ultrasound showed at least two antral follicles 2–8 mm in diameter, the stimulation was started with HMG 225 IU daily and letrozole 2.5 mg daily from the day of or day after oocyte retrieval. The authors stopped letrozole with follicle growth and added medroxyprogesterone acetate 10 mg daily if they suspected short luteal phase with impending menstruation. After the trigger, oocyte retrieval was performed in 36–38 hours. This study included 38 patients undergoing follicular stimulation. Twenty women did not have any viable embryos with the follicular phase minimal stimulation. Thirty women underwent luteal phase stimulation, and 13 women did not have viable embryos. Eventually 21 women had 23 frozen-thawed embryo transfer cycles resulting in 13 clinical pregnancies. The number of oocytes retrieved was significantly higher in luteal phase stimulation, but the number of top-quality and cryopreserved embryos was comparable among groups (both day 3 and blastocyst stage embryos were frozen) [15].

13.3   Luteal Phase Mild Stimulation

As discussed above, luteal phase mild stimulation can be a good alternative for women with DOR and/or ARA to obtain frozen embryos for delayed frozen-thawed embryo transfer. Unlike some others, we do recommend this protocol exclusively in ovulatory women with basal FSH >20 IU/L. Luteal phase elevation of endogenous progesterone keeps LH levels at reasonable levels of 2–8 IU/L. The FSH levels most of the time stay below 20 IU/L, which should help to prevent potential adverse effects of high FSH levels on oocyte and later on embryo quality.

As depicted in Fig. 13.1, the stimulation is started right after first P4 elevation is detected after performing a transvaginal ultrasound to assess the side and the measurements of the ovulating follicle and the antral follicle count. After the first E2, LH, and P4 levels are measured, the mild stimulation is started with recombinant FSH 150 IU daily. In this protocol, each time we do labs, we have to perform an ultrasound. This is to closely monitor E2, LH, and P4 progression while assessing the follicle response. When the P4 level starts decreasing below 3 ng/mL while having growing follicles above 13 mm in diameters, we start monitoring the patients daily. When the P4 drops below 1 ng/mL, the patients may start their menstrual period. At that time, we observe a boost in the follicle growth as well. It is very rare that these patients require low-dose antagonist dose. However, if antagonist is needed, then we may have to add highly purified HMG 75 IU to the regimen while decreasing the recombinant FSH down to 75 IU, or in some cases, we keep recom-

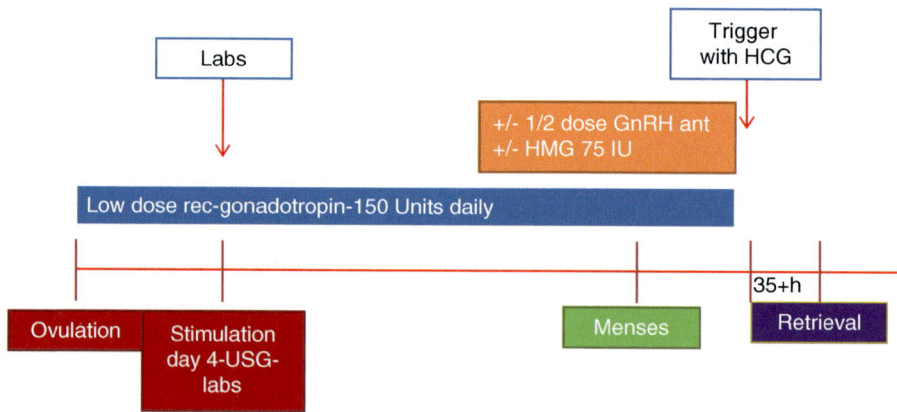

Luteal phase mild stimulation – when early LH surge cannot be prevented, when FSH is >20 IU/L in minimal stimulation with poor response to minimal stimulation
Total FSH dose/cycle 1500 IU while mostly no need for antagonist, consider hp-HMG, only when antagonist is used

Fig. 13.1 Luteal phase mild stimulation with a recombinant FSH

binant FSH at 150 IU as well. We trigger the final oocyte maturation with HCG with or without GnRH agonist. If P4 is still elevated, these patients benefit more from HCG trigger at 5000 IU or full 10,000 IU.

Oocyte retrieval is scheduled 35–35.5 hours after the trigger. Frequently, such women may start their menstrual bleeding at around the day of oocyte retrieval. We did not find this detrimental to the cycle outcome, and we do not use prophylactic antibiotics during the oocyte retrievals routinely. Having menstrual bleeding during the oocyte retrieval is not one of the indications for antibiotic prophylaxis at our center.

Similar to minimal stimulation cycles, we freeze embryos to provide the best chances for frozen-thawed embryo transfers in the future. In cases, requiring embryo biopsy for genetic testing, we have to watch them in culture until they reach the blastocyst stage. In other cases, we attempt to freeze stage-specific embryos to later synchronize the endometrium for either day 3 or day 5 stage. Like reported by others, we freeze all top-quality eight-cell stage embryos on day 3. Other embryos are taken toward the blastocyst stage for vitrification [15, 16].

13.4 Prolonged Ovarian Suppression and Estrogen Priming Followed by Mild Stimulation

This option is reserved as a last resort protocol for women with profound DOR within the spectrum of premature ovarian insufficiency (POI). These women show high basal FSH above 40 IU/mL and short cycles with short follicular and luteal phases. It is very frequent to observe multiple cystic follicles with increased E2 levels, which is typical for a pre-menopausal state. In such women, obtaining competent oocytes with minimal stimulation or luteal phase mild stimulation would not be possible.

As we discuss in the chapter on activation of ovarian cortex, prolonged suppression of both FSH and LH in such women still with some oocytes in their ovaries may be beneficial for natural stimulation of early folliculogenesis. The clinicians performing many medicated frozen-thawed embryo transfer cycles with ovarian suppression followed by estradiol use may note that after 2 weeks of GnRH agonist suppression followed by 12–14 days of estradiol treatment to develop the endometrial stripe, emergence of 2–6 mm antral follicles can be observed on the day of assessment of the endometrial lining before starting progesterone. Since minimal and mild stimulation protocols require accumulation of frozen embryos, we perform quite few frozen-thawed embryo transfers. We are inspired by observing increased 2–6 mm antral follicles in the ovaries of many women with DOR while performing their transvaginal ultrasounds primarily to make decisions about their endometrial stripe thickness and pattern. That was the reason that we called this mild stimulation alternative as FET (for frozen embryo transfer) protocol informally to be on the same page with our team members.

It has been shown that prolonged suppression of FSH and LH by using GnRH analogs can be useful in women with hypergonadotropic amenorrhea and also those with POI of genetic origin in terms of achieving spontaneous ovulation or response to gonadotropin treatment, respectively [17, 18]. Suppression may last from 4 to 12 weeks followed by estradiol use for priming of follicles. This approach may decrease the forced early follicle selection by high FSH and may restore responsiveness of follicles to FSH when needed perhaps through mitigation of both FSH and LH receptor desensitization at granulosa cell level. LH suppression may also relieve medullary pressure to the cortex via its ovarian stromal effects, which will be discussed in activation of ovarian cortex chapter.

13.4.1 Treatment Details

Figure 13.2 shows our prolonged ovarian suppression and estrogen priming mild stimulation protocol. Certainly, like minimal stimulation and luteal phase mild stimulation protocols, this protocol is highly customized for each patient especially in terms of durations of GnRH agonist and micronized estradiol use and the frequency of progesterone in oil injections to control LH when necessary.

We recommend this protocol in women younger than 40 years of age within the POI spectrum in terms of FSH levels and mostly undetectable AMH levels but still having some menstrual cycles. Menstrual cycles can either be spaced apart more than every 35 days or may be more frequent than every 24 days.

If there is no contraindication, patients start using combined birth control pills (OCPs) containing at least 30 mcg of ethinyl estradiol with the first day of their menses (cycle day 1 or 2). After about 8–10 days of OCP use, patients need a

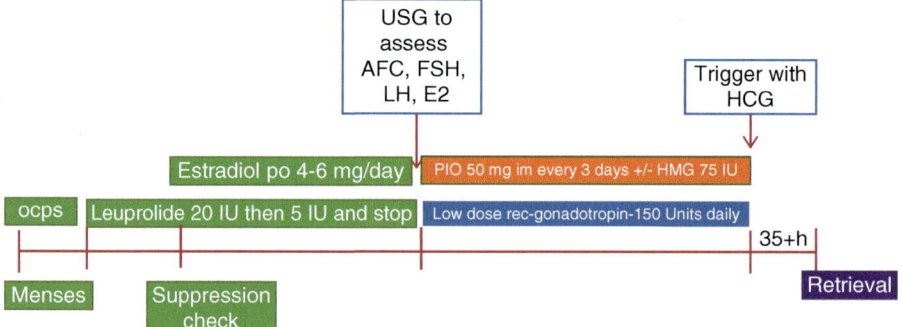

Long suppression protocol with E2 priming and mild stimulation – when high FSH (>20 IU/L) and LH (>10 IU/L) along with lack of response and embryo development as the issues Rec-FSH daily dose 150 units after several weeks of suppression and estrogen priming, im progesterone in oil use rather than antagonist to control LH if needed.

Fig. 13.2 Prolonged ovarian suppression, estrogen priming, and mild stimulation protocol

transvaginal ultrasound to assess for potential follicle cyst presence and laboratory tests to assess E2 and LH levels to start GnRH agonist, leuprolide acetate 20 IU daily. If they have E2 levels at or above 100 pg/mL combined with LH levels at or above 5 IU/L while seeing follicle(s) >8 mm, we delay starting GnRH agonist. If we start GnRH agonist with such findings, due to the initial flare effects of GnRH agonist, follicle cyst formation may happen. At times, these cysts are functional, and they may take up to 3 months for them to resolve. Therefore, it would be best to make sure that OCPs are showing at least some LH suppressing effects before we start GnRH agonist. In women with contraindications to use OCPs, we try oral medroxyprogesterone acetate 10–20 mg daily.

After 7–10 days of daily GnRH agonist use, OCPs are stopped, and patients continue with only leuprolide acetate 20 IU (1 mg) daily with the goal of suppressing LH to less than 1 IU/L. At that point, E2 will be suppressed to below 20 pg/mL unless patients develop functional ovarian cyst or follicle growth. Once achieved, the suppressed state may be maintained for another 2–4 weeks or longer while assessing the ovaries and E2 and LH levels weekly. Then when the emergence of 2–4 mm antral follicles are observed, oral daily micronized estradiol is started to keep E2 levels at 150 pg/mL or above to assure continued FSH suppression when the leuprolide acetate dose is dropped to 5 IU daily. Twice weekly transvaginal ultrasounds and E2 and LH levels are performed to assess further emergence of antral follicles 2–6 mm in size. When these are observed, both micronized estradiol and GnRH agonist are discontinued, and recombinant FSH at 150 IU daily dose is started. Transvaginal ultrasound and E2 and LH monitoring are started after the first 3 days of stimulation. When increasing LH levels >4 IU/L are observed, in order to avoid GnRH antagonist use and just like a frozen-thawed embryo transfer preparation, progesterone in oil injections (PIO) 50 mg intramuscularly every 3–4 days are started titrating to P4 and LH levels. Progesterone levels are kept at or above 3 ng/mL to prevent LH surge. Many patients may not need PIO at all, or all they need may be one to three doses.

Some patients do not show recovery of LH levels during the stimulation phase. If the endogenous LH levels are continuing to be below 1 IU/L, such women may need addition of hp-HMG to the protocol. Either recombinant FSH is decreased to 75 IU, and 75 IU daily HMG is added, or at times especially if FSH levels are also below 8 IU/L, 75 IU of HMG is added to the daily 150 IU dose of recombinant FSH. Although this may seem to be a compromise from the principles of mild stimulation, monitoring of FSH levels may help with this decision-making.

When the leading follicle size of 16–18 mm is reached, final oocyte maturation is triggered with HCG 5000–10,000 IU, and oocyte retrieval is performed at 35–35.5 hours. As in all minimal and mild stimulation cycles, fertilization method of choice (conventional IVF or intracytoplasmic sperm injection) and the embryo stage at vitrification are individualized per patient.

After the oocyte retrieval, since the patients show endogenous P4 increase, we offer an assessment of the ovaries in 2–3 days to start luteal phase mild stimulation if we see more 2–6 mm antral follicles. Therefore, we use the principles of dual or double stimulation in this protocol to take advantage of emergence of antral follicles. Unlike others, we do not start stimulation on the day or day after oocyte retrieval since we use HCG to trigger for final oocyte maturation especially in cases with P4 levels are still >3 ng/mL on the day of trigger or those with suppressed LH levels. We had witnessed that some antral follicles observed during the oocyte retrieval may just disappear 2–3 days after the oocyte retrieval suggesting that some may just be atretic follicles.

As we discuss in the activation of ovarian cortex chapter, using GnRH antagonist for prolonged suppression phase may have some additional merits. Currently the use of daily GnRH antagonist for prolonged suppression may increase the medication costs considerably. However, with the recent marketing of oral antagonist like elagolix, GnRH antagonist can be used for this indication in the near future.

13.5   Conclusion

In women with profound DOR associated with FSH increase above 20 IU/L at basal state or as tested during the minimal stimulation cycle, we recommend additional approaches to obtain competent oocytes for frozen embryo accumulation. These approaches are through luteal phase mild stimulation or prolonged suppression-estrogen priming-mild stimulation protocols as discussed in this chapter. Further refining of such protocols would be possible in the future by the use of medroxy-progesterone acetate to avoid LH surge when the luteal phase is short or by the use of oral antagonist to prevent flare effects of GnRH agonists.

References

1. Nahum R, Thong KJ, Hillier SG. Metabolic regulation of androgen production by human thecal cells in vitro. Hum Reprod. 1995;10(1):75–81.
2. Takao Y, Honda T, Ueda M, Hattori N, Yamada S, Maeda M, et al. Immunohistochemical localization of the LH/HCG receptor in human ovary: HCG enhances cell surface expression of LH/HCG receptor on luteinizing granulosa cells in vitro. Mol Hum Reprod. 1997;3(7):569–78.
3. Yong EL, Baird DT, Yates R, Reichert LE Jr, Hillier SG. Hormonal regulation of the growth and steroidogenic function of human granulosa cells. J Clin Endocrinol Metab. 1992;74(4):842–9.
4. Ludwig M, Katalinic A, Banz C, Schroder AK, Loning M, Weiss JM, et al. Tailoring the GnRH antagonist cetrorelix acetate to individual patients' needs in ovarian stimulation for IVF: results of a prospective, randomized study. Hum Reprod. 2002;17(11):2842–5.
5. Lainas T, Zorzovilis J, Petsas G, Stavropoulou G, Cazlaris H, Daskalaki V, et al. In a flexible antagonist protocol, earlier, criteria-based initiation of GnRH antagonist is associated with increased pregnancy rates in IVF. Hum Reprod. 2005;20(9):2426–33.
6. Jeppesen JV, Kristensen SG, Nielsen ME, Humaidan P, Dal Canto M, Fadini R, et al. LH-receptor gene expression in human granulosa and cumulus cells from antral and preovulatory follicles. J Clin Endocrinol Metab. 2012;97(8):E1524–31.
7. Winkler N, Bukulmez O, Hardy DB, Carr BR. Gonadotropin releasing hormone antagonists suppress aromatase and anti-Mullerian hormone expression in human granulosa cells. Fertil Steril. 2010;94(5):1832–9.

8. Muteshi C, Child T, Ohuma E, Fatum M. Ovarian response and follow-up outcomes in women diagnosed with cancer having fertility preservation: comparison of random start and early follicular phase stimulation – cohort study. Eur J Obstet Gynecol Reprod Biol. 2018;230:10–4.
9. Qin N, Chen Q, Hong Q, Cai R, Gao H, Wang Y, et al. Flexibility in starting ovarian stimulation at different phases of the menstrual cycle for treatment of infertile women with the use of in vitro fertilization or intracytoplasmic sperm injection. Fertil Steril. 2016;106(2):334–41 e1.
10. Sighinolfi G, Sunkara SK, La Marca A. New strategies of ovarian stimulation based on the concept of ovarian follicular waves: from conventional to random and double stimulation. Reprod Biomed Online. 2018;37(4):489–97.
11. Ubaldi FM, Capalbo A, Vaiarelli A, Cimadomo D, Colamaria S, Alviggi C, et al. Follicular versus luteal phase ovarian stimulation during the same menstrual cycle (DuoStim) in a reduced ovarian reserve population results in a similar euploid blastocyst formation rate: new insight in ovarian reserve exploitation. Fertil Steril. 2016;105(6):1488–95.e1.
12. Cimadomo D, Vaiarelli A, Colamaria S, Trabucco E, Alviggi C, Venturella R, et al. Luteal phase anovulatory follicles result in the production of competent oocytes: intra-patient paired case-control study comparing follicular versus luteal phase stimulations in the same ovarian cycle. Hum Reprod. 2018;33:1442.
13. Jin B, Niu Z, Xu B, Chen Q, Zhang A. Comparison of clinical outcomes among dual ovarian stimulation, mild stimulation and luteal phase stimulation protocols in women with poor ovarian response. Gynecol Endocrinol. 2018;34(8):694–7.
14. Wang N, Wang Y, Chen Q, Dong J, Tian H, Fu Y, et al. Luteal-phase ovarian stimulation vs conventional ovarian stimulation in patients with normal ovarian reserve treated for IVF: a large retrospective cohort study. Clin Endocrinol. 2016;84(5):720–8.
15. Kuang Y, Chen Q, Hong Q, Lyu Q, Ai A, Fu Y, et al. Double stimulations during the follicular and luteal phases of poor responders in IVF/ICSI programmes (Shanghai protocol). Reprod Biomed Online. 2014;29(6):684–91.
16. Kuang Y, Chen Q, Fu Y, Wang Y, Hong Q, Lyu Q, et al. Medroxyprogesterone acetate is an effective oral alternative for preventing premature luteinizing hormone surges in women undergoing controlled ovarian hyperstimulation for in vitro fertilization. Fertil Steril. 2015;104(1):62–70.e3.
17. Menon V, Edwards RL, Lynch SS, Butt WR. Luteinizing hormone releasing hormone analogue in treatment of hypergonadotrophic amenorrhoea. Br J Obstet Gynaecol. 1983;90(6):539–42.
18. Ishizuka B, Kudo Y, Amemiya A, Ogata T. Ovulation induction in a woman with premature ovarian failure resulting from a partial deletion of the X chromosome long arm, 46,X,del(X)(q22). Fertil Steril. 1997;68(5):931–4.

Chapter 14
Control of Luteinizing Hormone (LH)

Beverly G. Reed

14.1 Luteinizing Hormone: An Overview

Luteinizing hormone (LH) is a large glycoprotein that takes form as a heterodimer. It is secreted from the anterior pituitary in a pulsatile fashion. While its alpha-subunit is identical in structure to thyroid-stimulating hormone, follicle-stimulating hormone (FSH), and human chorionic gonadotropin (HCG), LH's beta-subunit is what makes it unique and allows for its biological in vivo activity [1, 2].

Ovarian follicles contain granulosa cells and theca cells, both of which are critical for follicular growth and maturation. Theca cells contain LH receptors, and under stimulation, these cells produce androgen precursor. Granulosa cells contain FSH receptors, and with stimulation, androgen precursor from the theca cells can be aromatized into estradiol [1, 2].

During assisted reproductive technology treatment (ART), emphasis has typically been placed on the use of FSH to promote follicular growth and development. This is because early in stimulation, granulosa cells in the ovarian follicle mainly contain FSH receptors. However, as the ovarian follicle grows, LH receptors also develop on the granulosa cells. Thus, LH becomes an important potential contributor to granulosa cell signaling. In women who have moderate levels of endogenous LH, emphasis on adding only FSH may be a reasonable strategy. However, women with low endogenous levels of LH or women who have ongoing exogenous LH suppression may need customization of their protocol to prevent follicular LH deprivation. Studies from women with hypogonadotropic hypogonadism have underlined the integral role that LH plays in follicular steroidogenesis [3–6]. If women with low endogenous FSH and LH are treated with recombinant FSH only, follicular growth can occur. However, the estradiol response is blunted possibly due to lack

B. G. Reed (✉)
IVFMD, Irving, TX, USA
e-mail: drreed@ivfmd.net

© Springer Nature Switzerland AG 2020
O. Bukulmez (ed.), *Diminished Ovarian Reserve and Assisted Reproductive Technologies*, https://doi.org/10.1007/978-3-030-23235-1_14

Fig. 14.1 Review of how too much or too little LH can affect an IVF cycle

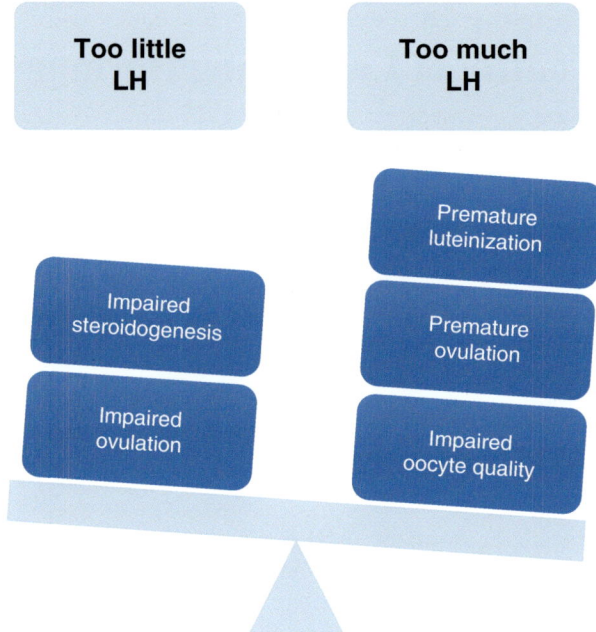

of androgen substrate from the theca cells, and the follicle may become incapable of luteinization and/or ovulation (Fig. 14.1). Hence, the importance of LH maintenance during IVF treatment cannot be ignored.

14.2   Avoidance of Pre-cycle Oral Contraceptives

While most of our minimal stimulation in vitro fertilization (IVF) patients have diminished ovarian reserve and would not be expected to have hypogonadotropic hypogonadism, we take this lesson from nature to help us apply the importance of LH presence during our treatment protocols and to help us avoid iatrogenic low LH. One of the most common practices we see that can cause LH suppression is the use of pretreatment oral contraceptive pills.

For traditional IVF, oral contraceptive pills prior to stimulation may have many advantages. First, they help prevent ovarian cysts prior to stimulation start, reduce the risk for ovarian hyperstimulation syndrome, and may even result in better cycle outcomes in certain high-responder patients [7–9]. Second, they allow for follicular synchronization, which ultimately increases the chances that the follicles will grow at an even pace throughout stimulation. Third, the use of oral contraceptive pills allows fertility clinics to schedule IVF cycles according to facility and embryologist availability and thus adds to convenience for both the clinic and the patient. All of these reasons make the use of oral contraceptive pills leading up to IVF stimulation very reasonable for patients who are expected to be normal or high responders.

However, the use of long-term oral contraceptive pills for patients with diminished ovarian reserve needs to be avoided. Oral contraceptive use has been shown to decrease ovarian volume, antral follicle count, and anti-Mullerian hormone (AMH) levels [10]. Since patients with diminished ovarian reserve are already low on all of these factors, the implementation of oral contraceptives can have a large detrimental effect. In addition, oral contraceptives reduce endogenous DHEA-S, testosterone, and serum insulin-like growth factor (IGF-1) levels [11–13]. At a time when many patients are eager to take fertility supplements such as DHEA, testosterone, and growth hormone, we feel that a better strategy is to avoid suppression of those important cofactors. Oral contraceptives and, more specifically, the progestin component of oral contraceptives are known to suppress endogenous LH [14, 15]. The length of suppression after cessation of oral contraceptives can vary, but since IVF stimulation is usually started approximately 3–4 days after oral contraceptives have been stopped, it is logical to expect some ongoing effects during the early portion of the stimulation. Since the early part of the stimulation is critical for optimizing the number of follicles that can be recruited for the cycle, we recommend complete avoidance of oral contraceptives altogether just before starting the stimulation. Alternatively, we recommend the use of estrogen priming. As discussed in the minimal stimulation chapter, the short-term use of oral contraceptives for a few days may be needed in some clinical scenarios. However, any such use is always after estrogen priming and followed by estrogen priming again before starting stimulation.

14.3 Estrogen Priming as an Alternative to Pre-cycle Oral Contraceptives

Estrogen suppresses endogenous FSH, which allows for the same follicular synchronization that oral contraceptives provide. But, unlike progestin use, estrogen use does not cause profound LH suppression. Hence, its use prior to minimal stimulation IVF is beneficial. Our estrogen priming protocol consists of initiating estradiol 4 mg orally starting approximately 3–4 days after ovulation as confirmed by a rise in the serum progesterone level [16]. The oral estradiol is discontinued at the time of menses in preparation for IVF stimulation start on cycle day 2 or 3.

14.4 The Importance of LH Monitoring

When we initially began implementing minimal stimulation IVF for patients with diminished ovarian reserve, we did not monitor LH levels. Unfortunately, at that time (2012–2014), we had a premature ovulation rate of 12% (unpublished data). We have learned that women with diminished ovarian reserve and/or advanced reproductive age tend to have a higher risk for premature ovulation when compared to normal or high responders [17]. At the same time, the standard fixed or flexible

GnRH antagonist protocols that are commonly used for the average patient are not applicable to our special patient population as mentioned in minimal stimulation IVF section.

Starting in 2015, we incorporated close LH monitoring during our minimal stimulation IVF cycles, which is started as early as day 4 of treatment with clomiphene citrate. Our premature ovulation rate dropped drastically from 12% in the years 2012–2014 to 0% in the years 2015–2016 ($p = 0.0017$, unpublished data, Fig. 14.2a). Our data shows that monitoring serum LH levels during the stimulation resulted in an overall earlier average initiation of GnRH antagonist when compared to previous years. The 2012–2014 group (which did not monitor LH) initiated GnRH antagonist on an average of stimulation day 8 versus an average of stimulation day 5.6 in the 2015–2016 group (which underwent LH monitoring, $p < 0.0001$, unpublished data, Fig. 14.2b). In addition, the group that underwent frequent LH monitoring used less GnRH antagonist overall (416 mcg versus 670 mcg, $p < 0.0001$, Fig. 14.2c).

14.5   When to Initiate GnRH Antagonist Treatment

To initiate monitoring of serum LH, we bring patients in immediately after their third day of stimulation for their first LH level. It is important to concurrently draw an estradiol serum level as this gives context on how to interpret the LH level (Fig. 14.3). If the LH level is low (≤ 5 IU/L), GnRH antagonist treatment is not yet begun. If the LH is >5 IU/L, the LH level is further interpreted according to the patient's serum estradiol level. In general, a follicle would need to have an estradiol exposure of >150 pg/mL for at least 36–40 hours to have the potential for premature ovulation. Therefore, if the estradiol is <150 pg/mL, the GnRH antagonist is withheld. If the estradiol level is above 150 pg/mL and the LH level is >5 IU/L, a half dose of a GnRH antagonist (125 mcg) is given immediately, and the patient is scheduled for a sonogram and repeat labs the next day. The sonogram can give further guidance on whether the GnRH antagonist needs to be continued at that time of the cycle. For example, if a sonogram shows several follicles measuring 16 mm, continuation with the GnRH antagonist is necessary since those follicles are likely capable of premature ovulation. However, if the sonogram demonstrates that all follicles are less than 12 mm, the GnRH antagonist can be safely held that day since smaller follicles are not likely to undergo premature luteinization and/or ovulation. At times, one can encounter LH levels at or above 10 IU/L, while the estradiol level is still less than 100 pg/mL. Rather than considering GnRH antagonist administration, we recognize that this could be an indicator of more severe diminished ovarian reserve and that we may need to consider what the FSH level is in such patients. If the LH level continues to be higher than 10 IU/L with low estradiol levels at another measurement, we assess FSH level. If the FSH level is above 20 IU/L, it is illogical to continue with that cycle as discussed in the minimal stimulation section.

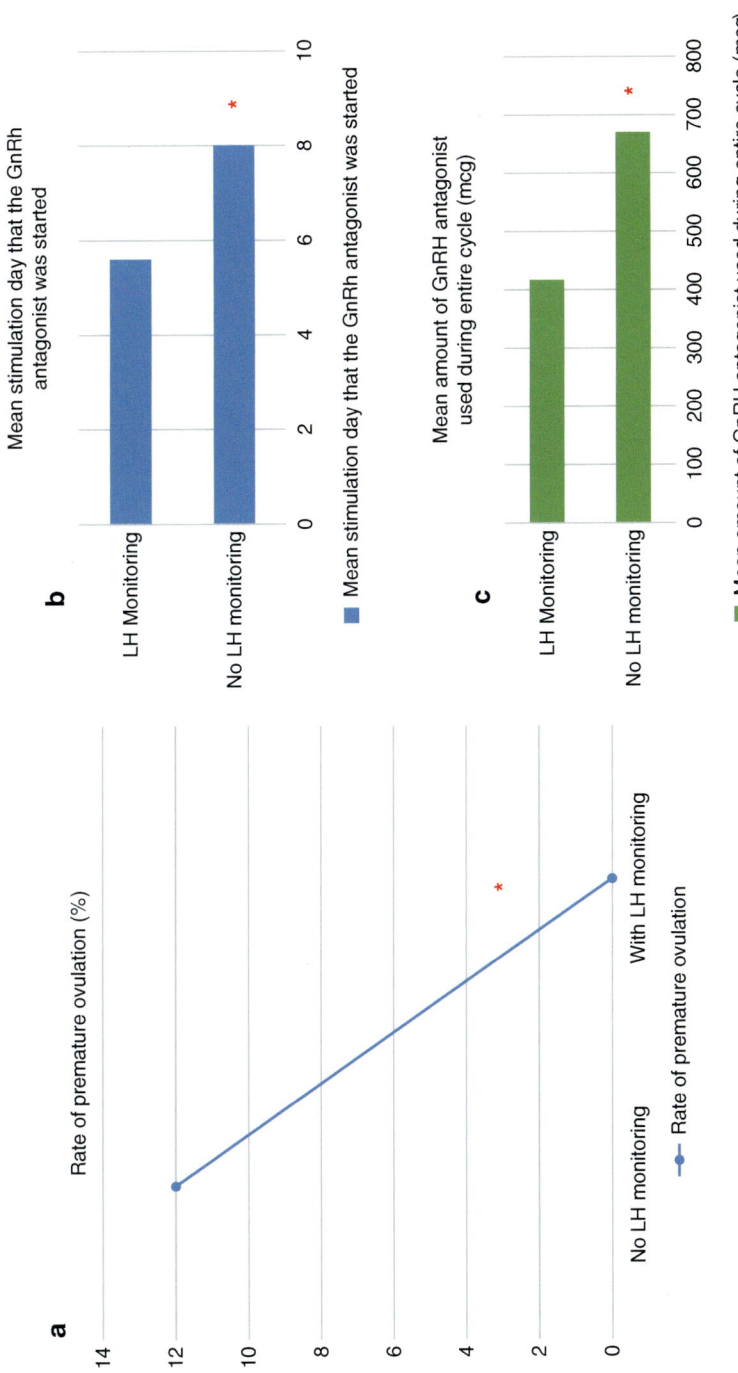

Fig. 14.2 (**a–c**) Based on retrospective unpublished data collected at University of Texas Southwestern Medical Center, Dallas, Texas. Eighty-eight patients underwent 129 minimal stimulation IVF cycles, and they were divided between two groups: patients who did not have LH monitoring and patients who had LH monitoring during their minimal stimulation IVF cycle. (**a**) The premature ovulation rate was eliminated once LH monitoring was incorporated ($p = 0.0017$). (**b**) The addition of LH monitoring resulted in earlier initiation of the GnRH antagonist on average when compared to no LH monitoring ($p < 0.0001$). (**c**) The group with LH monitoring required roughly only 2/3 of the amount of GnRH antagonist when compared to the group that did not undergo LH monitoring ($p < 0.0001$)

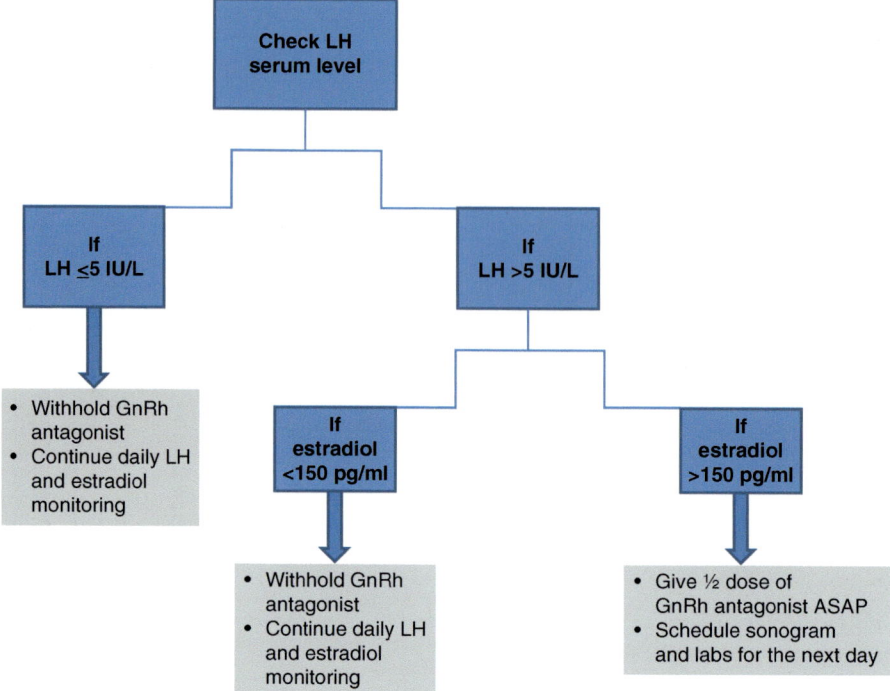

Fig. 14.3 Flowchart to assist in deciding when to start the GnRH antagonist during minimal stimulation IVF

14.6   Justification for Lower Doses of GnRH Antagonist

As described above, we seek to limit over-suppression of LH. A full dose of a GnRH antagonist is much more likely to contribute to over-suppression of LH. Early dose findings studies with GnRH antagonists demonstrated lower clinical pregnancy rates with either too high or too low of a dose resulting in inadequate LH suppression or over-suppression of LH [18–21]. Ultimately, a moderate dose (250 mcg) was recommended, but that dose has primarily been studied in a normal patient with average ovarian reserve. We suspect that patients with diminished ovarian reserve require lower doses and that avoidance of over-suppression may be beneficial. So, our strategy is to monitor intensely to avoid as much GnRH antagonist use as possible. On occasion, we have had patients who are able to complete an entire treatment cycle without the use of any GnRH antagonist. The majority of our patients are able to complete their stimulation using only half doses of GnRH antagonist once the medication is initiated. Once GnRH antagonist has been initiated in a treatment cycle, we continue LH monitoring to determine if the half dose of GnRH antagonist is sufficient. If the serum LH continues to trend up despite initiation of a half dose of GnRH antagonist with further estradiol increase and follicle growth, we may increase the GnRH antagonist to a full dose (250 mcg). But, rarely is that dose continued for the remainder of the stimulation. When initiating GnRH antagonist during the treatment cycle, we give consideration to adding highly purified human menopausal gonadotropin (HMG, Menopur, Ferring Reproductive Health) as a way to counteract the LH suppression with HCG-driven LH effect. While the use of recombinant LH would be appealing for this purpose, this product is not currently available in the United States. If GnRH antagonist is given early in the stimulation, we still administer HMG every other day. However, after day 5 of stimulation, if LH control requires daily antagonist, we may use daily HMG with alternating dosing of 75 IU and 150 IU every other day to minimize gonadotropin dose and to mitigate receptor desensitization.

14.7 Logistics and Practical Considerations for LH Monitoring and GnRH Antagonist Treatment

Of note, the patient must be willing to come for laboratory assessments early in the morning so that same day results and decisions can be made. She must also be willing to potentially undergo daily lab assessment. She needs to be readily available by phone in case urgent GnRH antagonist administration is needed. Should a patient not be reachable for medication instructions, premature ovulation or luteinization could occur.

In the United States, we have two choices for injectable GnRH antagonists: ganirelix (Antagon; Merck-Organon) or cetrorelix (Cetrotide; Merck Serono). Ganirelix comes in a prefilled syringe. While that is convenient for patients, it makes giving a half dose of medication more logistically complicated. Therefore, our preferred GnRH antagonist is cetrorelix due to its packaging. Cetrorelix comes as a powder in a vial that must be reconstituted with saline at the time of use. Once the medication has been reconstituted, the patient is able to withdraw only half of the medication from the vial, and the remaining half can be refrigerated and used for the next day. Please note that using a half dose in this manner represents off-label usage of the medication. Unlike ganirelix, cetrorelix requires refrigeration. Therefore, patients who will be leaving their home for work will need to bring their medication in a lunch cooler so that it is always accessible should it be needed.

14.8 Future LH Monitoring and LH Control Options

Alternative options for LH control in the future may include the use of progestins instead of GnRH antagonists. Previously, progestins could not be utilized in this fashion because it would have prematurely advanced endometrial receptivity and would have eliminated the option for a fresh transfer. However, as mentioned elsewhere in this textbook, we feel that a freeze-all approach is warranted with the use of daily clomiphene citrate due to untoward effects on the endometrial thickness. The widespread availability and usage of vitrification have allowed us to easily adopt this strategy. Therefore, we are now able to consider other options to control LH that were not previously considered due to negative endometrial effects. One recent study showed that medroxyprogesterone 10 mg orally controlled LH levels and allowed larger follicular development without premature ovulation in minimal stimulation IVF for poor responders [22].

Therefore, the use of a progestin during a freeze-all cycle could be a viable and more affordable alternative to GnRH antagonist use, and therefore, this is an area that warrants further study.

Another novel option could be to implement the use of an oral GnRH antagonist (elagolix, Orilissa, AbbVie) [23]. This medication is currently only FDA approved for the treatment of moderate to severe endometriosis pain, but recent studies are exploring new uses such as in the treatment of uterine fibroids [23, 24]. Consideration for the use of elagolix instead of injectable GnRH antagonists could be well embraced by patients who would likely appreciate less injections and a more affordable price. Hence, this should be a focus of future studies as well.

We hope that at some point, patients will have an option to purchase a monitor to check LH at home (similar to a glucometer). This would reduce the need for daily blood draws and would perhaps allow for even finer LH control.

Finally, we have had occasional patients in which the LH surge could not be reliably prevented. An alternative stimulation strategy is luteal phase stimulation. By waiting to start stimulation after the patient has already ovulated during her own cycle, a portion of the stimulation can be performed without the use of GnRH antagonist. However, it also involves close monitoring because as the progesterone level returns to low levels, ovulation can occur.

References

1. Carr BR, Blackwell R, Azziz R. Essential reproductive medicine. New York: McGraw-Hill Companies, Inc.; 2004.
2. Fritz M, Speroff L. Clinical gynecologic endocrinology & infertility. 8th ed. Philadelphia: Lippincott; 2011.
3. Shoham Z, Mannaerts B, Insler V, Coelingh-Bennink H. Induction of follicular growth using recombinant human follicle-stimulating hormone in two volunteer women with hypogonadotropic hypogonadism. Fertil Steril. 1993;59:738–42.
4. Group TERHLS. Recombinant human luteinizing hormone (LH) to support recombinant human follicle-stimulating hormone (FSH)-induced follicular development in LH- and FSH-deficient anovulatory women: a dose-finding study [1]. J Clin Endocrinol Metab. 1998;83:1507–14.
5. Couzinet B, Lestrat N, Brailly S, Forest M, Schaison G. Stimulation of ovarian follicular maturation with pure follicle-stimulating hormone in women with gonadotropin deficiency. J Clin Endocrinol Metab. 1988;66:552–6.
6. Strauss JF, Steinkampf MP. Pituitary-ovarian interactions during follicular maturation and ovulation. Am J Obstet Gynecol. 1995;172:726–35.

7. Wang L, Zhao Y, Dong X, Huang K, Wang R, Ji L, Wang Y, Zhang H. Could pretreatment with oral contraceptives before pituitary down regulation reduce the incidence of ovarian hyperstimulation syndrome in the IVF/ICSI procedure? Int J Clin Exp Med. 2015;8:2711–8.
8. Damario MA, Barmat L, Liu HC, Davis OK, Rosenwaks Z. Dual suppression with oral contraceptives and gonadotrophin releasing-hormone agonists improves in-vitro fertilization outcome in high responder patients. Hum Reprod. 1997;12:2359–65.
9. Farquhar C, Rombauts L, Kremer JA, Lethaby A, Ayeleke RO. Oral contraceptive pill, progestogen or oestrogen pretreatment for ovarian stimulation protocols for women undergoing assisted reproductive techniques. Cochrane Database Syst Rev. 2017;(5):CD006109.
10. Birch Petersen K, Hvidman HW, Forman JL, Pinborg A, Larsen EC, Macklon KT, Sylvest R, Andersen AN. Ovarian reserve assessment in users of oral contraception seeking fertility advice on their reproductive lifespan. Hum Reprod. 2015;30:2364–75.
11. Zimmerman Y, Eijkemans MJC, Coelingh Bennink HJT, Blankenstein MA, Fauser BCJM. The effect of combined oral contraception on testosterone levels in healthy women: a systematic review and meta-analysis. Hum Reprod Update. 2014;20:76–105.
12. Amiri M, Kabir A, Nahidi F, Shekofteh M, Ramezani Tehrani F. Effects of combined oral contraceptives on the clinical and biochemical parameters of hyperandrogenism in patients with polycystic ovary syndrome: a systematic review and meta-analysis. Eur J Contracept Reprod Health Care. 2018;23:64–77.
13. Phelan N, Conway SH, Llahana S, Conway GS. Quantification of the adverse effect of ethinylestradiol containing oral contraceptive pills when used in conjunction with growth hormone replacement in routine practice. Clin Endocrinol (Oxf). 2012;76:729–33.
14. Cohen BL, Katz M. Pituitary and ovarian function in women receiving hormonal contraception. Contraception. 1979;20:475–87.
15. Girmus RL, Wise ME. Progesterone directly inhibits pituitary luteinizing hormone secretion in an estradiol-dependent manner. Biol Reprod. 1992;46:710–4.
16. Reed BG, Babayev SN, Bukulmez O. Shifting paradigms in diminished ovarian reserve and advanced reproductive age in assisted reproduction: customization instead of conformity. Semin Reprod Med. 2015;33:169–78.
17. Reichman DE, Zakarin L, Chao K, Meyer L, Davis OK, Rosenwaks Z. Diminished ovarian reserve is the predominant risk factor for gonadotropin-releasing hormone antagonist failure resulting in breakthrough luteinizing hormone surges in in vitro fertilization cycles. Fertil Steril. 2014;102:99–102.
18. Huirne JAF, van Loenen ACD, Schats R, McDonnell J, Hompes PGA, Schoemaker J, Homburg R, Lambalk CB. Dose-finding study of daily GnRH antagonist for the prevention of premature LH surges in IVF/ICSI patients: optimal changes in LH and progesterone for clinical pregnancy. Hum Reprod. 2005;20:359–67.
19. Winkler N, Bukulmez O, Hardy DB, Carr BR. Gonadotropin releasing hormone antagonists suppress aromatase and anti-Müllerian hormone expression in human granulosa cells. Fertil Steril. 2010;94:1832–9.
20. Lee TH, Lin YH, Seow KM, Hwang JL, Tzeng CR, Yang YS. Effectiveness of cetrorelix for the prevention of premature luteinizing hormone surge during controlled ovarian stimulation using letrozole and gonadotropins: a randomized trial. Fertil Steril. 2008;90:113–20.
21. A double-blind, randomized, dose-finding study to assess the efficacy of the gonadotrophin-releasing hormone antagonist ganirelix (Org 37462) to prevent premature luteinizing hormone surges in women undergoing ovarian stimulation with recombinant follicle stimulating hormone (Puregon). The ganirelix dose-finding study group. Hum Reprod. 1998;13:3023–31.
22. Chen Q, Wang Y, Sun L, Zhang S, Chai W, Hong Q, Long H, Wang L, Lyu Q, Kuang Y. Controlled ovulation of the dominant follicle using progestin in minimal stimulation in poor responders. Reprod Biol Endocrinol. 2017;15:71.
23. Ezzati M, Carr BR. Elagolix, a novel, orally bioavailable GnRH antagonist under investigation for the treatment of endometriosis-related pain. Womens Health (Lond). 2015;11:19–28.
24. Carr BR, Stewart EA, Archer DF, et al. Elagolix alone or with add-Back therapy in women with heavy menstrual bleeding and uterine leiomyomas. Obstet Gynecol. 2018;132:1252–64.

Chapter 15
Preventing Premature Ovulation

Orhan Bukulmez

15.1   Introduction

The context of premature ovulation does not exactly refer to premature luteinization or unpreventable LH surge that is discussed in the previous section. This topic is rather more relevant to premature follicle rupture, which can be observed before the planned oocyte retrieval or at the time of the retrieval procedure itself.

In women with diminished ovarian reserve (DOR) and/or advanced reproductive age (ARA), after triggering for final oocyte maturation, even if the oocyte retrieval is attempted at the conventional time interval of 35–36 hours, disappearance of especially the follicles at or above 18 mm can be observed. At times, such follicles can be so fragile that even the gentle introduction of the transvaginal ultrasound probe may lead to rupture of the follicles in front of the operator's eyes. Other times, no follicles but only the fluid in the cul-de-sac can be observed leading to hopeless attempts of cul-de-sac fluid aspiration to find an oocyte. Considering the limited number of follicles in such patients and the corresponding small volume of fluid in the cul-de-sac, this attempt is usually unsuccessful and may potentially risk the case for especially bowel complications. Therefore, we mainly discuss preventive measures taken to prevent premature ovulation or follicle rupture, which is not associated with LH surge.

O. Bukulmez (✉)
Division of Reproductive Endocrinology and Infertility, Fertility and Advanced Reproductive Medicine Assisted Reproductive Technologies Program, Department of Obstetrics and Gynecology, University of Texas Southwestern Medical Center, Dallas, TX, USA
e-mail: Orhan.Bukulmez@UTSouthwestern.edu

© Springer Nature Switzerland AG 2020   195
O. Bukulmez (ed.), *Diminished Ovarian Reserve and Assisted Reproductive Technologies*, https://doi.org/10.1007/978-3-030-23235-1_15

15.2   Earlier Performance of Oocyte Retrieval After the Administration of Trigger Agent

The groups focusing on patients with DOR and poor ovarian response (POR) are well aware of the phenomenon of early follicle rupture not related to LH surge. Therefore, after triggering for final oocyte maturation with either gonadotropin-releasing hormone (GnRH) agonist or human chorionic gonadotropin (HCG), such practices schedule oocyte retrieval in 32–34 hours when the trigger agent was administered with follicle size ≥18 mm [1]. Some others administer HCG at 5000 IU when the leading follicle size exceeds 16 mm and the oocyte retrieval is performed 34 hours after the HCG administration to mitigate follicle rupture before follicle aspiration [2].

Triggering final oocyte maturation in women with ARA at or above the age of 43 years to prevent premature luteinization of the follicles not related to LH surge is also discussed in minimal stimulation chapter. There is some data supporting the administration HCG 10,000 IU when the leading follicle size is between 16 and 18 mm in conventional IVF stimulation cycles without changing the timing of the retrieval. This may also be relevant to younger DOR patients as well although with smaller follicle diameters, cytoplasmic immaturity may be an issue, which may impact proper embryo development [3].

On the other hand, at least from the studies in general IVF population, it is reported that the best time interval for oocyte retrieval after triggering for final oocyte maturation should be between 35 and 38 hours to get the most metaphase II oocytes [4]. In the former years of IVF, earlier oocyte retrievals were mainly performed to minimize the effects of unprevented LH surge before the era of GnRH agonist protocols and GnRH antagonist use. From the earlier days of IVF to now, the data suggest the optimal time interval to be 36 hours [5].

It was also suggested that if the oocyte retrieval was scheduled earlier than 36 hours after the triggering for final oocyte maturation, perhaps delayed denudation of the oocytes from their surrounding cumulus granulosa cells may compensate for the earlier retrieval in conventional IVF stimulation cases planned for intracytoplasmic injection (ICSI). This hypothesis was tested in a cohort study in women <38 years of age undergoing conventional IVF stimulation for ICSI, and the HCG trigger was administered with at least three follicles >17 mm. This retrospective study included retrieval time intervals between 34 and 38 hours after triggering but assessed in two groups whether the retrieval was done before or after 36 hours. Cumulus cell denudation time after the retrieval ranged between 5 minutes and 7 hours (mean 2.3 ± 1.3 hours). This was examined in two groups whether denudation was performed in less or more than 2 hours after the oocyte retrieval. As the time interval from HCG administration is extended beyond 36 hours, ICSI outcomes improved. Despite the similar proportion of metaphase II oocytes in each group, fertilization rates and clinical pregnancy rates with similar number and quality of the embryos transferred were higher in the group with oocyte retrieval performed beyond 36 hours as compared to those undergoing earlier oocyte retrievals.

Regardless of the HCG-retrieval interval, retrieval denudation interval did not show any impact on clinical pregnancy rates. In a similar fashion, denudation-ICSI interval (mean 1.2 ± 1.1 hours) did not affect ICSI outcome. The authors concluded that in patients with normal ovarian reserve undergoing ICSI, prolongation of the time for cumulus denudation while keeping the oocytes in culture or prolonging the ICSI time interval from denudation did not compensate the potential negative effects of performing oocyte retrievals earlier than 36 hours from the time of triggering for final oocyte maturation with HCG [6]. Certainly, many of such studies are from conventional IVF stimulation cycles and normal responders may not be relevant to minimal/mild stimulation or natural cycle approaches for women with POR, DOR, and/or ARA.

In the earlier years of our minimal stimulation IVF practice for patients with POR and DOR, we did observe disappearance of follicles or follicle collapse during the oocyte retrieval process if we sticked with the 36 hours interval from the time of HCG and/or GnRH agonist trigger. We then started to do the retrievals at 35 hours following the triggering. For some patients with oocyte maturation issues or problems in embryo progression after fertilization, we scheduled retrievals 35.5 hours after triggering. In patients with persistent early follicle collapse, performing oocyte retrievals as early as 34 hours may result in immature oocytes and issues with proper embryo progression. Therefore, we keep our retrieval times at 35 hours or 35.5 hours following the administration of the trigger agent. We take additional measures instead of doing earlier retrievals as described below.

15.3 Nonsteroidal Anti-inflammatory Agents

Indomethacin, one of the nonsteroidal anti-inflammatory drugs (NSAIDs), has been in use to prevent premature ovulation in IVF cycles [7]. Indomethacin found support especially in prevention of ovulation in natural cycles for IVF. This agent was shown to delay ovulation for a week when used as 50 mg orally three times daily for 7 days. Indomethacin is used in minimal stimulation IVF cycles at 50 mg dose provided on the day of GnRH agonist administration for triggering to prevent premature ovulation without adversely affecting LH surge-induced effects on oocyte maturation [1].

Inhibitory effects of indomethacin or aspirin on ovulation was first observed in rodents [8, 9]. It was then demonstrated that indomethacin does not prevent LH surge but acts directly on the ovary [10]. In pigs, it was reported that the inhibition of ovulation by the indomethacin given 24 hours after HCG trigger can be reversed by prostaglandin F2alpha administration [11].

In women, indomethacin at 50 mg orally three times daily used for 3 days or more started with the positive urinary LH testing was shown to delay ovulation without any ill effects on menstrual cycle length and FSH, LH, estradiol, and progesterone levels [12]. When used in modified natural IVF cycles as compared to the same treatment protocol without indomethacin use, while decreasing the rate of premature ovulation, indomethacin 50 mg orally three times daily started when follicles sizes reached 14 mm did not seem to have any adverse effects on embryo development and clinical pregnancy rates [13].

In summary, leukocytes, cytokines, and many inflammatory mediators including prostaglandins have a close relationship in the ovulation process [14]. NSAIDs, like indomethacin and ibuprofen, exert their actions by inhibiting the action of the cyclooxygenase enzymes (COX), which convert arachidonic acid to prostaglandin H2 (PGH2). Of the two isoforms, COX-1 and COX-2, COX-2 inhibition is the one thought to be involved in inhibiting the ovulation. The preovulatory rise in gonadotropins stimulates COX-2 in the granulosa cells, leading to an increase in PGH2 and other prostanoids. These in turn will act on granulosa and theca cells to induce secretion of matrix metalloproteinases (MMPs) that degrade the extracellular matrix, eventually leading to follicle rupture and ovulation [15]. LH surge itself induces this inflammatory cascade leading to follicle rupture through MMPs, which is inhibited by nonselective COX inhibitors like indomethacin and ibuprofen. However, such agents like ibuprofen may also have dose-related impact on platelet function which may resolve 24 hours after the last dose of ibuprofen [16].

In our practice, we use single 600 mg dose of oral ibuprofen, day after administration of HCG and/or GnRH analog, with lunch about 18 hours before the oocyte retrieval in select cases. These are typically women >40 years old with leading follicles >18 mm in sizes or with recent history of follicle rupture at the time of oocyte retrieval. We observed that ibuprofen single-dose regimen is adequate to prevent premature follicle rupture before or at the time of oocyte retrieval. In a small comparative within-patient study, 600 mg single dose of ibuprofen administered about 18 hours before oocyte retrieval was demonstrated to decrease the levels of interleukin (IL)-6, IL-8, eotaxin, granulocyte colony-stimulating factor, MMP-3, MMP-7, MMP-12, and MMP-13 as compared to the cycles of the same patients without ibuprofen use. Since in both consecutive cycles we did not observe premature follicle rupture in all patients with or without ibuprofen, at least this study shows that 600 mg single dose of ibuprofen does induce anti-inflammatory changes as reflected in the follicular fluid studies. We do not use higher doses or doses closer to the oocyte retrieval time to avoid potential bleeding tendency which may be associated with ibuprofen use [17, 18].

15.4 Conclusion

Prevention of premature ovulation or follicle rupture before or at the time of oocyte retrieval is an important issue affecting the oocyte yield especially in women with DOR and/or ARA undergoing minimal or mild stimulation protocols. We mainly discussed two strategies. One is planning oocyte retrieval earlier than the norm of 36 hours following the administration of the trigger agent. Some practitioners plan oocyte retrieval as early as 32 hours. However earlier retrievals can be associated with decrease in mature oocyte yield and embryo progression issues. Keeping the oocytes with their surrounding cumulus cells may not assist with mitigating such problems. NSAIDs have been use to prevent ovulation. Our preferred method of preventing premature ovulation is keeping oocyte retrieval time 35–35.5 hours after administration of the trigger agent while considering single oral dose of ibuprofen at 600 mg after lunch, about 18 hours before the oocyte retrieval procedure in select cases.

References

1. Zhang J, Chang L, Sone Y, Silber S. Minimal ovarian stimulation (mini-IVF) for IVF utilizing vitrification and cryopreserved embryo transfer. Reprod Biomed Online. 2010;21(4):485–95.
2. Mendez Lozano DH, Brum Scheffer J, Frydman N, Fay S, Fanchin R, Frydman R. Optimal reproductive competence of oocytes retrieved through follicular flushing in minimal stimulation IVF. Reprod Biomed Online. 2008;16(1):119–23.
3. Wu YG, Barad DH, Kushnir VA, Wang Q, Zhang L, Darmon SK, et al. With low ovarian reserve, Highly Individualized Egg Retrieval (HIER) improves IVF results by avoiding premature luteinization. J Ovarian Res. 2018;11(1):23.
4. Weiss A, Neril R, Geslevich J, Lavee M, Beck-Fruchter R, Golan J, et al. Lag time from ovulation trigger to oocyte aspiration and oocyte maturity in assisted reproductive technology cycles: a retrospective study. Fertil Steril. 2014;102(2):419–23.
5. Mansour RT, Aboulghar MA, Serour GI. Study of the optimum time for human chorionic gonadotropin-ovum pickup interval in in vitro fertilization. J Assist Reprod Genet. 1994;11(9):478–81.
6. Garor R, Shufaro Y, Kotler N, Shefer D, Krasilnikov N, Ben-Haroush A, et al. Prolonging oocyte in vitro culture and handling time does not compensate for a shorter interval from human chorionic gonadotropin administration to oocyte pickup. Fertil Steril. 2015;103(1):72–5.
7. Nargund G, Waterstone J, Bland J, Philips Z, Parsons J, Campbell S. Cumulative conception and live birth rates in natural (unstimulated) IVF cycles. Hum Reprod. 2001;16(2):259–62.
8. Armstrong DT, Grinwich DL. Blockade of spontaneous and LH-induced ovulation in rats by indomethacin, an inhibitor of prostaglandin biosynthesis. I. Prostaglandins. 1972;1(1):21–8.
9. Orczyk GP, Behrman HR. Ovulation blockade by aspirin or indomethacin – in vivo evidence for a role of prostaglandin in gonadotrophin secretion. Prostaglandins. 1972;1(1):3–20.
10. Sato T, Taya K, Jyujo T, Igarashi M. Ovulation block by indomethacin, an inhibitor of prostaglandin synthesis: a study of its site of action in rats. J Reprod Fertil. 1974;39(1):33–40.
11. Downey BR, Ainsworth L. Reversal of indomethacin blockade of ovulation in gilts by prostaglandins. Prostaglandins. 1980;19(1):17–22.
12. Athanasiou S, Bourne TH, Khalid A, Okokon EV, Crayford TJ, Hagstrom HG, et al. Effects of indomethacin on follicular structure, vascularity, and function over the periovulatory period in women. Fertil Steril. 1996;65(3):556–60.
13. Kadoch IJ, Al-Khaduri M, Phillips SJ, Lapensee L, Couturier B, Hemmings R, et al. Spontaneous ovulation rate before oocyte retrieval in modified natural cycle IVF with and without indomethacin. Reprod Biomed Online. 2008;16(2):245–9.
14. Bukulmez O, Arici A. Leukocytes in ovarian function. Hum Reprod Update. 2000;6(1):1–15.
15. Weiss G, Goldsmith LT, Taylor RN, Bellet D, Taylor HS. Inflammation in reproductive disorders. Reprod Sci. 2009;16(2):216–29.
16. Goldenberg NA, Jacobson L, Manco-Johnson MJ. Brief communication: duration of platelet dysfunction after a 7-day course of ibuprofen. Ann Intern Med. 2005;142(7):506–9.

17. Bou-Nemer L, Word A, Carr B, Bukulmez O. One dose of ibuprofen decreases levels of inter-leukins involved in ovulation in the follicular fluid of women undergoing minimalo stimulation in-vitro fertilization. Fertil Steril. 2017;108(3):e258.
18. Bou Nemer L, Shi H, Carr BR, Word RA, Bukulmez O. Effect of single-dose ibuprofen on follicular fluid levels of interleukins in poor responders undergoing in vitro fertilization. Syst Biol Reprod Med. 2019;65(1):48–53.

Chapter 16
Trigger Agents and Post-trigger Testing

John Wu, David Prokai, and Orhan Bukulmez

16.1 Trigger Agents

Human chorionic gonadotropin (hCG), a substitute for the endogenous mid-cycle surge of luteinizing hormone (LH), is the traditional trigger agent to induce final oocyte maturation for in vitro fertilization (IVF) cycles. This is because both hCG and LH stimulate the same LH receptor [1]. The principal difference lies in their half-lives where LH has a short circulating half-life of 30 minutes [2] in comparison to hCG with a prolonged half-life of approximately 37 hours [3]. Therefore, hCG is able to activate the entire cascade of ovarian hyperstimulation syndrome (OHSS) by sustaining multiple corpora lutea while inducing the vascular endothelial growth factor pathway [4, 5]. The risk of OHSS led to the use of GnRH agonists for the induction of LH surge as an alternative for exogenous hCG [6–8]. Previously, Nakano et al. exhibited that GnRH agonists were able to induce an LH surge [9]. GnRH-agonist-only trigger decreases the risk of OHSS significantly as compared to hCG-only trigger [10–12]. GnRH agonists can also induce a physiological-like LH and follicle-stimulating hormone (FSH) surge, which may result in better oocyte and embryo quality [13]. The additional FSH surge stimulates the resumption of oocyte meiosis, LH receptor formation, and cumulus expansion [14, 15]. Although the risk of OHSS is reduced, GnRH agonists alone induces luteolysis leading to a luteal phase defect, which has a negative effect on pregnancy rates in fresh embryo transfer cycles [16, 17].

J. Wu · D. Prokai · O. Bukulmez (✉)
Division of Reproductive Endocrinology and Infertility, Fertility and Advanced Reproductive Medicine Assisted Reproductive Technologies Program, Department of Obstetrics and Gynecology, University of Texas Southwestern Medical Center, Dallas, TX, USA
e-mail: Orhan.Bukulmez@UTSouthwestern.edu

© Springer Nature Switzerland AG 2020
O. Bukulmez (ed.), *Diminished Ovarian Reserve and Assisted Reproductive Technologies*, https://doi.org/10.1007/978-3-030-23235-1_16

16.2   Dual Trigger

A bolus of low-dose hCG combined with a GnRH agonist, called a dual trigger, was developed to improve oocyte maturation while providing sustained support for the luteal phase and decreasing the risk of OHSS [11, 18, 19]. The use of dual trigger increases the number of mature oocytes, fertilized embryos, and implantation and pregnancy rates in comparison to the use of hCG alone in normal and high responders [20]. The incidence of clinically significant OHSS is reduced to 0.5% [18]. We considered potential benefits of its use in women with expected POR undergoing minimal stimulation IVF which is followed by frozen embryo transfer (FET) as discussed in this book. We compared the minimal stimulation outcomes in patients with expected poor ovarian response (POR) undergoing minimal stimulation IVF with a freeze-all approach triggered with either hCG 10,000 units only or dual trigger with leuprolide 2 mg plus hCG 5000 units.

A first cycle analysis of 107 minimal stimulation IVF cycles was performed. All patients met ESHRE criteria for POR, defined as women age over 40 years, and/or with previous poor outcomes to conventional high-dose stimulation with ≤3 oocytes or with abnormal ovarian reserve tests anti-Mullerian hormone (AMH) < 1.1 ng/mL and/or total antral follicle count (TAFC) < 7 [21]. The primary outcome was the number of oocytes retrieved. The secondary outcomes were the number of mature metaphase II oocytes and the number of 2PN zygotes and whether any cleavage or blastocyst stage embryo was frozen. We were also interested to see whether dual trigger with leuprolide acetate and hCG resulted in a FSH surge as suggested in the literature in comparison to hCG-only trigger [13].

16.2.1   The Number of Oocytes Retrieved Was Comparable Between Single and Dual Trigger Groups

There were no significant differences in the baseline characteristics between the two groups (Table 16.1). There was a statistically significant difference in days of stimulation, total dose of gonadotropins, total antagonist dose (vials), peak follicle size (mm), pre-trigger P4 level (ng/mL), and percentage of patients that underwent

Table 16.1 Patient demographics and baseline characteristic (mean ± SD)

Characteristic	HCG trigger alone ($n = 55$)	Dual trigger ($n = 52$)	P value
Age at the time of the cycle (y)	38.36 ± 3.92	39.50 ± 3.05	0.10
Body mass index (kg/m^2)	26.39 ± 5.21	25.99 ± 5.43	0.70
Anti-Mullerian hormone (ng/mL)	0.74 ± 0.76	0.97 ± 0.92	0.16
Total antral follicle count (n)	7.78 ± 3.79	7.83 ± 5.17	0.96

Table 16.2 Characteristics and outcomes of ovarian stimulation (mean ± SD or % where applicable)

Variable	HCG trigger alone ($n = 55$)	Dual trigger ($n = 52$)	P value
Days of stimulation	**10.13 ± 1.29**	**10.98 ± 2.21**	**0.016**
Total gonadotropins (IU)	**500.45 ± 138.49**	**600.96 ± 229.71**	**0.007**
Total antagonist dose (vial)	**1.65 ± 0.89**	**2.66 ± 1.10**	**<0.001**
Peak follicle size (mm)	**21.99 ± 3.77**	**20.27 ± 2.88**	**0.009**
No of follicles ≥ 10 mm	4.25 ± 1.97	3.81 ± 1.92	0.24
No of follicles ≥ 14 mm	2.98 ± 1.41	2.81 ± 1.43	0.53
No follicles ≥ 16 mm	2.31 ± 1.25	2.13 ± 1.11	0.45
Pre-trigger E2 (pg/mL)	1082.56 ± 608.33 ($n = 54$)	926.35 ± 455.47	0.14
Pre-trigger LH (IU/L)	6.66 ± 4.23 ($n = 54$)	5.60 ± 3.16	0.15
Pre-trigger P4 (ng/mL)	**0.54 ± 0.35 ($n = 38$)**	**0.41 ± 0.21**	**0.033**
No of oocytes	2.69 ± 1.75	2.23 ± 1.35	0.10
No of MII	2.16 ± 1.27 ($n = 24$)	2.10 ± 1.27 ($n = 42$)	0.83
No of 2PN fertilization	2.09 ± 1.42	1.75 ± 1.33	0.20
ICSI (the remaining with conventional insemination)	**43.60%**	**80.80%**	**<0.001**
No of day 3 embryos frozen	1.57 ± 0.78 ($n = 7$)	1.13 ± 0.84 (n:8)	0.87
No of blastocyst stage embryos frozen	1.15 ± 1.13 ($n = 48$)	0.91 ± 1.18 (n:45)[a]	0.187
Any embryo frozen	67.27%	51.92%	0.12

[a]One patient with both day 3 and blastocyst stage embryos frozen

ICSI. However, no statistical differences were found for number of oocytes retrieved, MII oocytes, or the number of 2PN fertilized zygotes (Table 16.2). Further multivariate regression analysis confirmed that trigger type after adjusting for other independent variables was not found to be significant for predicting either the number of 2PN zygotes or the number of retrieved oocytes.

16.2.2 FSH Surge Is Induced by Dual Trigger in Minimal Stimulation Cycles

Pre- and post-trigger FSH levels were analyzed in 20 representative samples from both single and dual trigger patients. The patients triggered with hCG alone had an insignificant change in FSH levels, whereas the patients who underwent dual trigger showed an FSH surge as expected (Table 16.3). Therefore, an FSH surge induced by leuprolide trigger did not improve minimal stimulation IVF cycle outcome.

Table 16.3 Mean pre- and post-trigger FSH values to assess for FSH surge

Means	HCG trigger ($n = 10$)	Dual trigger ($n = 10$)	P value
Pre-trigger FSH (IU/L)	8.40	11.02	0.12
Post-trigger FSH (IU/L)	8.78	52.13	<0.001
Fold change	1.04	5.06	<0.001

16.3 Pre-trigger and Post-trigger Laboratory Testing

Testing the pre-trigger values of estradiol (E2) and progesterone (P4) may be predictive of the number of oocytes retrieved and the number of embryos developed [22]. Some authors suggest that the post-trigger E2 is predictive of live birth outcomes [23, 24], whereas others have not seen any differences [25, 26]. In women triggered with hCG alone, the levels of HCG and P4 are frequently checked the day after the trigger. These labs may help to assure medication compliance and potency as well. However, it was not clear if endocrinologic response to hCG trigger is predictive of minimal and mild stimulation outcomes in women with expected POR. To answer this question, we performed first cycle analysis of pre-trigger and post-trigger labs in minimal and mild stimulation cycles. Pre-trigger labs were from the day of hCG trigger, and post-trigger labs were assessed the day after trigger, in the morning.

16.3.1 Post-trigger FSH Levels

Our first cycle analysis of post- trigger FSH showed that the mean ± SD FSH levels were 11.4 ± 6.2 IU/L. FSH was found to be negatively correlated to the number of oocytes retrieved. As FSH levels increased, the number of oocytes retrieved decreased (Fig. 16.1). Elevated post-trigger FSH is likely due to endogenous FSH production reflecting severe diminished ovarian reserve with minimal contribution from the low-dose gonadotropins used in minimal and mild stimulation.

16.3.2 Pre- and Post-trigger E2, LH, and P4 and Post-trigger hCG Levels

We assessed the first cycle pre- and post-trigger data (E2, LH, P4, and post-trigger hCG) from minimal and mild stimulation cycles performed between 2016 and 2018 which involved 81 women. Both absolute values and fold change (post-trigger/pre-trigger ratios for E2, LH, and P4) were analyzed. The summary data is provided in Table 16.4. In regression models, only pre-trigger estradiol predicted the number of retrieved oocytes, which is in line with the published literature (Fig. 16.2).

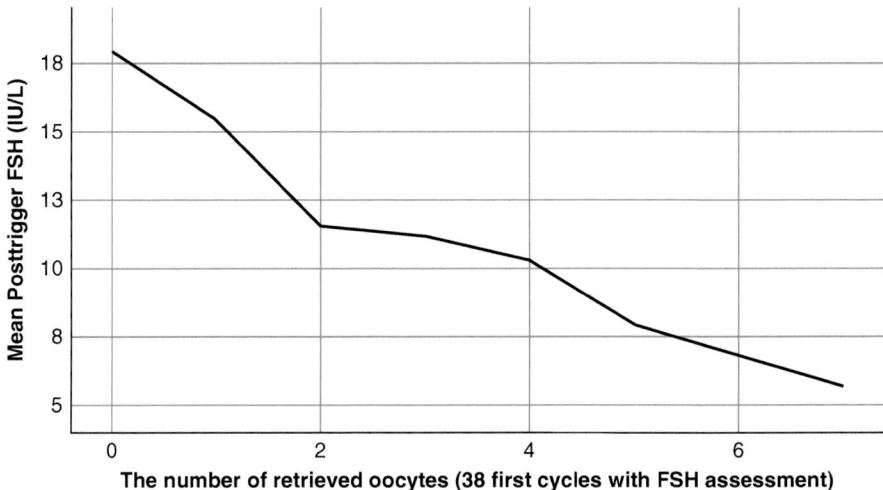

Fig. 16.1 The number of retrieved oocytes decreased with increasing post-trigger FSH levels

Table 16.4 First cycle parameters of minimal/mild stimulation treatment to assess pre- and post-trigger labs (81 patients; n, number of first cycles with the relevant data)

Parameters	Mean ± SD
Age (years)	39.6 ± 3.8
AMH (ng/mL)	1.07 ± 0.95
Total gonadotropin dose (IU)	672.5 ± 464.9
Pre-trigger E2 (pg/mL)	905.4 ± 439.0
Post-/pre-trigger E2 ratio	1.2 ± 0.2 (*n*:58)
Post-/pre-trigger P4 ratio	4.9 ± 3.6 (*n*:62)
Post-trigger HCG (IU/L)	268.9 ± 135.8 (*n*:61)
Retrieved oocytes	2.3 ± 1.7

SD standard deviation

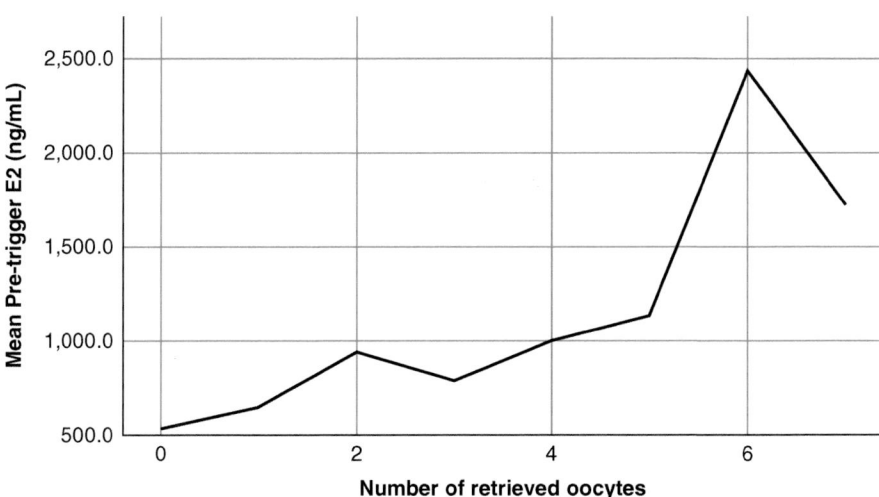

Fig. 16.2 The number of retrieved oocyte increased by increasing pre-trigger estradiol (E2) levels (first cycle analysis)

Post-trigger fold changes (post-trigger/pre-trigger ratios) of E2, LH, and P4 levels did not predict the number of oocytes retrieved in patients with expected POR undergoing minimal or mild stimulation. Some clinicians through personal/conference communications suggest that decreased E2 after trigger may be associated with an earlier ovulation in women with DOR/POR and the oocyte retrieval may be performed earlier than the planned time; however, this data has yet to be verified and published.

16.4   Conclusions

The use of dual trigger in minimal stimulation IVF for expected POR patients does not improve total oocyte or mature oocyte yield in contrast to various reports in normal responders even when accounting for age, BMI, AMH, total antral follicle count, and varying stimulation characteristics analyzed with multivariate regression. Although using a dual trigger has seemingly revolutionized conventional IVF by maintaining positive outcomes in stimulation cycles while minimizing risks of OHSS, the use of dual trigger in expected POR patients may not carry the same advantages. There is currently no evidence that the use of dual trigger improves stimulation outcomes in expected POR patients undergoing minimal stimulation IVF. Single trigger with hCG may be preferable due to the lower cost and improved patient comfort.

In terms of pre- and post-trigger labs in patients with DOR and/or ARA undergoing minimal and/or mild stimulation, only pre-trigger E2 levels seem to correlate with oocyte yield. Post-trigger fold changes of E2, LH, and P4 are not predictive of oocyte yield. Post-trigger hCG may be useful to demonstrate patient compliance; however, a simple home urine pregnancy test performed the day after hCG administration may provide a similar information and may be more convenient and less costly.

References

1. Pierce JG, Parsons TF. Glycoprotein protein hormones: structure and function. Ann Rev Biochem. 1981;50:465–95.
2. Schalch DS, Parlow AF, Boon RC, Reichlin S. Measurement of human luteinizing hormone in plasma by radioimmunoassay. J Clin Invest. 1968;47(3):665–78.
3. Faiman C, Ryan RJ, Zwirek SJ, Rubin ME. Serum FSH and HCG during human pregnancy and puerperium. J Clin Endocrinol Metab. 1968;28(9):1323–9.
4. Emperaire JC, Ruffie A. Triggering ovulation with endogenous luteinizing hormone may prevent the ovarian hyperstimulation syndrome. Hum Reprod. 1991;6(4):506–10.
5. Navot D, Bergh PA, Laufer N. Ovarian hyperstimulation syndrome in novel reproductive technologies: prevention and treatment. Fertil Steril. 1992;58(2):249–61.

6. Gonen Y, Casper RF, Jacobson W, Blankier J. Endometrial thickness and growth during ovarian stimulation: a possible predictor of implantation in in vitro fertilization. Fertil Steril. 1989;52(3):446–50.
7. Imoedemhe DA, Sigue AB, Pacpaco EL, Olazo AB. Stimulation of endogenous surge of luteinizing hormone with gonadotropin-releasing hormone analog after ovarian stimulation for in vitro fertilization. Fertil Steril. 1991;55(2):328–32.
8. Olivennes F, Fanchin R, Bouchard P, Taieb J, Frydman R. Triggering of ovulation by a gonadotropin-releasing hormone (GnRH) agonist in patients pretreated with a GnRH antagonist. Fertil Steril. 1996;66(1):151–3.
9. Nakano R, Mizuno T, Kotsuji F, Katayama K, Washio M, Tojo S. "Triggering" of ovulation after infusion of synthetic luteinizing hormone releasing factor (LRF). Acta Obstet Gynecol Scand. 1973;5(3):269–72.
10. Kol S. Luteolysis induced by a gonadotropin-releasing hormone agonist is the key to prevention of ovarian hyperstimulation syndrome. Fertil Steril. 2004;81(1):1–5.
11. Shapiro BS, Daneshmand ST, Garner FC, Aguirre M, Thomas S. Gonadotropin-releasing hormone agonist combined with a reduced dose of human chorionic gonadotropin for final oocyte maturation in fresh autologous cycles of in vitro fertilization. Fertil Steril. 2008;90(1):231–3.
12. Itskovitz-Eldor J, Kol S, Mannaerts B. Use of a single bolus of GnRH agonist triptorelin to trigger ovulation after GnRH antagonist ganirelix treatment in women undergoing ovarian stimulation for assisted reproduction, with special reference to the prevention of ovarian hyperstimulation syndrome: preliminary report: short communication. Hum Reprod. 2000;15(9):1965–8.
13. Griffin D, Feinn R, Engmann L, Nulsen J, Budinetz T, Benadiva C. Dual trigger with gonadotropin-releasing hormone agonist and standard dose human chorionic gonadotropin to improve oocyte maturity rates. Fertil Steril. 2014;102(2):405–9.
14. Andersen CY, Leonardsen L, Ulloa-Aguirre A, Barrios-De-Tomasi J, Moore L, Byskov AG. FSH-induced resumption of meiosis in mouse oocytes: effect of different isoforms. Mol Hum Reprod. 1999;5(8):726–31.
15. Eppig JJ. FSH stimulates hyaluronic acid synthesis by oocyte-cumulus cell complexes from mouse preovulatory follicles. Nature. 1979;281(5731):483–4.
16. Griesinger G, Diedrich K, Devroey P, Kolibianakis EM. GnRH agonist for triggering final oocyte maturation in the GnRH antagonist ovarian hyperstimulation protocol: a systematic review and meta-analysis. Hum Reprod Update. 2006;12(2):159–68.
17. Orvieto R, Rabinson J, Meltzer S, Zohav E, Anteby E, Homburg R. Substituting HCG with GnRH agonist to trigger final follicular maturation - A retrospective comparison of three different ovarian stimulation protocols. Reprod Biomed Online. 2006;13(2):198–201.
18. Shapiro BS, Daneshmand ST, Garner FC, Aguirre M, Hudson C. Comparison of "triggers" using leuprolide acetate alone or in combination with low-dose human chorionic gonadotropin. Fertil Steril. 2011;95(8):2715–7.
19. Griffin D, Benadiva C, Kummer N, Budinetz T, Nulsen J, Engmann L. Dual trigger of oocyte maturation with gonadotropin-releasing hormone agonist and low-dose human chorionic gonadotropin to optimize live birth rates in high responders. Fertil Steril. 2012;97(6):1316–20.
20. Lin MH, Shao-Ying Wu F, Kuo-Kuang Lee R, Li SH, Lin SY, Hwu YM. Dual trigger with combination of gonadotropin-releasing hormone agonist and human chorionic gonadotropin significantly improves the live-birth rate for normal responders in GnRH-antagonist cycles. Fertil Steril. 2013;100(5):1296–302.
21. Ferraretti AP, La Marca A, Fauser BCJM, Tarlatzis B, Nargund G, Gianaroli L, et al. ESHRE consensus on the definition of "poor response" to ovarian stimulation for in vitro fertilization: the Bologna criteria. Hum Reprod. 2011;26(7):1616–24.
22. Zhu H, Liu L, Yang L, Xue Y, Tong X, Jiang L, et al. The effect of progesterone level prior to oocyte retrieval on the numbers of oocytes retrieved and embryo quality in IVF treatment cycles: an analysis of 2,978 cycles. J Assist Reprod Genet. 2014;31(9):1183–7.

23. Kondapalli LA, Molinaro TA, Sammel MD, Dokras A. A decrease in serum estradiol levels after human chorionic gonadotrophin administration predicts significantly lower clinical pregnancy and live birth rates in in vitro fertilization cycles. Hum Reprod. 2012;27(9):2690–7.
24. Reljic M, Vlaisavljevic V, Gavric V, Kovacic B, Cizek-Sajko M. Value of the serum estradiol level on the day of human chorionic gonadotropin injection and on the day after in predicting the outcome in natural in vitro fertilization/intracytoplasmic sperm injection cycles. Fertil Steril. 2001;75(3):539–43.
25. Chiasson MD, Bates GW, Robinson RD, Arthur NJ, Propst AM. Measuring estradiol levels after human chorionic gonadotropin administration for in vitro fertilization is not clinically useful. Fertil Steril. 2007;87(2):448–50.
26. Huang R, Fang C, Wang N, Li L, Yi Y, Liang X. Serum estradiol level change after human chorionic gonadotropin administration had no correlation with live birth rate in IVF cycles. Eur J Obstet Gynecol Reprod Biol. 2014;178:177–82.

Chapter 17
Oocyte Retrieval

John Wu

17.1 Introduction

In 1970, Steptoe and Edwards successfully recovered oocytes for in vitro fertilization (IVF) via laparoscopy. Patients underwent laparoscopy 29–31 hours after hCG administration. At first, they used a syringe and needle for aspiration but noted that it was lacking which led to the development of an aspiration device. Through a medium bore needle acting as a sleeve, the aspiration needle was inserted for repeated entry into the abdominal cavity. Follicles, described as bluish, pink swellings, were penetrated separately with a maximum vacuum pressure of 120 mmHg to avoid damage to the oocytes [1]. This technique pioneered minimally invasive oocyte retrieval. Other techniques including the transabdominal ultrasound guided transvesical route followed [2] but were limited by the distance of the abdominal probe to the ovaries and complications from traversing the bladder [3].

Fifteen years later in 1985, Wikland and colleagues described the first transvaginal ultrasound-guided oocyte retrieval [4], which has remained the standard technique for its improved visualization, cost effectiveness, and fewer complications [5, 6]. The optimal oocyte retrieval techniques will be discussed in this chapter. Many of the techniques apply to all patients regardless of protocol; however, we will also address the specific differences in technique that may be preferable in minimal and/ or mild stimulation protocols used in women with diminished ovarian reserve (DOR) and/or advanced reproductive age (ARA).

J. Wu (✉)
Division of Reproductive Endocrinology and Infertility, Department of Obstetrics and Gynecology, The University of Texas Southwestern Medical Center, Dallas, TX, USA
e-mail: john.wu@utsouthwestern.edu

© Springer Nature Switzerland AG 2020
O. Bukulmez (ed.), *Diminished Ovarian Reserve and Assisted Reproductive Technologies*, https://doi.org/10.1007/978-3-030-23235-1_17

17.2   Anesthesia

Adequate anesthesia is an essential part of a successful oocyte retrieval. There are several approaches including local analgesia, regional analgesia, conscious sedation, and general anesthesia [7]. After weighing the risks and benefits of each method, the use of conscious sedation combining propofol, fentanyl, and midazolam is recommended. There is concern that the use of propofol has toxic effects on the ability of the oocytes to be fertilized in mice [8] and that propofol can be identified in the follicular fluid [9]. Nevertheless, propofol has no negative effect on fertilization rates, pregnancy rates, or live birth rates [10]. Due to its safety profile, quick induction properties, and minimal effects on clinical outcomes, conscious sedation with propofol is recommended as first-line anesthesia for minimal stimulation IVF. We recommend that induction with propofol occurs just prior to the introduction of the needle in order to minimize the exposure of the oocytes to anesthetic agents.

If no anesthesiologist is available, the use of local analgesia may be considered. Using a paracervical block with lidocaine may be employed; however, its effectiveness alone is questionable. In one study, 43% of women with a paracervical block reported the procedure as "very painful" or "painful"; nearly a third of the women required additional IV sedation during the procedure [11]. However, this is the most cost-effective method available.

17.3   Prevention of Infection

17.3.1   Prophylactic Antibiotics

The risk of post-procedure infection, such as pelvic inflammatory disease, is estimated to be 0.3% [12]. Prophylactic antibiotic treatment is controversial due to the low incidence of infectious complications following retrieval. A retrospective study comparing oocyte donors who received prophylactic antibiotics for oocyte retrieval reduced postoperative infection from 0.4% to 0.0% in the group receiving antibiotics [13]. Due to the minimal benefits of using universal antibiotic prophylaxis, we reserve prophylactic antibiotics for high-risk groups such as patients with endometriomas, history of pelvic inflammatory disease, hydrosalpinx, or a transuterine aspiration.

17.3.2   Cleansing of Vagina

Antiseptics such as povidone-iodine solution are toxic to oocytes, and evidence suggests that their use prior to retrieval may be associated with lower pregnancy rates in comparison to normal saline [14]. Thorough irrigation with sterile saline prior to needle puncture is adequate to clean the vagina and decrease bacterial load.

17.4   Equipment

17.4.1   Transvaginal Ultrasound

Transvaginal ultrasound-guided oocyte retrieval is considered standard of care. It improves imaging of the ovaries due to the close proximity of the probe to the structure of interest. Furthermore, transvaginal sonography employs the use of high-frequency sound waves via a specialized endovaginal probe (5/7.5 MHz) in comparison to the low-frequency transabdominal probe (3/3.5 MHz). The higher frequency improves visualization of nearby structures but decreases depth.

17.4.2   Needle

The most common needle sizes range from 16 to 20 gauge. Advantages of larger lumen needles include increased stiffness for easier follicle puncture and higher oocyte recovery rates. Advantages of thinner needles include less damage to the cumulus-oocyte complex, less pain, and less bleeding.

An important consideration for needle size and tubing length is the concept of dead space. With larger lumen needles and longer tubing, there is an increased potential for dead space which translates into requiring more follicular fluid to be aspirated before follicular fluid enters the collecting tubule. Prolonged residence of aspirate in the dead space may lead to loss of oocytes or exposure of the oocytes to toxic conditions [15].

We recommend a single lumen 17-gauge needle. There are commercially available double lumen needles purposed for flushing. One lumen is for the introduction of the flushing media, while the other is for the aspiration of the follicular fluid.

The use of needle guides is imperative for effective and safe retrievals. Both disposable and reusable needle guides are commercially available. A needle guide is secured along the transvaginal probe through which the needle can be placed (Fig. 17.1). This allows the surgeon to direct the needle with accuracy. Furthermore, it allows the needle tip to be visualized at all times. If the needle tip cannot be seen, the needle should be removed and the needle guide should be inspected to ensure secure placement on the probe.

17.4.3   Vacuum

Using a vacuum system for stable negative pressures is essential (Fig. 17.2). The typical range is between 80 and 300 mmHg; however, we recommend a lower pressure < 140 mmHg. Higher pressures above 180 mmHg may damage the oocyte [16]. Increasing the aspiration pressure will increase the velocity of the fluid and thus increase the shear forces on the cumulus-oocyte complex [15]. The

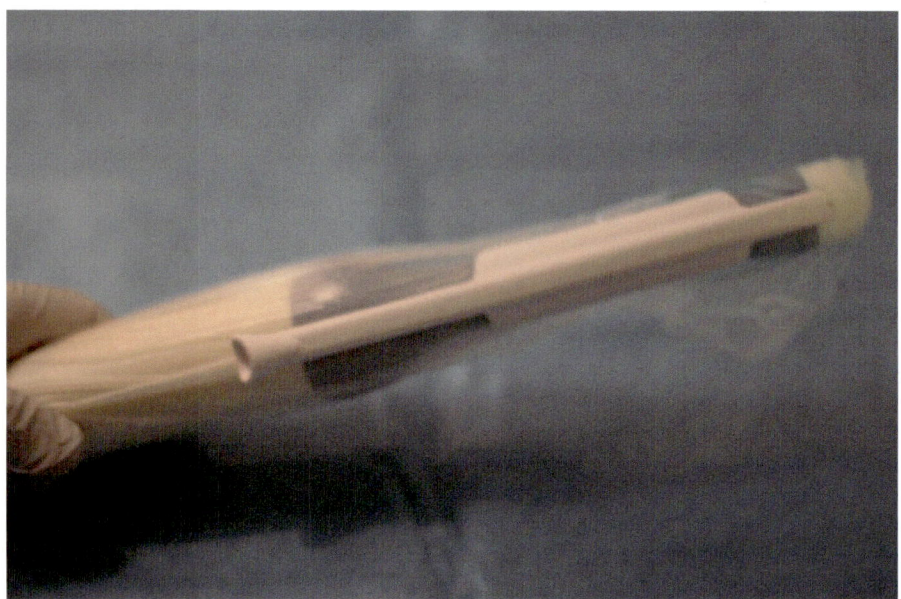

Fig. 17.1 Transvaginal ultrasound probe with disposable needle guide

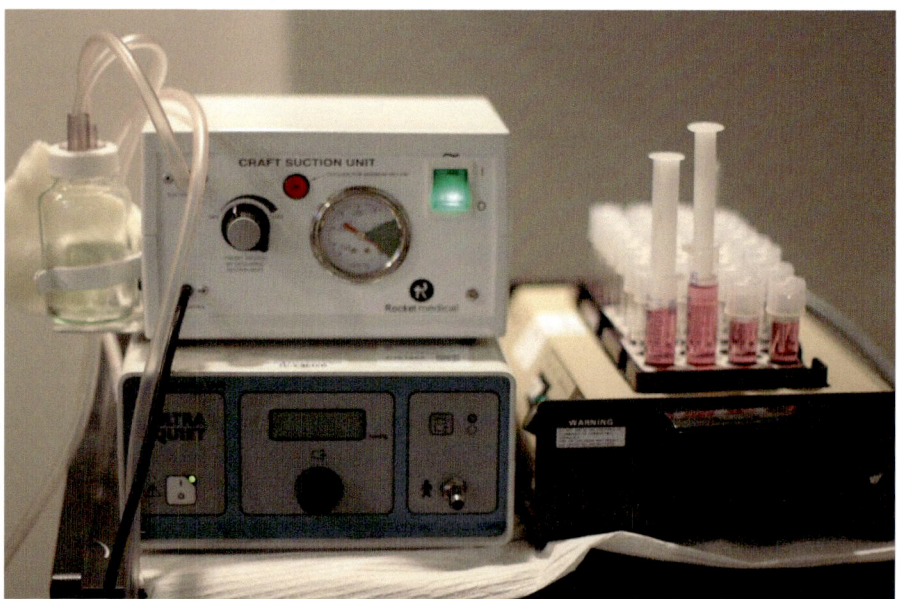

Fig. 17.2 Mechanical aspiration system

use of a manual syringe is not recommended due to the unknown pressures exerted and the increased risk for damaged oocytes [17].

17.5   Technique

17.5.1   Patient Positioning

The patient is placed in dorsal lithotomy position in Allen stirrups prior to induction of anesthesia to minimize the exposure of the oocytes to anesthetic agents. The patient should be situated at the end of the operating table, to allow for maximal maneuverability of the ultrasound probe. However, care must be taken to ensure that the sacrum is fully supported by the operating bed.

17.5.2   Bladder Decompression

Patients should empty their bladder prior to oocyte retrieval to decrease risk of needle puncture of the bladder. If the bladder is noted to be full during the initial ultrasound, the bladder should be drained with a catheter. No antibiotics are necessary if catheterization is performed.

17.5.3   Fixation of the Ovary

Using the ultrasound probe, the ovary must be fixed against the pelvic sidewall to ensure successful puncture. If the ovary is not adequately fixed, the needle may further displace the ovary rather than puncture the ovary. Care must be made to ensure that no vessels, bowel, and/or bladder is in between the vaginal wall and the ovary. Color Doppler may be employed to identify vascularity. If the ovary cannot be adequately fixed against the pelvic sidewall, an assistant may provide abdominal pressure to help fix the ovary.

17.5.4   Needle Entry

Faster needle entry should be employed to increase position accuracy and decrease tissue damage. Robotic studies show that the puncture force required and tissue displacement both decrease as the insertion velocity of the needle increases in biological tissues [18]. Thus, it is desirable to enter the follicles with as much velocity as safely possible. For difficult entries in which the ovary is displaced with needle force or the wall of the follicle stretches, drilling into the follicle with gentle rotation may be employed. However, this likely increases the size of the hole in the follicle wall which is less desirable due to potential loss of the oocyte between the follicle wall and the needle. The depth of entry should be approximately two-thirds of the total follicular depth to ensure that the needle is in the follicle for a safe and effective aspiration.

17.5.5 Follicle Curetting

Some practitioners do not move the needle once it is entered into the follicle, while others employ a technique called follicle curetting. This technique involves rotating the needle inside the follicle after complete aspiration of the follicular fluid. Dahl et al. found that follicular curetting significantly increased oocyte yield [19]. An additional benefit may be the result of preventing needle obstruction by a collapsed wall or debris.

17.5.6 Follicle Size

Studies have shown that there is a high rate of oocyte recovery in follicles with a mean diameter greater than 12 mm on sonography [20]. Therefore, we attempt to aspirate all follicles >10 mm (Fig. 17.3).

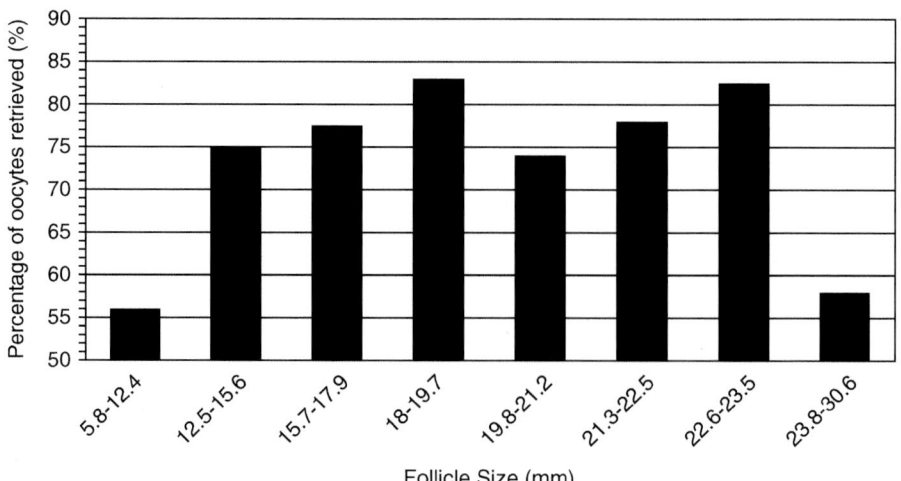

Fig. 17.3 Percentage of follicles from which an oocyte was obtained as function of follicle size. (Modified from Wittmaack et al. [20])

17.5.7   Flushing of Follicles in Minimal and Mild Stimulation Cycles

Follicular flushing has been shown to increase the likelihood of recovering a retained oocyte. Bagtharia and Haloob demonstrated that 40% of oocytes are obtained with a single aspiration, whereas 82% of oocytes could be recovered with two flushes, and up to 97% of oocytes could be retrieved with up to four flushes [21]. In minimal stimulation cycles, it is imperative to obtain every single oocyte due to the low number of expected oocytes per cycle.

The principle of flushing is to replace the follicle with additional fluid to flush out the oocyte. After the follicle is aspirated, the needle is left in place because removal of the needle from the follicle precludes flushing. Flushing requires an assistant to exchange tubes and flush, being careful to prevent introduction of air into the system (Fig. 17.4). The amount of flushing media to inject can be determined visually, attempting to fill the collapsed follicle to its original size or based on the size of follicle (Table 17.1). Flushing should be repeated until the oocyte is recovered or the follicle has lost its integrity and no longer expands with flushing. Most follicles will be retrieved within the first couple

Fig. 17.4 Oocyte collection and flushing

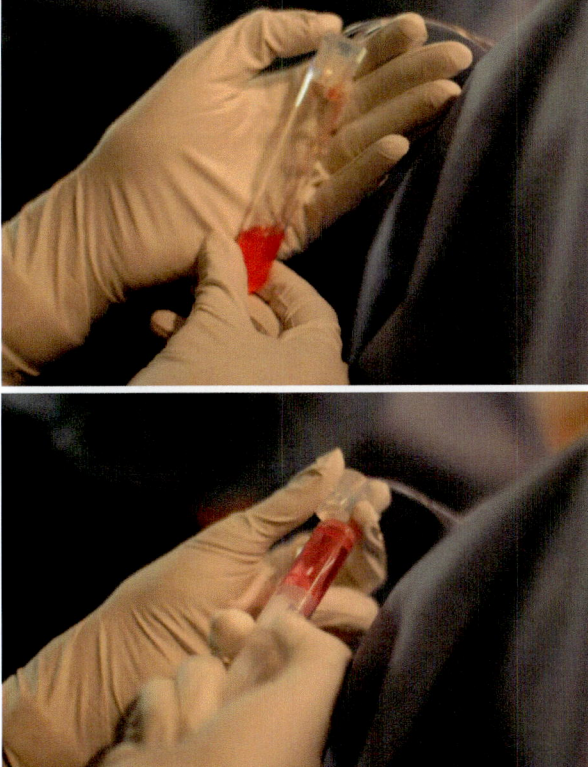

Table 17.1 Amount of flush
per follicle size

Average diameter (mm)	Media flush (mL)
10	0.5
12	1.0
14	1.5
16	2.0
18	3.0
20	4.0
22	5.5
24	7.0

flushes; however, it may take upward of ten flushes for a single follicle! Oocytes collected by flushing do result in embryos and eventual live birth.

17.5.8 Application of Vacuum Pressure

During introduction of the needle into the follicle, there is an increase in the internal pressure of the follicle. Thus, during needle puncture, there may be loss of follicular fluid and possibly the oocyte between the wall of the follicle and the needle. Therefore, vacuum pressure should be applied prior to and during follicle puncture. Furthermore, after the follicle is aspirated, negative pressure is created within the follicle. If the needle is removed without vacuum pressure, there will be backflow from the tubing into the follicle, and once again the oocyte may be pulled back into the follicle. Accordingly, when leaving the follicle, vacuum pressure should be maintained to prevent backflow [22].

17.6 Complications

Although rare, complications of oocyte retrieval include injury to pelvic organs, hemorrhage, and infection. The most common complication is minor vaginal bleeding occurring in 1.4–18.4% of all punctures [23]. Tips to decrease risk of hemorrhage include minimizing movement of the needle in the vaginal wall which may cause vaginal tearing and reducing the number of vaginal and ovarian punctures. The majority of vaginal bleeding can be treated with application of pressure and if necessary topical agents and rarely suture.

Intra-abdominal bleeding likely occurs after all retrievals, even after uncomplicated retrievals. Dessole et al. estimated that 230 mL of blood loss at 24 hours is normal after an uncomplicated retrieval [24]. Intra-abdominal hemorrhage following transvaginal oocyte retrieval occurs in 0.07–0.08% of punctures [25, 26]. Hemoperitoneum may result due to puncture of pelvic vessels such as the iliac, uterine, and ovarian vessels. Risk of hemorrhage increases in patients with coagulopathy and difficult cases in which transuterine routes must be utilized.

The risk of pelvic infection is reported between 0.01% and 0.6% [27]. The risk of infection is due to introducing pathogenic microorganisms into the peritoneal cavity from the vagina. The risk is further potentiated in the presence of pelvic inflammatory disease, hydrosalpinges, and chronic inflammation such as endometriosis [28]. Pelvic infections after transvaginal oocyte retrieval often present as pelvic abscesses [29]. The use of prophylactic antibiotics may decrease rates of infection, but the absolute risk of pelvic infection is rare; thus we recommend antibiotics for high-risk patients such as those with pelvic inflammatory disease, endometriosis, or hydrosalpinges.

17.7 Conclusion

Over time, the process of oocyte retrieval has been enhanced to improve outcomes. Although the majority of clinicians perform oocyte retrievals similarly, i.e., transvaginal needle aspiration, there still are variations in practice including type of anesthesia, prophylactic antibiotics, and equipment. In minimal stimulation for the diminished ovarian reserve patient, the number of oocytes expected is much lower than conventional stimulation in normo- and high responders; thus the use of follicular flushing is recommended to ensure the maximal number of oocytes retrieved per cycle.

References

1. Steptoe P, Edwards R. Laparoscopic recovery of preovulatory human oocytes after priming of ovaries with gonadotrophins. Lancet [Internet]. 1970 Apr 4 [cited 2018 Nov 15];295(7649):683–9. Available from: https://www.sciencedirect.com/science/article/pii/S0140673670909232?via%3Dihub.
2. Lenz S. Percutaneous oocyte recovery using ultrasound. Clin Obstet Gynaecol [Internet]. 1985 Dec [cited 2018 Nov 15];12(4):785–98. Available from: http://www.ncbi.nlm.nih.gov/pubmed/3914383.
3. Ashkenazi J, Ben David M, Feldberg D, Shelef M, Dicker D, Goldman JA. Abdominal complications following ultrasonically guided percutaneous transvesical collection of oocytes for in vitro fertilization. J In Vitro Fert Embryo Transf [Internet]. 1987 Dec [cited 2018 Nov 15];4(6):316–8. Available from: http://www.ncbi.nlm.nih.gov/pubmed/3437215.
4. Wikland M, Enk L, Hamberger L. Transvesical and transvaginal approaches for the aspiration of follicles by use of ultrasound. Ann N Y Acad Sci [Internet]. 1985 [cited 2018 Nov 15];442:182–94. Available from: http://www.ncbi.nlm.nih.gov/pubmed/3893266.
5. Feldberg D, Goldman JA, Ashkenazi J, Shelef M, Dicker D, Samuel N. Transvaginal oocyte retrieval controlled by vaginal probe for in vitro fertilization: a comparative study. J Ultrasound Med [Internet]. 1988 Jun 1 [cited 2018 Nov 15];7(6):339–43. Available from: http://doi.wiley.com/10.7863/jum.1988.7.6.339.
6. Cohen J, Debache C, Pez JP, Junca AM, Cohen-Bacrie P. Transvaginal sonographically controlled ovarian puncture for oocyte retrieval for in vitro fertilization. J In Vitro Fert Embryo Transf [Internet]. 1986 Oct [cited 2018 Nov 16];3(5):309–13. Available from: http://www.ncbi.nlm.nih.gov/pubmed/3537171.

7. Vlahos NF, Giannakikou I, Vlachos A, Vitoratos N. Analgesia and anesthesia for assisted reproductive technologies. Int J Gynecol Obstet [Internet]. 2009 Jun 1 [cited 2018 Nov 19];105(3):201–5. Available from: https://www.sciencedirect.com/science/article/pii/S002072920900040X.

8. Tatone C, Francione A, Marinangeli F, Lottan M, Varrassi G, Colonna R. An evaluation of propofol toxicity on mouse oocytes and preimplantation embryos. Hum Reprod [Internet]. 1998 Feb [cited 2018 Nov 19];13(2):430–5. Available from: http://www.ncbi.nlm.nih.gov/pubmed/9557852.

9. Coetsier T, Dhont M, Sutter P De, Merchiers E, Versichelen L, Rosseel MT. Propofol anaesthesia for ultrasound guided oocyte retrieval: accumulation of the anaesthetic agent in follicular fluid. Hum Reprod [Internet]. 1992 Nov 1 [cited 2018 Nov 19];7(10):1422–4. Available from: https://academic.oup.com/humrep/article/664652/Propofol.

10. Goutziomitrou E, Venetis CA, Kolibianakis EM, Bosdou JK, Parlapani A, Grimbizis G, et al. Propofol versus thiopental sodium as anaesthetic agents for oocyte retrieval: a randomized controlled trial. Reprod Biomed Online [Internet]. 2015 Dec [cited 2018 Nov 19];31(6):752–9. Available from: https://linkinghub.elsevier.com/retrieve/pii/S1472648315004253.

11. Hammarberg K, Wikland M, Nilsson L, Enk L. Patients' experience of transvaginal follicle aspiration under local anesthesia. Ann N Y Acad Sci [Internet]. 1988 Oct 1 [cited 2018 Nov 19];541(1 In Vitro Fert):134–7. Available from: http://doi.wiley.com/10.1111/j.1749-6632.1988.tb22249.x.

12. Roest J, Mous H, Zeilmaker G, Verhoeff A. The incidence of major clinical complications in a Dutch transport IVF programme. Hum Reprod Update [Internet]. 1996 Jul 1 [cited 2018 Nov 19];2(4):345–53. Available from: https://academic.oup.com/humupd/article-lookup/doi/10.1093/humupd/2.4.345.

13. Weinreb EB, Cholst IN, Ledger WJ, Danis RB, Rosenwaks Z. Should all oocyte donors receive prophylactic antibiotics for retrieval? Fertil Steril [Internet]. 2010 Dec 1 [cited 2018 Nov 19];94(7):2935–7. Available from: https://www.sciencedirect.com/science/article/pii/S001502821000926X?via%3Dihub.

14. van Os HC, Roozenburg BJ, Janssen-Caspers HA, Leerentveld RA, Scholtes MC, Zeilmaker GH, et al. Vaginal disinfection with povidone iodine and the outcome of in-vitro fertilization. Hum Reprod [Internet]. 1992 Mar [cited 2018 Nov 19];7(3):349–50. Available from: http://www.ncbi.nlm.nih.gov/pubmed/1587940.

15. Rose BI. Approaches to oocyte retrieval for advanced reproductive technology cycles planning to utilize in vitro maturation: a review of the many choices to be made. J Assist Reprod Genet [Internet]. 2014 Nov [cited 2018 Nov 29];31(11):1409–19. Available from: http://www.ncbi.nlm.nih.gov/pubmed/25212532.

16. Hashimoto S, Fukuda A, Murata Y, Kikkawa M, Oku H, Kanaya H, et al. Effect of aspiration vacuum on the developmental competence of immature human oocytes retrieved using a 20-gauge needle. Reprod Biomed Online [Internet]. 2007 Jan 1 [cited 2018 Nov 26];14(4):444–9. Available from: https://www.sciencedirect.com/science/article/pii/S1472648310608917?via%3Dihub.

17. Cohen J, Avery S, Campbell S, Mason BA, Riddle A, Sharma V. Follicular aspiration using a syringe suction system may damage the zona pellucida. J In Vitro Fert Embryo Transf [Internet]. 1986 Aug [cited 2018 Nov 30];3(4):224–6. Available from: http://www.ncbi.nlm.nih.gov/pubmed/3760658.

18. Mahvash M, Dupont PE. Fast needle insertion to minimize tissue deformation and damage. IEEE Int Conf Robot Autom ICRA [proceedings] IEEE Int Conf Robot Autom [Internet]. 2009 Jul 6 [cited 2018 Nov 29];2009:3097–3102. Available from: http://www.ncbi.nlm.nih.gov/pubmed/21399738.

19. Dahl SK, Cannon S, Aubuchon M, Williams DB, Robins JC, Thomas MA. Follicle curetting at the time of oocyte retrieval increases the oocyte yield. J Assist Reprod Genet [Internet]. 2009 Jun [cited 2018 Nov 29];26(6):335–9. Available from: http://www.ncbi.nlm.nih.gov/pubmed/19548079.

20. Wittmaack FM, Kreger DO, Blasco L, Tureck RW, Mastroianni L, Lessey BA. Effect of follicular size on oocyte retrieval, fertilization, cleavage, and embryo quality in in vitro fertilization cycles: a 6-year data collection. Fertil Steril [Internet]. 1994 Dec 1 [cited 2018 Nov 29];62(6):1205–10. Available from: https://www.sciencedirect.com/science/article/pii/S00150 28216571866?via%3Dihub.
21. Bagtharia S, Haloob A. Is there a benefit from routine follicular flushing for oocyte retrieval? J Obstet Gynaecol (Lahore) [Internet]. 2005 May 2. [cited 2018 Nov 26];25(4):374–376. Available from: http://www.tandfonline.com/doi/full/10.1080/01443610500118970.
22. Horne R, Bishop CJ, Reeves G, Wood C, Kovacs GT. Aspiration of oocytes for in-vitro fertilization [Internet]. Vol. 2, Human reproduction update. 1996 [cited 2018 Nov 29]. Available from: https://pdfs.semanticscholar.org/cca0/988ca5db0b8487a22e3755a9f21e3c1d524e.pdf.
23. El-Shawarby SA, Margara RA, Trew GH, Lavery SA. A review of complications following transvaginal oocyte retrieval for in-vitro fertilization. Hum Fertil [Internet]. 2004 Jun 3 [cited 2018 Nov 30];7(2):127–33. Available from: http://www.tandfonline.com/doi/full/10.1080/146 47270410001699081.
24. Dessole S, Rubattu G, Ambrosini G, Miele M, Nardelli GB, Cherchi PL. Blood loss following noncomplicated transvaginal oocyte retrieval for in vitro fertilization. Fertil Steril [Internet]. 2001 Jul 1 [cited 2018 Nov 30];76(1):205–6. Available from: https://www.sciencedirect.com/science/article/pii/S0015028201018581?via%3Dihub.
25. Dicker D, Ashkenazi J, Feldberg D, Levy T, Dekel A, Ben-Rafael Z. Severe abdominal complications after transvaginal ultrasonographically guided retrieval of oocytes for in vitro fertilization and embryo transfer. Fertil Steril [Internet]. 1993 Jun [cited 2018 Nov 30];59(6):1313–5. Available from: http://www.ncbi.nlm.nih.gov/pubmed/8495784.
26. Bennett SJ, Waterstone JJ, Cheng WC, Parsons J. Complications of transvaginal ultrasound-directed follicle aspiration: a review of 2670 consecutive procedures. J Assist Reprod Genet [Internet]. 1993 Jan [cited 2018 Nov 30];10(1):72–7. Available from: http://www.ncbi.nlm. nih.gov/pubmed/8499683.
27. Bodri D, Guillén JJ, Polo A, Trullenque M, Esteve C. Complications related to ovarian stimulation and oocyte retrieval in 4052 oocyte donor cycles [Internet]. Vol. 17. 2008 [cited 2018 Dec 3]. Available from: www.rbmonline.com/Article/3310.
28. Moini A, Riazi K, Amid V, Ashrafi M, Tehraninejad E, Madani T, et al. Endometriosis may contribute to oocyte retrieval-induced pelvic inflammatory disease: report of eight cases{1}. J Assist Reprod Genet [Internet]. 2005 Aug [cited 2018 Dec 3];22(7–8):307–9. Available from: http://link.springer.com/10.1007/s10815-005-6003-2.
29. Benaglia L, Somigliana E, Iemmello R, Colpi E, Nicolosi AE, Ragni G. Endometrioma and oocyte retrieval–induced pelvic abscess: a clinical concern or an exceptional complication? Fertil Steril [Internet]. 2008 May 1 [cited 2018 Dec 3];89(5):1263–6. Available from: https://www.sciencedirect.com/science/article/pii/S001502820701206X?via%3Dihub.

Chapter 18
Fertilization: Conventional IVF Versus ICSI

Karla Saner Amigh

18.1 Normal Mammalian Gamete Development

Male and female gamete cells are unique because they are the only haploid cells in the body. Thus they are the only cells that go through the process of meiosis. The timing and gaps between meiotic events vary significantly for male and female gametes. A closer look at some of these differences can provide some insight as to why reproductive aging in particular has such an adverse effect on oocyte, and subsequent embryo, quality.

Male and female germ cells originate from primordial germ cells in very early embryonic development, where they develop into either oogonia in females or spermatogonia in males. In females, oogonia mitotically reproduce to a peak number around seven million cells while still in utero. A large number of these oogonia undergo atresia, while the remaining oogonia become encapsulated by follicular cells to form primordial follicles and go through the first meiotic division to become primary oocytes. At birth, a female has somewhere between 200,000 and 400,000 of these primary oocytes which are at the meiotic prophase I stage. These primary oocytes will stay at this stage until hormonal signals in puberty cause resumption of meiosis I. The primordial follicles are recruited in groups of about 50 follicles daily in a continual process through unknown mechanisms. The initial growth of these early follicles is a long process of several months, at which time most of the follicles will undergo atresia. Usually somewhere between five and ten of the early follicles will be rescued from atresia and continue to grow. The number of primordial follicles that develop, or are recruited, varies from cycle to cycle, but numbers will decrease with advancing reproductive age. Each cohort of rescued primordial follicles will resume meiosis with further

K. S. Amigh (✉)
Fertility & Advanced Reproductive Medicine Clinic at University of Texas Southwestern
Medical Center, Dallas, TX, USA
e-mail: karla.saner@utsouthwestern.edu

© Springer Nature Switzerland AG 2020
O. Bukulmez (ed.), *Diminished Ovarian Reserve and Assisted Reproductive Technologies*, https://doi.org/10.1007/978-3-030-23235-1_18

nuclear and cytoplasmic development when signaled by circulating FSH levels that begin in puberty after years of senescence. Some oocytes may stay at meiotic prophase for up to 50 years! Overall, only about 400 oocytes fully mature during a woman's reproductive life span [1].

In males, spermatogonia migrate to the fetal testes early in development, where they remain in the seminiferous tubules until puberty. While females are born with all of the oocytes that they will ever have, male spermatogonia utilize a different pathway to create gametes. A spermatogonia cell will undergo a mitotic division to produce two new cells: a primary spermatocyte and a spermatogonial stem cell. The spermatogonial stem cells allow males to continue producing sperm for most of their lives under normal circumstances. These "immortal" stem cells can explain how men who withstand testicular trauma or the use of chemotherapeutic agents may regain sperm production over time, as it only requires a small number of stem cells to survive and repopulate.

The other cell created during the mitotic division, the primary spermatocyte, will undergo meiosis I to produce two haploid secondary spermatocytes. The two secondary spermatocytes will then each undergo meiosis II and give rise to four spermatids. Immature spermatids then go through a maturation process called spermiogenesis as they progress through the male reproductive tract to morphologically differentiate into mature sperm. Thus, each spermatogonia cell eventually yields four sperm cells, allowing the testes to produce billions or trillions of sperm in a lifetime, unlike the ~400 eggs a woman will produce.

18.2   History of Intracytoplasmic Sperm Injection (ICSI)

Shortly after the initial successes of in vitro fertilization (IVF) were reported in the late 1970s [2–4], it became apparent that there was a need to broaden the indications for assisted reproductive technology (ART) treatment as it was originally applied to women with only tubal factor infertility. The role of sperm was almost taken for granted. However, as IVF became more widely adopted, it came to light that male factor issues were a major component of infertility, inviting a new focus on treating sperm issues. Male factor infertility was a major focus of study throughout the 1980s, with a great deal of attention paid to the spermatozoa and the oocyte-spermatozoan interaction.

One of the earliest indications for poor sperm quality in IVF was low concentration of sperm. Early attempts to simply concentrate the specimen, either by adding more sperm to the insemination dish or lowering the insemination volume of the culture, were ineffective [5]. Attention then turned to the oocyte, in an attempt to make it more amenable to sperm penetration. Experiments to manipulate the zona pellucida were attempted, including applying acidic Tyrode's solution to the zona to create a hole for the sperm to enter and mechanically creating a hole or split in the zona. Unfortunately these experiments either showed very poor to no fertilization or high polyspermy rates [6–8].

The earliest successes with circumventing total fertilization failure were with a procedure involving subzonal injection of sperm into the perivitelline space of the oocyte, the area between the zona pellucida and the actual oocyte, which was referred to as SUZI [9, 10]. While attempting to refine and improve the SUZI technique, investigators in Brussels unintentionally created a new technique that would revolutionize ART treatments. The investigators noted when they were attempting to inject the sperm into the perivitelline space, they would sometimes unintentionally pierce the oolemma and inject the sperm directly into the cytoplasm of the oocyte. They noted when this "accident" occurred and were surprised to discover that these accidentally injected eggs had close to 100% fertilization rates! They began calling this procedure ICSI, which is short for intracytoplasmic sperm injection. The researchers continued to perform both SUZI and ICSI on patients and waited until they had four pregnancies from this procedure before they published the first successful series of ICSI cases in 1992 [11]. These cases used ejaculated sperm with poor semen parameters that had previously failed conventional insemination and SUZI procedures. After this fortuitous incidental discovery, further work was done to refine the ICSI technique. Subsequent studies regarding the positioning of the oocyte during injection helped create one of the most universally adopted IVF protocols used worldwide today [12–14].

The next frontier to tackle was men with no sperm in the ejaculate. ICSI has been successfully applied to patients with both obstructive and nonobstructive azoospermia [15]. For cases of obstructive azoospermia, where spermatogenesis is normal, sperm can be surgically retrieved in an outpatient procedure from either the epididymis or testes. Surgically retrieved sperm can be used fresh if coordinated with the oocyte retrieval or frozen for future use. Sperm can be extracted from the epididymis through either microsurgical sperm aspiration (MESA) or percutaneous epididymal sperm aspiration (PESA). Epididymal sperm is normally motile.

Nonobstructive azoospermia is a more difficult problem to treat due to the etiology of the azoospermia. Nonobstructive azoospermia is often due to spermatogenic failure. Failure of the testes to make significant amounts of sperm can be induced by chemotherapeutic or radiologic treatments but can also be caused by abnormal steroid hormone production or genetic defects. In such cases it is sometimes possible to find small amounts of sperm in the testes. Sperm retrieval techniques include extraction via either testicular sperm extraction (TESE) using a needle or opening the testicle(s) and using a microscope to visually dissect dilated seminiferous tubules (micro TESE) [16], which are then further dissected by laboratory staff to search for viable sperm. Sperm derived directly from the testes are typically nonmotile or weakly motile, as they have not gone through the maturation process that occurs as sperm naturally progress through the epididymis. Using nonmotile sperm is technically more challenging for embryologists as they must try to make a determination that a sperm is indeed alive although immotile. While success rates with nonmotile testicular sperm are low, the advent of ICSI made it possible to attempt pregnancy with their own genetic material in these patients.

ICSI is a physiological side step, effectively eliminating the need for motile spermatozoa or the sperm-oocyte interaction at the cell surface level. ICSI is also invasive, as it requires breakage of the oolemma and addition of an entire spermatozoan into the cytoplasm of the oocyte [14]. Due to these inherently nonphysiological interventions, it is reasonable and prudent to question the safety of ICSI. Numerous studies have examined the effects of ICSI on everything from miscarriage rates to minor and major birth defects. By design, ICSI is a procedure utilized by a cohort seeking medical intervention to achieve pregnancy. Thus, it is impossible to separate ICSI effects from infertility effects. While data on over 25 years of ICSI is mostly reassuring, there is one caveat. The potential for a male factor infertility issue, typically through a Y-chromosome microdeletion, is real. While this potential defect could cause issues for male offspring, when faced with that risk versus not having a biological child, couples overwhelmingly choose to accept this risk. Overall, the general consensus is that ICSI is an effective and safe treatment option, especially for male factor infertility [17].

18.3   Indications for ICSI

As described in the previous section, ICSI was initially developed in the early 1990s for patients who had severely abnormal semen parameters or cycles with previous total fertilization failure with conventional insemination. Since its inception, ICSI has become widely adopted for many uses including the aforementioned male factor infertility, unexplained infertility, preimplantation genetic testing, frozen gametes, serodiscordant couples, and advanced maternal age and poor responders, among others.

18.3.1   Unexplained Infertility

Unexplained infertility is a diagnosis given to approximately 20–30% of couples who present for infertility evaluation. After a full battery of tests for both partners, a diagnosis of "unexplained" is frustrating for patients to hear. These patients are often younger and have no obvious reason for not becoming pregnant, and many will start with less invasive treatment plans, such as intrauterine insemination (IUI). After several failed rounds of IUI (and months of time), the physician and patient may make the decision to move to IVF. The next decision to be made is conventional insemination versus ICSI. ICSI use has increased dramatically for all indications, from 36.4% in 1996 to 76.2% in 2012 [18]. However, there is much debate over whether ICSI should be used in all cases [19]. In cases with no obvious etiology and normal semen parameters, it is reasonable to at least consider an ICSI/IVF split, especially if there is a history of failed IUI. Data from each cohort of treated eggs may yield insight for possible subsequent treatments.

18.3.2   Preimplantation Genetic Testing

Preimplantation genetic testing (PGT) is a commonly used technique to deselect embryos for transfer. Genetic testing of embryos through next generation sequencing yields results that allow clinics to remove likely abnormal embryos from the transfer queue. The test relies on embryologists removing a small number of trophectoderm cells from each embryo (embryo biopsy). These cells get sent to a specialized sequencing lab for testing and interpretation. ICSI is conventionally applied in PGT cases to theoretically avoid any potential contamination from sperm cells that may be adhered to the outside of the zona pellucida. However, there is no evidence to support the exclusive use of ICSI for PGT. Several publications have examined the insemination method for PGT-A (testing for aneuploidy) embryos and have demonstrated no significant differences in aneuploidy rates in embryos derived from ICSI versus conventional insemination [20–23].

18.3.3   Frozen Gametes

Due to ultrastructural changes in the membranes and acrosome of human sperm, coupled with typically low sperm quantities for frozen anonymous donor sperm, ICSI is commonly performed when using frozen sperm for IVF. However, frozen sperm has been used with some success for decades for intrauterine insemination when sperm number is not a limiting factor [24, 25]. Frozen donor oocytes are a relatively new addition to IVF protocols. Use of frozen, rather than fresh, donor oocytes provides a number of logistical advantages to both the patient and donor. Oocyte donors can complete their donations on their own time table and do not have to consider logistics of the recipient or synchronization with the recipient's cycle. Frozen donor oocytes can be quarantined per FDA guidelines in the same manner as frozen donor sperm, and frozen oocytes can be distributed worldwide to multiple recipients. Based on the published data [26–28] at this time, most commercial egg banks do recommend ICSI as the insemination method of choice for frozen oocytes.

18.3.4   Serodiscordant Couples

Patients of reproductive age living with chronic viral illness often desire pregnancy. However, these patients do require special considerations to avoid potential viral transmission to their partner and/or their offspring. Most commonly, patients with human immunodeficiency virus (HIV), hepatitis B (HBV), or hepatitis C (HCV) require risk-reducing strategies in order to achieve a successful outcome for all parties involved – patient, partner, and offspring. Both the American Society for Reproductive Medicine (ASRM) and the European Society of Human Reproduction and Embryology (ESHRE) have published guidelines for treating patients with infectious disease [29, 30]. Both entities recommend processing potentially infectious specimens in dedicated laboratory space when specimens of noninfected patients are not in the laboratory to avoid potential cross-contamination. For many IVF laboratories, space is at a premium, and this may prove difficult. Good tissue practice also requires any potentially infectious frozen gametes, which would include any specimens for which infectious disease screening is not completed, to be stored in separate liquid nitrogen tanks or stored in vapor phase tanks in quarantined areas.

For HIV-infected males with a seronegative female partner, it is recommended that the disease be stable with undetectable viral load in serum for at least 1 year prior to pregnancy attempts. Semen samples can then be processed and checked via polymerase chain reaction (PCR) for viral load, which may differ between serum and semen samples. Appropriately washed semen specimens that show no viral load can be used for intrauterine insemination (IUI), IVF, or IVF/ICSI [31]. To date, there are no published reports of infection to a mother or child in over 8000 IUI cycles using washed sperm with undetectable viral load. Similarly, for HBV- and HCV-infected males with seronegative female partners, it is imperative that efforts are made to stabilize and hopefully reduce viral load prior to fertility trials. It is crucial for patients to have established care with an infectious disease specialist who can guide patients and their fertility specialists through this process from their perspective. Additionally, prophylactic measures should be taken by the female partner and gradient washed sperm be used for insemination. No PCR testing of the final washed specimen is recommended at this time for HBV- or HCV-positive men.

For virus-positive females, appropriate preconception counseling is imperative so that patients carefully consider the potential for vertical transmission of virus to the fetus during pregnancy, or to the child during birth, or both. Medical management can significantly reduce, but not eliminate, this risk. There are no special laboratory considerations for IUI semen processing for virus-positive females with uninfected male partners. For IVF treatment, isolation from other patient samples is recommended. ICSI is also the insemination method most suited for these couples. Virus has been detected in both aspirated follicular fluid and cumulus cells. Therefore, removal of the potentially infectious cumulus cells and washing and moving denuded oocytes to fresh media can reduce although not completely eliminate infection potential.

18.4 Diminished Ovarian Reserve (DOR) and Advanced Reproductive Age (ARA)

Age is the main limiting factor for female fertility and good reproductive outcomes. As more and more women delay childbearing until their late 30–40s [32], the need for assisted reproduction via IVF increases. Conventional stimulation protocols were historically created and honed for young women with normal to high ovarian reserve. Aging oocytes, due to a number of intrinsic and extrinsic factors, require special considerations in the IVF laboratory. Many clinics have adopted an "ICSI-all" protocol, as this can streamline both the IVF and andrology laboratory workflow when all samples for all patients are treated in the same fashion. Proponents of this approach cite evidence indicating that ICSI does not provide a disadvantage over conventional insemination when used for non-male factor infertility [33–35].

Patients with aging oocytes require special considerations in the IVF laboratory. It is well documented that disturbances in the meiotic spindle, a crucial cellular organelle comprised of spindle fibers that move and segregate chromosomes during nuclear division, can adversely affect all aspects of embryo development [36–38]. The meiotic spindle cannot be observed with the standard inverted microscope typically used for ICSI. Noninvasive polarization microscopy (i.e., PolScope) can be used in conjunction with a standard ICSI microscope to visualize meiotic spindles in oocytes. Studies with the PolScope have demonstrated that oocytes from older patients [39] and poor-responder patients [40] have lower fertilization rates and overall lower success rates than younger patients. However, PolScope use requires denudation of oocytes, hence is only useful for guidance with ICSI. Aging oocytes with substandard meiotic spindles would likely benefit from conventional insemination rather than risking further spindle disruption from ICSI.

Similarly, the competence of the oocyte regarding cytoplasmic maturation and oocyte degeneration are also factors to consider. Studies examining the ICSI technique and cytoplasmic maturation indicate that oocyte cytoplasm becomes more viscous as the oocyte reaches maturity [41, 42]. This allows penetration of the oolemma to occur without complete loss of cytoplasm, which would cause immediate oocyte degeneration. While the overall oocyte degeneration rate during ICSI is typically low, patients with fragile eggs due to DOR and/or ARA would likely benefit from conventional insemination over ICSI in the absence of male factor issues, in part to avoid potential oocyte degeneration.

Oocyte development within the ovarian follicle requires bidirectional cross talk between the cumulus cells surrounding the oocyte and oocyte itself [43]. Conventional insemination methods keep the cumulus-oocyte complex intact longer. A sibling oocyte study comparing IVF versus ICSI in patients with no known male factor issues showed a higher number of available embryos for transfer or freeze and a lower oocyte degeneration rate in conventionally inseminated oocytes [44]. A larger, retrospective study consisting of women aged 40 years and over yielded similar results, with more available embryos in the IVF group over ICSI [21].

Conventional insemination for non-male factor cases is used less and less frequently, likely due to patient pressures. If it can be done, why not? The easy answer for practitioners faced with this question is to simply move forward with ICSI. With more and more patients presenting with combinations of DOR and ARA, it may be worthwhile for physicians to build an "ICSI versus conventional insemination for DOR/ARA" module into their IVF consultation. Women with DOR/ARA may benefit from conventional insemination for several reasons. First, the cumulus-oocyte complex in maintained intact overnight, instead of denuding these cells from the oocyte within just a few hours of egg retrieval. Allowing these cells to remain with the oocyte likely allows more eggs to reach maturity and subsequently fertilize, as opposed to oocytes that are stripped for ICSI and discarded if immature. Second, ICSI is an aggressive method of fertilization with subtle but potentially significant differences between operators. For patients with advanced reproductive age, small details such as amount of aspirated oocyte cytoplasm or aggressive cumulus cell denudation may be the difference between a viable embryo or not [45]. Conventional insemination reduces the chance of oocyte degeneration due to rough handling during ICSI.

Overall, patients with diminished ovarian reserve and/or advanced reproductive age can still be suitable candidates for minimal stimulation protocols, but their care plan, especially in the IVF laboratory, needs to be carefully scrutinized. Patients who benefit from minimal stimulation protocols for ovarian stimulation will have oocytes that can benefit from minimal manipulation in the laboratory [46]. Quick and careful handling of these delicate oocytes, along with standard conventional insemination methods in the absence of a clear male factor issue can help in the long-term goal of achieving a family for this patient population.

18.5   Conclusion

Development of the ICSI procedure revolutionized the practice of IVF. ICSI is now the gold standard implemented worldwide for treatment of male factor infertility with excellent outcomes. The application of the ICSI technique has become more widespread, with uses far beyond just male factor issues. However, for DOR/ARA patients with lower quantities of potentially more delicate oocytes, it is prudent to consider conventional insemination as a first-line treatment in the absence of male factor infertility.

References

1. Yanagimachi R. Intracytoplasmic injection of spermatozoa and spermatogenic cells: its biology and applications in humans and animals. Reprod Biomed Online. 2005;10(2):247–88.
2. Steptoe PC, Edwards RG. Birth after the reimplantation of a human embryo. Lancet. 1978;312(8085):366.
3. Lopata A, et al. Pregnancy following intrauterine implantation of an embryo obtained by in vitro fertilization of a preovulatory egg. Fertil Steril. 1980;33(2):117–20.
4. Jones HW, et al. Three years of in vitro fertilization at Norfolk. Fertil Steril. 1984;42(6):826–34.
5. O'Neill CL, et al. Development of ICSI. Reproduction. 2018;156(1):F51–8.
6. Kiessling AA, et al. Fertilization in trypsin–treated oocytes. Ann N Y Acad Sci. 1988;541(1):614–20.
7. Gordon JW, et al. Fertilization of human oocytes by sperm from infertile males after zona pellucida drilling. Fertil Steril. 1988;50(1):68–73.

8. Cohen J, et al. Treatment of male infertility by in vitro fertilization: factors affecting fertilization and pregnancy. Acta Eur Fertil. 1984;15(6):455–65.
9. Fishel S, et al. Twin birth after subzonal insemination. Lancet. 1990;335(8691):722–3.
10. Palermo G, et al. Induction of acrosome reaction in human spermatozoa used for subzonal insemination. Hum Reprod. 1992;7(2):248–54.
11. Palermo G, et al. Pregnancies after intracytoplasmic injection of single spermatozoon into an oocyte. Lancet. 1992;340(8810):17–8.
12. Palermo GD, et al. Development and implementation of intracytoplasmic sperm injection (ICSI). Reprod Fertil Dev. 1995;7(2):211–7; discussion 217–8.
13. Nagy ZP, et al. The influence of the site of sperm deposition and mode of oolemma breakage at intracytoplasmic sperm injection on fertilization and embryo development rates. Hum Reprod. 1995;10(12):3171–7.
14. Simopoulou M, et al. Making ICSI safer and more effective: a review of the human oocyte and ICSI practice. In Vivo. 2016;30(4):387–400.
15. Palermo GD, et al. Fertilization and pregnancy outcome with intracytoplasmic sperm injection for azoospermic men. Hum Reprod. 1999;14(3):741–8.
16. Schlegel PN. Testicular sperm extraction: microdissection improves sperm yield with minimal tissue excision. Hum Reprod. 1999;14(1):131–5.
17. Schlegel PN. Debate: is ICSI a genetic time bomb? No: ICSI is safe and effective. J Androl. 1999;20(1):18–22.
18. Boulet SL, et al. Trends in use of and reproductive outcomes associated with intracytoplasmic sperm injection trends and outcomes of intracytoplasmic sperm injection trends and outcomes of intracytoplasmic sperm injection. JAMA. 2015;313(3):255–63.
19. Orief Y, Dafopoulos K, Al-Hassani S. Should ICSI be used in non-male factor infertility? Reprod Biomed Online. 2004;9(3):348–56.
20. Feldman B, et al. Pre-implantation genetic diagnosis—should we use ICSI for all? J Assist Reprod Genet. 2017;34(9):1179–83.
21. Tannus S, et al. The role of intracytoplasmic sperm injection in non-male factor infertility in advanced maternal age. Hum Reprod. 2017;32(1):119–24.
22. Coates A, et al. Use of suboptimal sperm increases the risk of aneuploidy of the sex chromosomes in preimplantation blastocyst embryos. Fertil Steril. 2015;104(4):866–72.
23. Palmerola KL, et al. Minimizing mosaicism: assessing the impact of fertilization method on rate of mosaicism after next-generation sequencing (NGS) preimplantation genetic testing for aneuploidy (PGT-A). J Assist Reprod Genet. 2019;36(1):153–7.
24. Byrd W, et al. Intrauterine insemination with frozen donor sperm: a prospective randomized trial comparing three different sperm preparation techniques. Fertil Steril. 1994;62(4):850–6.
25. Ford WC, Mathur RS, Hull MG. Intrauterine insemination: is it an effective treatment for male factor infertility? Baillieres Clin Obstet Gynaecol. 1997;11(4):691–710.
26. Kazem R, et al. Cryopreservation of human oocytes and fertilization by two techniques: in-vitro fertilization and intracytoplasmic sperm injection. Hum Reprod. 1995;10(10):2650–4.
27. Gook DA, et al. Intracytoplasmic sperm injection and embryo development of human oocytes cryopreserved using 1,2-propanediol. Hum Reprod. 1995;10(10):2637–41.
28. Li XH, et al. Cryopreserved oocytes of infertile couples undergoing assisted reproductive technology could be an important source of oocyte donation: a clinical report of successful pregnancies. Hum Reprod. 2005;20(12):3390–4.
29. Ethics Committee of American Society for Reproductive Medicine. Human immunodeficiency virus (HIV) and infertility treatment: a committee opinion. Fertil Steril. 2015;104(1):e1–8.
30. Shenfield F, et al. Taskforce 8: ethics of medically assisted fertility treatment for HIV positive men and women. Hum Reprod. 2004;19(11):2454–6.
31. Zamora MJ, et al. Semen residual viral load and reproductive outcomes in HIV-infected men undergoing ICSI after extended semen preparation. Reprod Biomed Online. 2016;32(6):584–90.
32. Adamson GD, et al. International Committee for Monitoring Assisted Reproductive Technology: world report on assisted reproductive technology, 2011. Fertil Steril. 2018;110(6):1067–80.

33. Aboulghar MA, et al. Intracytoplasmic sperm injection and conventional in vitro fertilization for sibling oocytes in cases of unexplained infertility and borderline semen. J Assist Reprod Genet. 1996;13(1):38–42.
34. Fishel S, et al. Should ICSI be the treatment of choice for all cases of in-vitro conception? Hum Reprod. 2000;15(6):1278–83.
35. Nyboe Andersen A, Carlsen E, Loft A. Trends in the use of intracytoplasmatic sperm injection marked variability between countries. Hum Reprod Update. 2008;14(6):593–604.
36. Pickering SJ, et al. Cytoskeletal organization in fresh, aged and spontaneously activated human oocytes. Hum Reprod. 1988;3(8):978–89.
37. Battaglia DE, Klein NA, Soules MR. Changes in centrosomal domains during meiotic maturation in the human oocyte. Mol Hum Reprod. 1996;2(11):845–51.
38. Wang W-H, et al. The spindle observation and its relationship with fertilization after intracytoplasmic sperm injection in living human oocytes. Fertil Steril. 2001;75(2):348–53.
39. De Santis L, et al. Polar body morphology and spindle imaging as predictors of oocyte quality. Reprod Biomed Online. 2005;11(1):36–42.
40. Korkmaz C, et al. Effects of maternal ageing on ICSI outcomes and embryo development in relation to oocytes morphological characteristics of birefringent structures. Zygote. 2015;23(4):550–5.
41. Palermo GD, et al. Oolemma characteristics in relation to survival and fertilization patterns of oocytes treated by intracytoplasmic sperm injection. Hum Reprod. 1996;11(1):172–6.
42. Krause I, et al. Characterization of the injection funnel during intracytoplasmic sperm injection reflects cytoplasmic maturity of the oocyte. Fertil Steril. 2016;106(5):1101–6.
43. Turchi D, et al. Oocyte maturation: gamete-somatic cells interactions, meiotic resumption, cytoskeletal dynamics and cytoplasmic reorganization. Hum Reprod Update. 2015;21(4):427–54.
44. Ming L, et al. Higher abnormal fertilization, higher cleavage rate, and higher arrested embryos rate were found in conventional IVF than in intracytoplasmic sperm injection. Clin Exp Obstet Gynecol. 2015;42(3):372–5.
45. Sfontouris IA, et al. Live birth rates using conventional in vitro fertilization compared to intracytoplasmic sperm injection in Bologna poor responders with a single oocyte retrieved. J Assist Reprod Genet. 2015;32(5):691–7.
46. Babayev SN, Park CW, Bukulmez O. Intracytoplasmic sperm injection indications: how rigorous? Semin Reprod Med. 2014;32(04):283–90.

Chapter 19
Embryo Culture: Cleavage Versus Blastocyst Stage

Zexu Jiao

19.1 Introduction

The primary goal of embryo culture is to provide an optimal environment for gametes and resulting embryos in order to obtain healthy, good-quality embryos with a maximal potential for implantation and ultimately live birth. Since the early days of embryo culture in vitro, numerous approaches have been taken in attempts to improve implantation rates, including advancements in culture technologies and transfer of embryos at different developmental stages. Traditionally, cleavage stage embryos were transferred on day 2 or 3, but over the past decade, there has been an increasing trend to transfer blastocysts on day 5 or 6. In this chapter, we will review embryo culture systems and the effectiveness of cleavage vs blastocyst stage transfer, followed by discussion of the optimal embryo culture and transfer strategy in diminished ovarian reserve (DOR) patients.

19.2 Human Preimplantation Embryo Development

In humans, fertilization usually occurs in the ampullary-isthmic portion of the oviduct. After completing fertilization with fusion of the pronuclei during syngamy, the zygote has a diploid complement of chromosomes and then undergoes a series of cleavage divisions that culminate with a major wave of embryonic genome activation (EGA) between the four- and eight-cell stages. Following EGA, the embryo undergoes compaction to form a morula and then enters the uterus, which is

Z. Jiao (✉)
Division of Reproductive Endocrinology & Infertility, Fertility and Advanced Reproductive Medicine Assisted Reproductive Technologies Program, Department of Obstetrics and Gynecology, University of Texas Southwestern Medical Center, Dallas, TX, USA
e-mail: Zexu.Jiao@utsouthwestern.edu

© Springer Nature Switzerland AG 2020
O. Bukulmez (ed.), *Diminished Ovarian Reserve and Assisted Reproductive Technologies*, https://doi.org/10.1007/978-3-030-23235-1_19

approximately 3 days after fertilization. Subsequent cell divisions lead to the development of a blastocyst that comprises a fluid-filled blastocyst cavity and an inner cell mass (ICM), surrounded by trophectoderm (TE) cells. The ICM gives rise to tissues of the embryo proper, and TE will eventually form the placenta and extraembryonic tissue. The blastocyst rests freely in the uterine cavity for about 2 or 3 days, during which time it derives nutrients secreted by the uterine glands and increases slightly in size. On about the sixth day after fertilization, the uterus secretes enzyme that dissolves the zona pellucida (ZP) surrounding the blastocyst, allowing implantation to begin. The process of implantation, leading to the successful establishment of a pregnancy, must be carefully coordinated in time and in place (Fig. 19.1).

19.3 Embryo Culture

The human embryo culture is a complex subject. There are many variables to consider when culturing human embryos *in vitro*. These factors may be environmental, like laboratory air quality and temperature; physical, like the types of incubators used; or chemical, like the type of culture media (Table 19.1). All of these factors

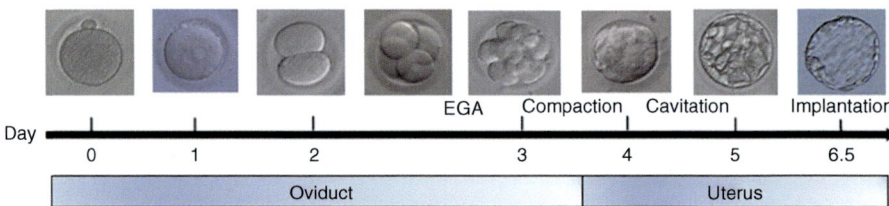

Fig. 19.1 Human preimplantation embryo development, EGA (embryonic genome activation)

Table 19.1 Factors in the laboratory that affect human embryo development *in vitro*	
	Air quality (purity, presence of VOCs)
	Light (intensity, wavelengths)
	Temperature (incubators, laboratory)
	pH of culture media and CO_2 concentration
	O_2 (low O_2 vs atmospheric O_2)
	Gas used (mix, purity)
	Incubator (type, number, management)
	Culture media (type, composition)
	Albumin type in media
	Osmolality in culture media
	Oil overlay
	Contact materials used (toxicity)
	Embryo density (number of embryos/drop, drop volume)
	Pipetting (times and speed of pipetting action)
	Micromanipulation (ICSI, biopsy, AH)
	Embryologist (number, skill level)
	Quality control and quality assurance

are required to be in harmony in order to achieve the optimal conditions for the growth of human embryos until the point of transfer.

19.3.1 Air Quality

Poor laboratory air quality is a recognized hazard to the culture of human embryos. While little is known about the actual components that effect these changes, Cohen et al. have postulated that four different categories of pollutants are involved: volatile organic compounds (VOCs); small inorganic molecules such as N_2O, SO_2 and CO; substances derived from building materials (i.e., adhesives and floor tiles); and other polluting compounds (i.e., pesticides, aerosols) [1].

In order to avoid the negative effects of poor air quality, careful consideration should be given to the site and the location of human IVF laboratory. In addition, an appropriate design of the laboratory is essential. The use of the lowest VOC emitting products for all construction materials is recommended. Positive pressure airflow in the laboratory coupled with the use of air purification systems and appropriate in-line filters for incubators will help to minimize the level of airborne contaminants and improve the outcomes. Furthermore, laboratory personnel can also introduce VOCs in the form of perfumes and deodorants; hence, discretion is required [2]. Finally, the use of oil overlay may be an effective way of limiting the impact of any diverse environmental factors.

19.3.2 Light

In IVF lab, embryos are exposed to both microscope and ambient light. Visible light has been shown to be an additional stress and has a deleterious effect on mammalian gamete and embryo development *in vitro* [3]. It is prudent to work in low illumination and to minimize the amount of time and observation made on gametes and embryos under the microscope. Light can also degrade the integrity of tissue culture media, so ideally media should be kept in the dark.

19.3.3 Temperature

Temperature is another variable of the culture system that impacts various aspects of gamete and embryo function, most notably meiotic spindle stability [4] and possibly embryo metabolism [5]. Maintaining temperature stability around 37 °C is important for the oocyte, followed by the cleavage stage embryo, with increased thermo-tolerance increasing after compaction [2]. Most laboratories set their equipment to run at 37 °C. Using an incubator with stringent temperature control and recovery is important. In addition, avoiding overuse of the incubators is critical to prevent temperature variations. Ambient air temperature can affect how temperature is maintained when embryos are outside of the incubator. Microscope stage warmers and incubator chambers also differ in their ability to hold the temperatures constant at 37 °C. So laboratories should set their thermostats to 71 °F and above and use solid-viewing surface microscope stages with a temperature of >37.5 °C on the warming stage.

19.3.4 pH and Carbon Dioxide (CO_2)

In mammals, the pH shifts from an alkaline environment in the oviduct (7.60 ± 0.01) to an acidic environment in the uterus (6.96 ± 0.01) [6]. Although embryos can develop over a range of media pH, it appears that pH set at or near 7.3 may provide adequate conditions for embryo growth in a static laboratory environment [7–9]. Media pH is primarily determined by the bicarbonate concentration in the media and the CO_2 concentration of the culture incubator. Therefore, it is advisable to use a CO_2 concentration of between 6% and 7% to yield a media pH of around 7.3. To properly monitor CO_2 level, digital CO_2 analysis units are preferred over a liquid-based system such as Fyrite. pH shows a dynamic pattern and is also influenced by specific media components such as lactate, pyruvate, and amino acids. Thus, directly assessing the pH of culture media within a laboratory's own culture is prudent as part of a rigorous quality control program. A simple and reliable method of checking the pH of a medium is to use color standards; however, this requires the presence of phenol red in the medium. Use of a pH meter is generally considered a more accurate mean of assessing pH. The analysis of media pH is best performed with a blood gas analyzer or with an optical device inside the incubator.

19.3.5 Oxygen (O_2)

Although the atmospheric level of O_2 at sea level is approximately 20.9%, physiological O_2 levels are lower; they vary in different parts of the reproductive tract, typically from 2% to 8% [10, 11]. Human embryo culture has traditionally used an atmosphere of around 20% O_2. More recently, increasing evidence suggests that culture in a low O_2 concentration improves preimplantation embryo development, implantation, and pregnancy rate [12, 13]. Of note, the vast majority of studies on lower O_2 levels for embryo culture have focused on 5%. However, the optimum O_2 concentration for human embryo development has yet to be elucidated, and further, it is unclear whether stage-specific differences exist [2].

19.3.6 Incubator

Incubator selection and management is critical for the success of an IVF program. In considering the type of incubator to be used, the overriding aim is to minimize disturbance to the embryos' environment and conditions, specifically temperature and pH. There are many types of incubators available for human IVF embryo culture.

Box-type incubators have been long used for clinical IVF and were later adapted to smaller box-type incubators. More recently, mini-benchtop incubators have been developed. Such incubators allow for direct heat between the chamber and culture vessel and a direct flow of premixed gas and therefore minimize changes in temperature and pH. Most recently, such chambers have evolved to include time-lapse capability, facilitating the constant monitoring of embryos without interrupted embryo culture [14]. To date, there is no clear consensus as to a superior incubator type, although the efficacy and environmental stability rely heavily on incubator use and management. This reinforces the need for strict quality control as well as proper management of laboratory IVF incubators to optimize their functions and maximize outcomes.

19.3.7 Culture Media

The media that are used to culture human preimplantation embryos is an important factor for the success rates of IVF/ICSI (intracytoplasmic sperm injection). In the first decade of human IVF, the culture media ranged from simple salt solutions such as Earle's or Tyrode's solutions to complex media intended for tissue culture such as HamF10. All of them were usually supplemented with different sources of proteins, mostly with fetal or maternal serum. Nowadays, as the industry expanded, numerous commercially culture media are available that contain various components including salts, energy substrates, serum supplements, amino acids, buffer solutions, antibiotics, vitamins, nucleotides, growth factors, and others. Such media can be used either as a sequential system, with different compositions for days 1–3 and 3–6, or as a single medium, used for the whole culture period [15]. Today, with the advent of time-lapse microscopy, the media designed specifically for the purpose of uninterrupted embryo culture have been shown to be effective [16]. Despite all these changes in culture media, it is still unclear whether the composition of the media affects embryo quality and implantation rates and which culture media leads to the best IVF/ICSI success rates [17]. With technological improvements and new approaches to assess embryo metabolism, morphokinetics, and other means of viability assessment, there remains the possibility that media formulations may still be further refined and improved to benefit embryo development and clinical outcomes.

19.3.8 Embryo Density

The number of embryos cultured per drop must also be considered. During IVF, embryos can be cultured either singly or in groups. Culturing embryos singly allows the history of each embryo to be traced. The benefit of group culture is that embryo produces autocrine or paracrine factors that promote development of both itself and surrounding embryos. Culture of embryos in small volumes enables these factors to reach sufficient concentrations to have an impact. Several studies indicate that extended group culture of embryos may be beneficial for human preimplantation embryo development and that the number of embryos per drop and/or incubation volume seems to be an important factor in determining IVF outcome [18, 19].

19.4 Cleavage Stage Versus Blastocyst Stage

The initial success of clinical IVF was compromised by suboptimal culture conditions, resulting in impaired embryo development and frequently arrested around the eight-cell stage. Consequently, it became the paradigm to transfer human embryos to the uterus asynchronously on days 1, 2, or 3. Indeed, it was advocated that if the laboratory conditions were not optimized, then embryos should be transferred back to the uterus as soon as possible to avoid suboptimal conditions. Improvements in embryo culture media formulations, combined with increases in efficiency and safety of the overall culture system, have led directly to a significant increase on the development and viability of the preimplantation embryo (for both cleavage and blastocyst transfers).

Over the past decade, there has been an increasing trend toward transferring embryos at blastocysts stage. Blastocyst transfer could be advantageous because the timing of exposure of the embryo to the uterine environment is more analogous to a natural cycle. In addition, extended embryo culture to the blastocyst stage permits embryo self-selection that has successfully initiated their EGA on day 3 [20, 21]. Moreover, growing embryos to the blastocyst stage is the most suitable for patients in need of genetic analyses.

Despite the above potential advantages of extended culture, there are also some theoretical disadvantages. First, there is a risk of losing some embryos because of the difference between the in vitro culture and uterine environment. These embryos might not survive the challenges of extended culture but might have survived in vivo if transferred on day 3. The consequence of this disadvantage is an increased likelihood that no embryo will be available for either transfer or freezing and further assisted reproduction cycles will be required [21, 22]. Second, there are concerns regarding its safety, particularly regarding whether any harm is caused when culturing embryos in vitro beyond EGA. Moreover, the longer duration of embryo incubation has raised concerns regarding fetal safety, such as increased preterm birth and birth defects [23, 24].

Currently, embryo transfer at blastocyst stage has become the strategy of choice for most clinics worldwide, with the aim of achieving a healthy singleton live birth and so minimizing the number of multiple births and their associated complications, while still maintaining pregnancy rates per transfer. This has been achieved by carrying out a single blastocyst transfer instead of single-embryo transfer on the cleavage stage. However, when considering a change in clinical practice, any potential benefit of the intervention should be weighed against the possible worse neonatal outcomes and increased costs. Subsequently, the question raised is what are the benefits and harms of blastocyst stage transfer when compared to cleavage stage embryo transfer?

Direct comparisons between the two stages of embryo development appear to support the use of blastocyst transfers in a clinical practice. Women who undergo fresh blastocyst transfers achieve higher live birth rates compared with those who receive fresh cleavage stage transfers [25]. However, in the few studies that report cumulative pregnancy rates after fresh and frozen transfers, no significant difference was found. Cleavage stage transfer is associated with greater numbers of embryos available for freezing, and blastocyst transfer is associated with increased number of cycles with no embryos to transfer [26, 27]. The American Society for Reproductive Medicine has voiced concern over the use of the blastocyst transfer method for assisted reproduction. They conclude that:

1. Evidence supports blastocyst transfer in "good prognosis" patients. Consideration is warranted to the transfer of a single embryo given the high risk of multiples in these patients
2. Blastocyst or cleavage stage embryos can be used for unselected or poor prognosis patients as the pregnancy/live birth rates are not significantly different; however, in these populations, there is a higher risk of embryos not progressing to blastocyst stage resulting in fewer/no embryos available for transfer [28].

When considering obstetric outcomes associated with blastocyst embryo transfer, the available evidence suggests an increased risk of perinatal mortality, preterm birth, and delivery of a large-for-gestational-age neonate, with a reduced risk of delivery of a small-for-gestational-age neonate [29]. However, as the quality of the evidence for the primary outcomes is low, additional well-designed randomized controlled trials are still needed before robust conclusions can be drawn. Further well-designed studies are warranted to evaluate the outcomes for blastocyst transfer including cumulative live birth rate after fresh and frozen transfers, perinatal mortality and severe perinatal morbidity, and longer-term follow-up of offspring outcomes.

19.5 What Stage Should Embryo Be Cultured and Transferred in Patients with Diminished Ovarian Reserve (DOR)?

There is an ongoing debate on identifying patients who would benefit from blastocyst culture and transfer. Blastocyst transfer may prove beneficial in several groups of patients, such as those with repeated implantation failures; women with uterine abnormalities that preclude multiple pregnancies, thus requiring more careful selection for single-embryo transfer; patients suspected of defects in oocyte quality, thus requiring embryos to be assessed for a more extended period of in vitro development; patients needing embryo biopsy for genetic selection; and lastly patients undergoing replacement of supernumerary embryos frozen at the blastocyst stage. Currently, most studies have analyzed the benefit of blastocyst transfer in good prognosis patients [30]. It is not clear whether this technique would benefit DOR patients.

DOR is an important limiting factor for the success of any treatment modality for infertility, which indicates a reduction in quantity and quality of oocytes especially in women with advanced reproductive age. DOR may be age related as seen in advanced years of reproductive life or may occur in young women due to diverse etiological factors. Deciding on blastocyst transfer depends on a minimum number of follicles, fertilized eggs, or eight-cell embryos on day 3. In unselected IVF patients, it was shown that the risk of cycle cancellation rate in a systematic blastocyst transfer policy may be as high as 27% [31]. A threshold of four good embryos on day 3 appeared to avoid blastocyst transfer cancellation in patients under 38 years of age [32]. An intermediate policy of having a minimum of four fertilized eggs had a cancellation rate of 10.1% for blastocyst transfer [33]. Given the attrition seen at each stage of the IVF process, the quantitative challenge presented by retrieving fewer oocytes is an obvious factor resulting in the higher blastocyst transfer cancellation in DOR patients [25]. In the University of Texas Southwestern Medical Center, for DOR patients without preimplantation genetic testing request, all good-quality embryos can be cryopreserved on day 3. For the remaining embryos, we further monitor their growth and development. Then any additional good-quality blastocysts are cryopreserved on day 5 or day 6 as reported by others [34, 35].

A number of studies have also suggested that patients with evidence of follicular depletion also exhibit reduced oocyte quality. This conclusion is logical given the fact that most patients with DOR are at an advanced reproductive age when oocyte quality is also compromised. Indeed, both depletion of the follicular pool and reduction in oocyte quality are physiologic events that accompany female aging [36, 37]. However, a recent study demonstrates that young poor responders have equivalent aneuploidy rates and blastulation potential as age-matched controls with normal ovarian reserve [38]. Thus, it appears that young DOR patients may exhibit a different phenotype than older DOR patients. There is currently not enough prospective data to make conclusions regarding how age affects the efficiency of blastocyst transformation among DOR patients. However, the clinicians should be mindful that younger patients with DOR might exhibit similar performance per embryo as their age-matched controls.

The success of blastocyst culture and transfer depends on adequate follicle recruitment by using controlled ovarian stimulation. Various treatment protocols have been proposed that are targeted at DOR patients, aiming to increase their ovarian response. The wide range of utilization of ovarian stimulation protocols reinforces the concern regarding the impact of stimulation protocol on oocyte quality in this cohort of women. The real focus in these patients should be on strategies to obtain oocytes with genetic and cytoplasmic competence rather than on strategies to obtain more than three oocytes. So far, there is insufficient evidence to support the routine use of any particular intervention either for pituitary downregulation, ovarian stimulation or adjuvant therapy in the management of DOR patients. More robust data from good-quality RCTs with relevant outcomes, such as blastocyst transformation rate, implantation rate, and live birth rate, are needed [39].

Furthermore, there are some considerations regarding the costs of the different transfer strategies. It is currently unclear which strategy is more cost-effective due to the poor reporting of data for cumulative pregnancy rate and early pregnancy losses of the two different strategies. However, if a cost-effectiveness analysis were to be done for cleavage stage transfers, the cost should also include the additional embryo freezing and subsequent frozen-thaw ETs if these have not been included in the cost of the cycle. For blastocyst stage transfer, one should consider the higher rates of cycle cancellation, as there may be no embryos for transfer or no embryos to freeze. Therefore, these DOR patients may need further cycles of stimulation and oocyte retrieval [26]. Moreover, the costs should take into account the additional laboratory staff and equipment required for blastocyst stage culture and transfer [28].

19.6 Conclusion

In summary, a great dilemma exists whether to apply blastocyst culture and transfer to DOR patients, who present with reduced number of oocyte and embryos. The debate would be better addressed if we had more data on the outcomes, costs, and the burden on the patients who need additional transfers of cleavage stage embryos. We should also consider the burden of performing additional controlled ovarian stimulation and oocyte retrieval cycles due to the higher cancellation rates with blastocyst stage culture and transfer. The development of culture technology, cryopreservation technology, and controlled ovarian stimulation strategies may provide the necessary tools for optimal embryo culture and transfer strategy in DOR patients.

References

1. Cohen J, Gilligan A, Esposito W, Schimmel T, Dale B. Ambient air and its potential effects on conception in vitro. Hum Reprod. 1997;12(8):1742–9.
2. Wale PL, Gardner DK. The effects of chemical and physical factors on mammalian embryo culture and their importance for the practice of assisted human reproduction. Hum Reprod Update. 2016;22(1):2–22.
3. Noda Y, Goto Y, Umaoka Y, Shiotani M, Nakayama T, Mori T. Culture of human embryos in alpha modification of Eagle's medium under low oxygen tension and low illumination. Fertil Steril. 1994;62(5):1022–7.
4. Sun XF, Zhang WH, Chen XJ, Xiao GH, Mai WY, Wang WH. Spindle dynamics in living mouse oocytes during meiotic maturation, ageing, cooling and overheating: a study by polarized light microscopy. Zygote. 2004;12(3):241–9.
5. Leese HJ, Baumann CG, Brison DR, McEvoy TG, Sturmey RG. Metabolism of the viable mammalian embryo: quietness revisited. Mol Hum Reprod. 2008;14(12):667–72.
6. Hugentobler S, Morris DG, Kane MT, Sreenan JM. In situ oviduct and uterine pH in cattle. Theriogenology. 2004;61(7–8):1419–27.
7. Dale B, Menezo Y, Cohen J, DiMatteo L, Wilding M. Intracellular pH regulation in the human oocyte. Hum Reprod. 1998;13(4):964–70.
8. Phillips KP, Leveille MC, Claman P, Baltz JM. Intracellular pH regulation in human preimplantation embryos. Hum Reprod. 2000;15(4):896–904.
9. Squirrell JM, Lane M, Bavister BD. Altering intracellular pH disrupts development and cellular organization in preimplantation hamster embryos. Biol Reprod. 2001;64(6):1845–54.

10. Ottosen LD, Hindkaer J, Husth M, Petersen DE, Kirk J, Ingerslev HJ. Observations on intrauterine oxygen tension measured by fibre-optic microsensors. Reprod Biomed Online. 2006;13(3):380–5.

11. Fischer B, Bavister BD. Oxygen tension in the oviduct and uterus of rhesus monkeys, hamsters and rabbits. J Reprod Fertil. 1993;99(2):673–9.

12. Dumoulin JC, Meijers CJ, Bras M, Coonen E, Geraedts JP, Evers JL. Effect of oxygen concentration on human in-vitro fertilization and embryo culture. Hum Reprod. 1999;14(2):465–9.

13. Bahceci M, Ciray HN, Karagenc L, Ulug U, Bener F. Effect of oxygen concentration during the incubation of embryos of women undergoing ICSI and embryo transfer: a prospective randomized study. Reprod Biomed Online. 2005;11(4):438–43.

14. Meseguer M, Rubio I, Cruz M, Basile N, Marcos J, Requena A. Embryo incubation and selection in a time-lapse monitoring system improves pregnancy outcome compared with a standard incubator: a retrospective cohort study. Fertil Steril. 2012;98(6):1481–9.e10.

15. Gardner DK, Lane M. Culture and selection of viable blastocysts: a feasible proposition for human IVF? Hum Reprod Update. 1997;3(4):367–82.

16. Hardarson T, Bungum M, Conaghan J, Meintjes M, Chantilis SJ, Molnar L, et al. Noninferiority, randomized, controlled trial comparing embryo development using media developed for sequential or undisturbed culture in a time-lapse setup. Fertil Steril. 2015;104(6):1452–9.e1–4.

17. Mantikou E, Youssef MA, van Wely M, van der Veen F, Al-Inany HG, Repping S, et al. Embryo culture media and IVF/ICSI success rates: a systematic review. Hum Reprod Update. 2013;19(3):210–20.

18. Rebollar-Lazaro I, Matson P. The culture of human cleavage stage embryos alone or in groups: effect upon blastocyst utilization rates and implantation. Reprod Biol. 2010;10(3):227–34.

19. Spyropoulou I, Karamalegos C, Bolton VN. A prospective randomized study comparing the outcome of in-vitro fertilization and embryo transfer following culture of human embryos individually or in groups before embryo transfer on day 2. Hum Reprod. 1999;14(1):76–9.

20. Oatway C, Gunby J, Daya S. Day three versus day two embryo transfer following *in vitro* fertilization or intracytoplasmic sperm injection. Cochrane Database Syst Rev. 2004;2:CD004378.

21. Glujovsky D, Blake D, Farquhar C, Bardach A. Cleavage stage versus blastocyst stage embryo transfer in assisted reproductive technology. Cochrane Database Syst Rev. 2012;7:CD002118.

22. Racowsky C, Jackson KV, Cekleniak NA, Fox JH, Hornstein MD, Ginsburg ES. The number of eight-cell embryos is a key determinant for selecting day 3 or day 5 transfer. Fertil Steril. 2000;73(3):558–64.

23. Braakhekke M, Kamphuis EI, Mol F, Norman RJ, Bhattacharya S, van der Veen F, et al. Effectiveness and safety as outcome measures in reproductive medicine. Hum Reprod. 2015;30(10):2249–51.

24. Maheshwari A, Kalampokas T, Davidson J, Bhattacharya S. Obstetric and perinatal outcomes in singleton pregnancies resulting from the transfer of blastocyst-stage versus cleavage-stage embryos generated through *in vitro* fertilization treatment: a systematic review and meta-analysis. Fertil Steril. 2013;100(6):1615–21.e1–10.

25. Glujovsky D, Farquhar C, Quinteiro Retamar AM, Alvarez Sedo CR, Blake D. Cleavage stage versus blastocyst stage embryo transfer in assisted reproductive technology. Cochrane Database Syst Rev. 2016;6:CD002118.

26. Glujovsky D, Farquhar C. Cleavage-stage or blastocyst transfer: what are the benefits and harms? Fertil Steril. 2016;106(2):244–50.

27. Martins WP, Nastri CO, Rienzi L, van der Poel SZ, Gracia C, Racowsky C. Blastocyst vs cleavage-stage embryo transfer: systematic review and meta-analysis of reproductive outcomes. Ultrasound Obstet Gynecol. 2017;49(5):583–91.

28. Practice Committees of the American Society for Reproductive Medicine, the Society for Assisted Reproductive Technology. Blastocyst culture and transfer in clinical-assisted reproduction: a committee opinion. Fertil Steril. 2013;99(3):667–72.

29. Martins WP, Nastri CO, Rienzi L, van der Poel SZ, Gracia CR, Racowsky C. Obstetrical and perinatal outcomes following blastocyst transfer compared to cleavage transfer: a systematic review and meta-analysis. Hum Reprod. 2016;31(11):2561–9.
30. Holden EC, Kashani BN, Morelli SS, Alderson D, Jindal SK, Ohman-Strickland PA, et al. Improved outcomes after blastocyst-stage frozen-thawed embryo transfers compared with cleavage stage: a Society for Assisted Reproductive Technologies Clinical Outcomes Reporting System study. Fertil Steril. 2018;110(1):89–94.e2.
31. Van der Auwera I, Debrock S, Spiessens C, Afschrift H, Bakelants E, Meuleman C, et al. A prospective randomized study: day 2 versus day 5 embryo transfer. Hum Reprod. 2002;17(6):1507–12.
32. Papanikolaou EG, D'Haeseleer E, Verheyen G, Van de Velde H, Camus M, Van Steirteghem A, et al. Live birth rate is significantly higher after blastocyst transfer than after cleavage-stage embryo transfer when at least four embryos are available on day 3 of embryo culture. A randomized prospective study. Hum Reprod. 2005;20(11):3198–203.
33. Emiliani S, Delbaere A, Vannin AS, Biramane J, Verdoodt M, Englert Y, et al. Similar delivery rates in a selected group of patients, for day 2 and day 5 embryos both cultured in sequential medium: a randomized study. Hum Reprod. 2003;18(10):2145–50.
34. Kuang Y, Chen Q, Fu Y, Wang Y, Hong Q, Lyu Q, et al. Medroxyprogesterone acetate is an effective oral alternative for preventing premature luteinizing hormone surges in women undergoing controlled ovarian hyperstimulation for *in vitro* fertilization. Fertil Steril. 2015;104(1):62–70. e3.
35. Kuang Y, Chen Q, Hong Q, Lyu Q, Ai A, Fu Y, et al. Double stimulations during the follicular and luteal phases of poor responders in IVF/ICSI programmes (Shanghai protocol). Reprod Biomed Online. 2014;29(6):684–91.
36. Shapiro BS, Richter KS, Harris DC, Daneshmand ST. Influence of patient age on the growth and transfer of blastocyst-stage embryos. Fertil Steril. 2002;77(4):700–5.
37. Meldrum DR, Casper RF, Diez-Juan A, Simon C, Domar AD, Frydman R. Aging and the environment affect gamete and embryo potential: can we intervene? Fertil Steril. 2016;105(3):548–59.
38. Morin SJ, Patounakis G, Juneau CR, Neal SA, Scott RT Jr, Seli E. Diminished ovarian reserve and poor response to stimulation in patients <38 years old: a quantitative but not qualitative reduction in performance. Hum Reprod. 2018;33:1489.
39. Fasouliotis SJ, Simon A, Laufer N. Evaluation and treatment of low responders in assisted reproductive technology: a challenge to meet. J Assist Reprod Genet. 2000;17(7):357–73.

Chapter 20
Endometrial Considerations for Minimal Stimulation

John Wu

20.1 Introduction

Whereas much of the considerations in IVF are given to the embryo, an essential but often overlooked aspect of reproduction is the endometrium. In 1907, Hitchmann and Adler made the original observation of histologic changes in the endometrium, undergoing biphasic changes. Following, Frankel and Meyer noted that the cyclic endometrial changes were correlated to the preovulatory and postovulatory follicle. Finally, in 1950, Noyes established endometrial dating by histology. Unfortunately, research regarding the endometrium has led to little change in clinical practice over the years. In terms of implantation and pregnancy rates, endometrial thickness and pattern remain the two most important factors. A 2014 systematic review and meta-analysis of 22 studies found that an endometrial thickness of ≤ 7 mm resulted in a statistically significantly lower clinical pregnancy rate of 23.3% versus 48.1% [1]. Similarly, a uniformly hyperechoic endometrium pattern has been associated with lower implantation and pregnancy rates [2, 3]. In this chapter we will explore the effects of minimal stimulation protocols on the endometrium.

20.2 Anatomy of the Endometrium

The endometrium consists of two layers, the upper stratum functionalis and lower stratum basalis. The functionalis allows for the implantation of the embryo, therefore it is the site of proliferation, secretion, and ultimately desquamation. The

J. Wu (✉)
Division of Reproductive Endocrinology & Infertility, Fertility and Advanced Reproductive Medicine Assisted Reproductive Technologies Program, Department of Obstetrics and Gynecology, University of Texas Southwestern Medical Center, Dallas, TX, USA
e-mail: john.wu@utsouthwestern.edu

© Springer Nature Switzerland AG 2020
O. Bukulmez (ed.), *Diminished Ovarian Reserve and Assisted Reproductive Technologies*, https://doi.org/10.1007/978-3-030-23235-1_20

basalis does not shed during menses and provides regenerative endometrium from endometrial stem cells. On transvaginal ultrasonography, the gold standard of endometrial lining measurement, a distinct multilayer pattern develops in the late proliferative phase, commonly described as the trilaminar pattern. This distinct pattern is formed by the basalis layers (hyperechoic) of the anterior and posterior endometrial layers, the stratum functionalis (hypoechoic) of the anterior and posterior layers, and a central hyperechoic line formed at the central cavity.

20.3   The Normal Menstrual Cycle

To understand the effects of minimal stimulation on the endometrium, one must first understand the endometrium in a normal menstrual cycle. The endometrial menstrual cycle can be viewed in two distinct phases, the proliferative phase and the secretory phase. The proliferative phase is associated with ovarian follicle growth (follicular phase) and increasing levels of estrogen. During this phase the stratum basalis regenerates the superficial layer of compact epithelial cells and intermediate layer of spongiosa. The endometrial glands begin to proliferate in response to hormones, namely, estrogen. At first, the glands are narrow and tubular, lined by low columnar epithelial cells. During proliferation, the endometrium grows from approximately 0.5 mm to 5.0 mm in height of a single layer. This growth is achieved by the proliferation of glands; an influx of ions, water, and amino acids; and re-expansion of the stroma.

With ovulation, the appearance of subnuclear intracytoplasmic glycogen vacuoles occurs. The changes seen in the secretory phase are secondary to the effects of progesterone being produced in mass quantities by the corpus luteum. Remarkably, the total endometrial height is fixed at its preovulatory extent despite continued availability of estrogen, likely due to an increase in 17β-hydroxysteroid dehydrogenase activity within the endometrium which converts bioactive estradiol to a less potent estrone [4]. The once narrow and tubular glands now are tortuous and secretory. The radial arteries become intensely coiled, and the stroma becomes edematous under the direction of progesterone. These changes reach their maximum about 7 days after ovulation. It is during the secretory phase that the window of implantation occurs, approximately 7–10 days after ovulation [5].

20.4   The Effects of Controlled Ovarian Stimulation on the Endometrium

Controlled ovarian stimulation (COS) protocols aim to produce a cohort of oocytes using high-dose gonadotropins allowing for the development of multiple embryos. The optimal number of oocytes retrieved per stimulation cycle is fiercely debated due to the challenge in balancing the advantages of supernumerary embryos and the risks of ovarian hyperstimulation syndrome and the negative effects of supraphysiologic hormones, i.e., estrogen and progesterone on the endometrium. It is well documented that COS leads to advanced development of the endometrium which may result in an alteration in the window of implantation and thus affect pregnancy rates [6]. Numerous studies now support that high serum progesterone (>1.5 ng/mL) on the day of trigger is associated with a decreased pregnancy rate (31% vs 19%) [7]. Due to the adverse effects of hyperstimulation on the endometrium, some argue that milder stimulation protocols may be more natural and have fewer effects upon the endometrium.

20.5   Clomiphene Citrate

Clomiphene citrate is a selective estrogen receptor modulator with variable agonistic-antagonistic effects on estrogen receptor-rich tissues including the hypothalamus, pituitary, ovary, and uterus. As an ovulation induction agent, it binds to estrogen receptors in the hypothalamus, disrupting the normal regulatory negative feedback of estrogen. In response to a perceived lack of estrogen, the anterior pituitary releases follicle-stimulating hormone to act upon the ovary to produce follicles. However, clomiphene citrate can also bind to estrogen receptors in other tissues, namely, the endometrium. At the level of the endometrium, clomiphene citrate acts as a competitive antagonist resulting in a detrimental effect on the endometrial thickness and pattern [8]. Further studies show that clomiphene citrate inhibits the recruitment of steroid receptor coactivator-1 and thereby ERα transactivation in human endometrial epithelial cells [9]. Others report that clomiphene citrate induces ubiquitination and degradation of ERα in Ishikawa cells [10].

20.5.1   The Effects of Clomiphene Citrate on Endometrial Thickness

The majority of literature regarding the negative effects of clomiphene citrate on the endometrial thickness is extrapolated from ovulation induction cycles with clomiphene citrate for intrauterine insemination. The use of clomiphene citrate is limited to 5 days in these instances, so the effects are minimal. However, when used for minimal stimulation, high doses of clomiphene citrate (100 mg) are given daily until the day of trigger. In a retrospective analysis of 230 cycles, it was found that the endometrial thickness was significantly thinner in minimal stimulation cycles (7.3 mm vs 12.9 mm). This occurred despite supraphysiologic levels of estrogen in the minimal stimulation group. The negative effect of clomiphene citrate was best illustrated when comparing endometrial thickness between minimal stimulation and

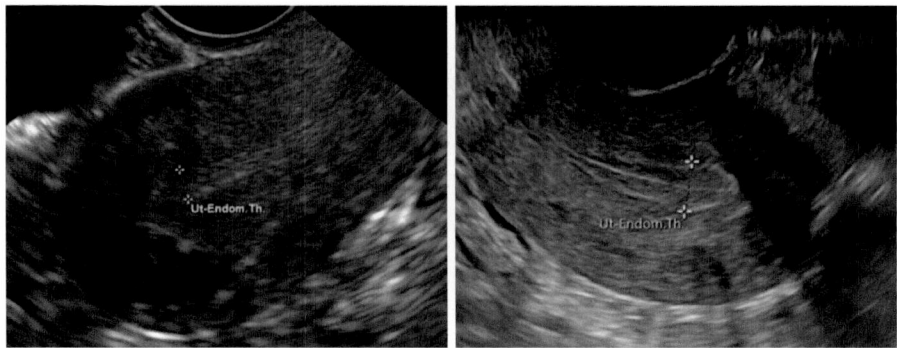

Fig. 20.1 Endometrial thickness (EMT) minimal stimulation (left; E$_2$ 781 pg/mL; EMT 4.0 mm) versus frozen embryo transfer (right; E$_2$ 296 pg/mL; EMT 8.8 mm) in the same patient

their subsequent frozen embryo transfers (7.62 mm vs 10.3 mm), despite lower estradiol levels during the transfer cycles [11] (Fig. 20.1). This suggests that these patients have the potential to have thick endometrial lining, but clomiphene citrate limits its growth during minimal stimulation.

20.5.2   The Effect of Clomiphene Citrate on Histomorphology

Underlying the effects of clomiphene citrate on endometrial thickness is its effects on endometrial differentiation at the cellular level. In endometrial samples obtained from patients undergoing minimal stimulation vs conventional stimulation at the time of oocyte retrieval, we noted stark differences. After minimal stimulation, small undifferentiated glands are dispersed in a sea of polygonal stromal cells. The glands remain narrow and tubular, as expected during the early-to-mid-proliferative phase. In contrast, large tortuous glands of secretory epithelium are the major component of endometrium after conventional stimulation (Fig. 20.2). Furthermore, histomorphometric analyses reveal an increased number of glands per cross-sectional area, along with decreased gland diameter and epithelial height suggesting decreased secretory differentiation with minimal stimulation (Table 20.1).

20.5.3   The Effect of Clomiphene Citrate on Gene Expression

We also observed profound differences in endometrial gene expression between minimal and conventional stimulation. Specifically, 3.4% (723 of 20,764 genes) are significantly differentially expressed. Surprisingly, RNA sequencing does not reveal significant changes in the estrogen receptor or its co-regulators nor in classic proliferation-associated genes in the endometrium such as *cyclinA* and *cMyc* or

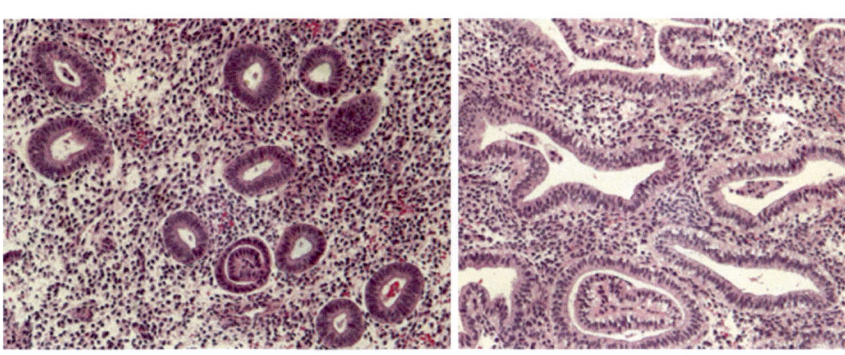

Fig. 20.2 H&E staining of endometrial biopsy samples from minimal stimulation (left) vs conventional stimulation (right)

Table 20.1 Morphometric analysis of endometrial biopsy samples

	Minimal stimulation	Conventional stimulation	P
Number of glands per mm^2	68 ± 21.2	33 ± 5.1	0.003
Gland volume fraction (%)	19.9 ± 2.4	41.5 ± 6.4	<0.0001
Average max gland diameter (μm)	64.7 ± 5.9	159.5 ± 25.2	0.001
Average gland height (μm)	17.2 ± 1.9	21.2 ± 1.4	0.002

antiproliferative genes such as *p27Kip1*. Perhaps, one of the most interesting pathways differentially expressed in the endometrium is that of WNT/β- catenin signaling which is known to be involved in endometrial proliferation. WNT7A is expressed by the luminal epithelium and is a diffusible factor that triggers cell proliferation [12]. Acting on the underlying stroma, WNT7A binds to the receptor Frizzled that phosphorylates the intracytoplasmic protein Dishevelled. When phosphorylated, Dishevelled inactivates glycogen synthase kinase β, turning off the breakdown of β-catenin by ubiquitination. The accumulation of β-catenin induces cell proliferation associated with endometrial growth.

Several WNT inhibitory genes are differentially expressed in minimal stimulation including *NOTUM, WISE/SOST, WIF-1, SFRP1*, and *SFRP4*. Secreted Frizzled-related proteins (sFRPs) antagonize Wnt signaling at the receptor level. Overexpression of sFRP4 and treatment with recombinant sFRPP4 protein inhibits endometrial cancer cell growth in vitro [13]. In endometrial samples comparing minimal stimulation to conventional stimulation, stromal-derived sFRP1 and sFRP4 were increased dramatically in endometrium obtained from clomiphene citrate-treated cycles. Immunofluorescence localized sFRPs to the endometrial stroma with notable accumulation directly underlying the glands, perhaps indicating paracrine signaling between the stroma and glands (Fig. 20.3). This is consistent with the current understanding that estrogen-induced stromal factors are required for epithelial proliferation. Estradiol increases epithelial cell proliferation when cocultured with stroma, but it does not increase proliferation in epithelial cells cultured in the absence of stromal cells.

Fig. 20.3 Immunofluores-
cent staining of minimal
stimulation endometrial
biopsy with anti-SFRP4
(40×)

The exact mechanism in which estrogen induces endometrial proliferation via stromal signaling has not been fully elucidated. Studies show that E2-induced IGF-1 results in epithelial proliferation. RNA sequencing of minimal versus conventional stimulation did not show any differences in gene expression for IGF-1 mRNA. However, binding proteins IGFBP4 and IGFBP5 were increased significantly with clomiphene citrate, which may indicate that clomiphene citrate induces binding proteins to prevent IGF-1 action of the glandular epithelium. Although the exact mechanisms are not established, it is likely that clomiphene citrate not only directly antagonizes epithelial cell growth but also alters stromal factors necessary for paracrine signaling to support endometrial gland proliferation.

20.6   Conclusions

Whereas there is a growing trend toward frozen embryo transfer in conventional IVF due to embryo-endometrial desynchronization, there is little evidence regarding minimal stimulation with the use of clomiphene citrate. Some may argue that the effects of clomiphene citrate on pregnancy rates in ovulation induction cycles with intrauterine insemination are minimal. However, it is difficult to extrapolate its effects on the endometrium during minimal stimulation with prolonged use. With a long half-life of 5 days, the effects of clomiphene citrate may linger even after the medication has been stopped, thus continually effecting the endometrium possibly during the window of implantation. Understanding that the endometrium is affected during minimal stimulation IVF is important when interpreting previous studies utilizing fresh transfer minimal stimulation protocols [14]. The evidence regarding endometrial thickness, histomorphology, and gene expression suggest that there is a severe delay in endometrial gland maturation. Whereas conventional stimulation leads to embryo-endometrial desynchronization due to early advancement, minimal stimulation causes severe delay. Thus, it is recommended that embryos are frozen after minimal stimulation to be transferred later when the endometrium can be adequately prepared to maximize pregnancy rates.

References

1. Kasius A, Smit JG, Torrance HL, Eijkemans MJC, Mol BW, Opmeer BC, et al. Endometrial thickness and pregnancy rates after IVF: a systematic review and meta-analysis. Hum Reprod Update [Internet]. 2014 [cited 2018 Aug 27];20(4):530–41. Available from: http://www.ncbi. nlm.nih.gov/pubmed/24664156.
2. Coulam CB, Bustillo M, Soenksen DM, Britten S. Ultrasonographic predictors of implantation after assisted reproduction. Fertil Steril [Internet]. 1994 [cited 2019 Mar 8];62(5):1004–10. Available from: https://www.sciencedirect.com/science/article/pii/S0015028216570654?via% 3Dihub.
3. Potlog-Nahari C, Catherino WH, McKeeby JL, Wesley R, Segars JH. A suboptimal endometrial pattern is associated with a reduced likelihood of pregnancy after a day 5 embryo transfer. Fertil Steril [Internet]. 2005 [cited 2019 Mar 8];83(1):235–7. Available from: https://www. sciencedirect.com/science/article/pii/S0015028204024501?via%3Dihub.
4. Gurpide E, Gusberg SB, Tseng L. Estradiol binding and metabolism in human endometrial hyperplasia and adenocarcinoma. J Steroid Biochem [Internet]. 1976 [cited 2019 Mar 8];7(11–12):891–6. Available from: http://www.ncbi.nlm.nih.gov/pubmed/1025366.
5. Wilcox AJ, Baird DD, Weinberg CR. Time of implantation of the conceptus and loss of pregnancy. N Engl J Med [Internet]. 1999 [cited 2019 Mar 8];340(23):1796–9. Available from: http://www.ncbi.nlm.nih.gov/pubmed/10362823.
6. Kolb BA, Najmabadi S, Paulson RJ. Ultrastructural characteristics of the luteal phase endometrium in patients undergoing controlled ovarian hyperstimulation. Fertil Steril [Internet]. 1997 [cited 2019 Mar 8];67(4):625–30. Available from: https://www.sciencedirect.com/science/ article/pii/S0015028297813568?via%3Dihub.
7. Bosch E, Labarta E, Crespo J, Simón C, Remohí J, Jenkins J, et al. Circulating progesterone levels and ongoing pregnancy rates in controlled ovarian stimulation cycles for in vitro fertilization: analysis of over 4000 cycles. Hum Reprod [Internet]. 2010 [cited 2019 Mar 8];25(8):2092–100. Available from: http://www.ncbi.nlm.nih.gov/pubmed/20539042.
8. Nakamura Y, Ono M, Yoshida Y, Sugino N, Ueda K, Kato H. Effects of clomiphene citrate on the endometrial thickness and echogenic pattern of the endometrium. Fertil Steril [Internet]. 1997 [cited 2018 Aug 27];67(2):256–60. Available from: http://www.ncbi.nlm.nih.gov/ pubmed/9022599.
9. Amita M, Takahashi T, Tsutsumi S, Ohta T, Takata K, Henmi N, et al. Molecular mechanism of the inhibition of estradiol-induced endometrial epithelial cell proliferation by clomiphene citrate. Endocrinology [Internet]. 2010 [cited 2018 Aug 27];151(1):394–405. Available from: http://www.ncbi.nlm.nih.gov/pubmed/19934375.
10. Amita M, Takahashi T, Igarashi H, Nagase S. Clomiphene citrate down-regulates estrogen receptor-α through the ubiquitin-proteasome pathway in a human endometrial cancer cell line. Mol Cell Endocrinol [Internet]. 2016 [cited 2017 Aug 29];428:142–7. Available from: http:// www.ncbi.nlm.nih.gov/pubmed/27033325.
11. Reed BG, Wu JL, Nemer LB, Carr BR, Bukulmez O. Use of clomiphene citrate in minimal stimulation in vitro fertilization negatively impacts endometrial thickness: an argument for a freeze-all approach. JBRA Assist Reprod [Internet]. 2018 [cited 2019 Mar 8];22(4):355–62. Available from: http://www.ncbi.nlm.nih.gov/pubmed/30264948.
12. Tulac S, Nayak NR, Kao LC, Van Waes M, Huang J, Lobo S, et al. Identification, characterization, and regulation of the canonical Wnt signaling pathway in human endometrium. J Clin

Endocrinol Metab [Internet]. 2003 [cited 2018 Aug 29];88(8):3860–6. Available from: https://academic.oup.com/jcem/article-lookup/doi/10.1210/jc.2003-030494.

13. Carmon KS, Loose DS. Secreted frizzled-related protein 4 regulates two Wnt7a signaling pathways and inhibits proliferation in endometrial cancer cells. Mol Cancer Res [Internet]. 2008 [cited 2017 Sep 8];6(6):1017–28. Available from: http://www.ncbi.nlm.nih.gov/pubmed/18567805.

14. Zhang J, Chang L, Sone Y, Silber S. Minimal ovarian stimulation (mini-IVF) for IVF utilizing vitrification and cryopreserved embryo transfer. Reprod Biomed Online [Internet]. 2010 [cited 2019 Mar 19];21(4):485–95. Available from: https://www.sciencedirect.com/science/article/pii/S1472648310004426?via%3Dihub.

Chapter 21
Frozen Embryo Transfer Preparation

David Prokai and Orhan Bukulmez

21.1 Frozen-Thawed Embryo Transfer (FET) Cycle

The use of embryo cryopreservation and subsequent frozen embryo transfer (FET) has expanded dramatically over the past few years. From 2006 to 2012, the number of autologous FET cycles reported to Society for Assisted Reproductive Technology (SART) in the United States increased by 82.5%, whereas fresh cycle starts increased by only 3.1% [1]. A number of factors have led to the increased utilization of embryo cryopreservation. There has been improved cryopreservation techniques that reduced embryo cryo-damage which have increased post-thaw survival rates [2]. There has also been a large push on behalf of professional organizations like the American Society for Reproductive Medicine (ASRM) toward the increased use of elective single-embryo transfers (eSET) to reduce the incidence of multiple gestations [3]. In some countries, there may also be government-imposed limitations on the number of embryos to be transferred. Increased usage of GnRH agonist "triggers" to prevent ovarian hyperstimulation syndrome (OHSS) in high responders have also increased the number of frozen cycles. This is secondary to the fact that fresh transfers following GnRH triggers were shown to have lower implantation rates compared to conventional human chorionic gonadotropin (hCG) triggers [1]. Additionally, for patients needing preimplantation genetic testing (PGT), embryo freezing may become a necessity to allow for the biopsy results to return [4]. Also, due to emerging evidence for potentially improved obstetric outcomes, some providers and clinics have switched to a so-called "freeze-all" approach where they have moved away from fresh transfers completely [1]. Lastly, several stimulation parameters have been noted to be associated with lower pregnancy rates in fresh

D. Prokai · O. Bukulmez (✉)
Division of Reproductive Endocrinology & Infertility, Fertility and Advanced Reproductive Medicine Assisted Reproductive Technologies Program, Department of Obstetrics and Gynecology, University of Texas Southwestern Medical Center, Dallas, TX, USA
e-mail: Orhan.Bukulmez@UTSouthwestern.edu

© Springer Nature Switzerland AG 2020
O. Bukulmez (ed.), *Diminished Ovarian Reserve and Assisted Reproductive Technologies*, https://doi.org/10.1007/978-3-030-23235-1_21

transfer cycles: premature progesterone elevation prior to trigger, fluid in the endo-metrial cavity, and poor endometrial development [5]. Any or a combination of these factors may lead a provider to turn away from a fresh transfer and move toward embryo cryopreservation and then an FET at a later point.

For our minimal stimulation approaches, employing embryo cryopreservation strategies is a necessity. Stimulation protocols that use clomiphene citrate or letro-zole for more than 5 consecutive days may require "freeze-all" and subsequent FET due to deficiencies in the development of the endometrium as discussed in this book. For women with diminished ovarian reserve (DOR), the embryo yield from each cycle may be as few as 1–2 and their total embryo yield from multiple cycles may be less than 5–10. Given the enormous time, emotional, and financial invest-ment in these embryos, the care and attention to detail that must be paid during the FET cycle equals if not surpasses the attention given during the ovarian stimulation phase. Each embryo is "precious" and it is far more costly and time consuming in the long run to have to go through another stimulation cycle rather than cancelling an FET cycle if there is any concern regarding endometrial development or hor-mone levels.

With that being said, the most effective way of preparing the endometrium is still debated in the literature. The most recent Cochrane database systematic review from 2017 did not find sufficient evidence to recommend one regimen over another [6]. Several options have emerged and the protocols used vary by clinic. In this chapter, we will review the existing data regarding the various methods and review the pros and cons of each method. Additionally, we will review our clinic approach and rationale toward our endometrial preparation and transfer strategies.

21.2   Artificial Cycle (AC) FET

We will begin with a discussion of using exogenous estrogen administration to grow the endometrial lining followed by progesterone addition for luteal phase support. This type of cycle allows the careful titration of estradiol (E2) levels toward a desired target, and for high-volume clinics, it gives the ability to predict the date of embryo thaw, making this the regimen of choice for many centers. Developed in order to synchronize donors and recipients in oocyte donor programs, this was the first method of endometrial preparation described [7].

21.2.1   Estrogen Supplementation

Fundamental toward the growth of the endometrial lining in an artificial embryo transfer is the administration of exogenous E2 in order to prepare the endometrial lining for progesterone initiation and subsequent embryo transfer. A few key things must be considered in regard to estrogen supplementation: the duration of administration, the route of administration, dosage, and fixed versus escalating dosage.

Regarding the duration of E2 administration, there is no consensus on the optimal duration. Still, a study by Borini et al. does illustrate a few crucial points [8]. This study randomized oocyte recipient to the administration of escalating doses of oral E2 (2–6 mg daily) over a time period of 5–76 days. The patients were divided into five groups based on the duration of treatment (<10 days, 11–20 days, 21–30 days, 31–40 days, and >40 days). Notably, there was no significant difference in pregnancy and implantation rates between groups. However, the group with <10 days of E2 administration had a higher rate of miscarriages (41%), $p < 0.05$ versus groups that have longer E2 treatment (11–20 days, 15%), and (>40 days, 1%). This study seems to indicate that extended durations of E2 treatment do not meaningfully alter endometrial receptivity but that supplementation over too brief of a period (<10 days) is associated with higher miscarriage rate. Importantly, several limitations of this study must be considered. Most important among them is the retrospective nature of the study, and all the cycles considered were oocyte donation cycles; thus it cannot be extrapolated that the findings would hold true for patients using their own oocytes which may not be of the same quality as those obtained from young donors.

A later cohort observational study examined this question, but this time, it included patients using their own embryos, and they also examined the effect that GnRH agonist downregulation may play in regard to duration of supplementation and clinical outcomes. They found that clinical pregnancy rate (CPR) was highest without downregulation and with E2 supplementation of <20 days compared to >20 days (25.6% vs 16.7%; $P = 0.037$), and interestingly, they did not find a difference in CPR for <20 days and >20 days when downregulation was used (32.6% vs 31.9%, $P = 0.825$) [9]. Another large retrospective study found that even if the optimal endometrial thickness was reached, initiating progesterone prior to 9 days of E2 treatment resulted in diminished pregnancy rates [10]. Taken together, these studies seem to show a trend toward approximately 12–16 days of E2 supplementation prior to progesterone start as the "sweet spot." It is well known that the rising E2 levels during the follicular phase induce histologic and morphologic changes in the endometrium while leading to the formation of progesterone receptors [11, 12]. Thus it is not unreasonable to extrapolate that a certain critical duration of E2 exposure is needed in order to fully develop the most ideal complement of progesterone receptors to ensure ideal receptivity.

In regard to the route of administration of E2 (oral tablets, transdermal patches, vaginal preparations, and intramuscular injections), no study that we know of has directly compared the methods in terms of endometrial lining thickness and ongoing pregnancy rate. Nonetheless, carefully examining several studies by comparing the reported peak E2 levels and the reported endometrial thickness on the day of progesterone start shows that oral versus transdermal seems to be comparable [13–16]. Thus without a head-to-head trial, the evidence suggests that there is no difference between the modes of administration for E2 in regard to ongoing pregnancy rate in artificial cycles. This leaves it up to the choice of the physician/practice or patient preference. One important factor to consider though is the metabolism of E2 if taken via the oral route [17]. The first-pass hepatic metabolism can be avoided by opting for transdermal, intramuscular, or vaginal route [17, 18]. This might be of particular benefit in patients taking medications that are known to enhance estradiol metabolism if taken orally (most notoriously some antiepileptic medications) [19]. Additionally, some studies have suggested that the transdermal route may give the most steady dosing of E2 which may be the preferred method for endometrial receptivity given its similarity to steady physiologic dosing [18]. Lastly, some have suggested that E2 should be given in gradually increasing doses such that it mimics the rise in E2 produced by the dominant follicle in a natural cycle. The largest retrospective study thus far examining constant E2 dosing versus increasing E2 dosing showed no difference in live birth rate between the two regimens [14].

21.2.1.1 Monitoring During E2 Addition

One key question regarding monitoring during E2 administration is whether or not a GnRH agonist is being employed to prevent follicular recruitment or inadvertent LH surge/ovulation. The use of GnRH agonist downregulation affords the highest degree of control over the timing of embryo transfer and also minimizes the risk of premature ovulation which, as several studies reported, is in the range of 2–4% [20, 21]. Two trials examined cycles with and without the use of GnRH agonist and found comparable outcomes between the two treatment strategies [20, 22]. Of note, these trials included good prognosis patients and did not have any advanced reproductive age (ARA) patients listed in their demographics. Therefore, despite lack of evidence showing clear benefit, our center uses GnRH agonist downregulation in AC-FET in our DOR and ARA patients. We feel that higher resting gonadotropin levels and impaired ovarian feedback mechanisms associated with DOR make these patients more apt to recruit follicles and ovulate during exogenous E2 administration. If GnRH agonist is not used, it is import that the administration of E2 begins shortly after menses (at least before cycle day 4) to prevent unintended follicular recruitment [23].

Our approach to AC-FET is as follows: if a patient has no contraindications to oral contraceptive pills (OCPs), they start on continuous OCPs with at least 30 mcg of ethinyl estradiol at the onset of menses. During this time on OCPs, if the patient has not had a cavity evaluation with saline infusion sonogram and/or a mock embryo transfer, this can be accomplished once their menstrual bleeding subsides. After at least 7 days of OCPs, the patient is started on leuprolide acetate (Lupron®, TAP Pharmaceuticals, North Chicago, IL, United States) 1.0 mg (20 IU) daily. There is overlap of about 7 days of OCPs and leuprolide acetate to prevent GnRH agonist-associated flare. Then OCPs are stopped, and the patient is instructed to call the clinic with the first day of menses. Typically, the patient is called in on cycle day 4–5 while continuing leuprolide acetate 1.0 mg daily. Lupron can also be started in luteal phase to avoid OCPs. During the ultrasound assessment for suppression, the endometrial lining is checked to ensure that the lining is thin (<4 mm) and the ovaries are suppressed with no growing follicles. On this day, E2 level and LH levels are checked to ensure hypothalamic suppression. We define suppression as E2 <50 pg/ml and LH <2.5 mIU/mL. Once the suppression is confirmed, a step-up or "cascade" E2 regimen is begun. With the initiation of E2 dose, leuprolide acetate dose is decreased to 0.25 mg daily. The typical starting dose is oral micronized E2 2 mg (17ß-Estradiol, Estrace®, Teva Pharmaceuticals, Sellersville, PA) for 4 days, followed by 4 mg for 4 days, and then 6 mg for 4 days. If estradiol patches are used, then the typical regimen is 1 patch (100 μg, Minivelle) every other day (qod)×2 days, then 2 patches qod ×4days, then 3 patches qod ×4 days and lastly 4 patches qod×4days. At each escalation of E2 dosing, the E2 and LH serum levels are checked to ensure continued suppression and appropriately rising E2 levels. Special attention is paid to a steady progressive rise in E2 level, and fluctuating, dropping or erratic E2 levels are grounds for cycle cancellation for fears of harming the microarchitecture of the developing endometrium. Once at least 12–14 days of E2 exposure are achieved, a lining check ultrasound is performed to assess endometrial thickness. A thickness of >7 mm and trilaminar configuration is considered the most optimal (see section below on Endometrial Lining). We also assess if there are intense sub-endometrial contractions totally changing the thickness and the pattern of the endometrial stripe. Importantly, mild contractions are usually observed during the E2 phase of the cycle.

With satisfactory lining development, progesterone in oil injections or vaginal micronized progesterone capsules are started. On the day of progesterone start, GnRH agonist is discontinued. The E2 dose is also decreased slightly to the next "step-down" (i.e., 6 mg – >4 mg or 4 mg – >2 mg). This combination of E2 and progesterone are continued with a check in the levels of both of these hormones no sooner than 2 days later and adjustments to the E2 and progesterone can be made prior to the embryo thaw and transfer. The transfer is then performed according to the stage embryo frozen for that patient. On the day of transfer, E2 and progesterone levels are again checked to ensure that proper serum levels are achieved. Depending on the method, vaginal versus intramuscular (IM) progesterone, the desired serum levels will differ. With IM progesterone, a target level of 12–15 ng/ mL is considered optimal, while with vaginal progesterone, the target levels is in the 8–10 ng/mL range. Occasionally, vaginal progesterone will be added in if serum levels with IM progesterone are not adequate. Once stable dosing is found for E2 and progesterone, they are continued until the day of first human chorionic gonadotropin (HCG) level. HCG level is typically assessed 9 days or 11 days after the FET for blastocyst and day 3 cleavage stage embryos, respectively. We monitor HCG progression every 48 hours for at least one to two occasions to ensure appropriate doubling. Then, with appropriate rise in HCG levels, we schedule the first obstetric ultrasound at 6-week gestational age. We continue E2 and progesterone supplementation until the 10th week of pregnancy (Fig. 21.1).

An alternative approach that is used by our clinic if Lupron suppression is incomplete or ineffective is the use of consecutive doses of GnRH antagonist at the onset

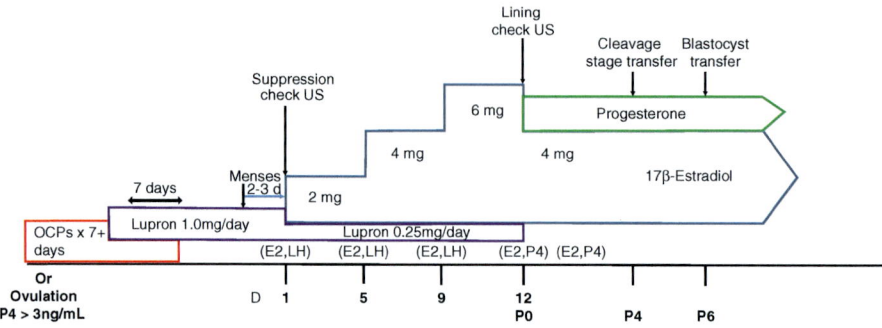

Fig. 21.1 Artificial cycle – FET. Luteal Lupron (GnRH agonist) and OCP –> Lupron start illustrated

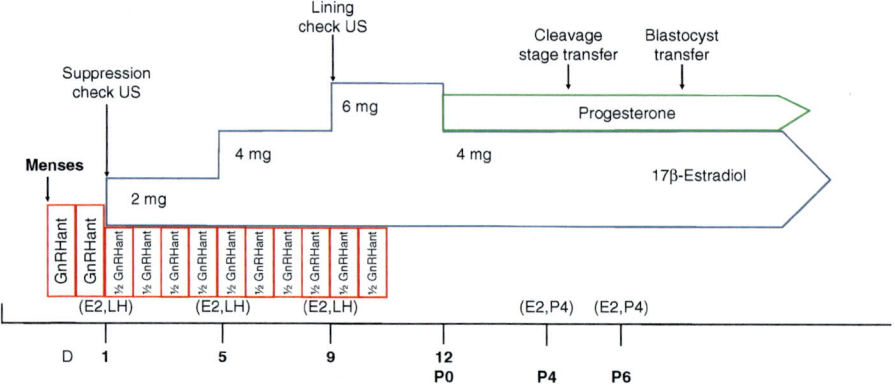

Fig. 21.2 Artificial cycle – FET. GnRH Antagonist Cycle Protocol illustrated

of menses. Full doses (250 mcg daily) of antagonist are given after the onset of menses and the patient presents for ultrasound to ensure a thin endometrial stripe and no follicular activity. GnRH antagonist is given at "half dose" amounts and the estrogen dosing is begun as described above. Half doses of GnRh antagonist are continued until the E2 level is >150 pg/ml at which level follicular recruitment is unlikely. The remainder of the FET protocol is the same as the luteal/OCP/leuprolide acetate FET protocol as described above (Fig. 21.2.).

21.2.2   Endometrial Lining (Stripe)

In addition to carefully monitoring the progressive rise of E2 levels during the FET cycle, the most important checkpoint prior to starting progesterone is the assessment of the endometrial lining appearance and sonographic thickness.

Classically, a thin endometrial lining has been defined as both <7 mm and <8 mm in frozen-thaw embryo transfer cycles [24–29]. The reported incidence of thin lining in assisted reproductive technology (ART) cycles ranges between 1.5% and 9.1% [24, 26–29]. Theories regarding the impact of thin endometrium and poor ART outcomes involve possible poor growth of the endometrial glandular epithelium, decreased vascular endothelial growth factor (VEGF), poor vascular development, higher uterine blood flow impedance, and the oxidative effects of close vascular supply [30].

Select studies have looked at the impact of endometrial lining thickness specifically for FET. Findings of one such study found that the lowest pregnancy rates were associated with endometrial lining thickness of <7 mm and >14 mm and significantly higher rates of clinical pregnancy and subsequent live birth were achieved with endometrial thickness in the 9–14 mm range [25]. One of the largest studies to date examined whether each millimeter of decreasing endometrial thickness resulted in decreased pregnancy and live birth rates. This analysis of the large Canadian ART Registry (CARTR-BORN database) included a total of 20,114 frozen-thawed embryo transfer cycles from the time period of January 1, 2013, to December 31, 2015 [31]. Their findings showed that for FET cycles, both clinical pregnancy and live birth rates decreased with each millimeter below 7 mm, with no significant difference in miscarriage rates for each decreased millimeter. Most interesting in this analysis was the findings of diminishing but not markedly decreased pregnancy rates for even very low endometrial thickness levels. The study found live birth rates of 28.4, 27.4, 23.7, 15, and 21.2% and for endometrial thickness ≥8 mm, 7–7.9 mm, 6–6.9 mm, 5–5.9 mm, and 4–4.9 mm, respectively [31]. The slight increase in live birth rates for the 4–4.9 mm group likely represents a statistical artifact due to small number of transfers in this group, but nonetheless it does illustrate that even with decrease in endometrial thickness all the way down to <5 mm, pregnancy is possible. This study can be cited as a valuable counseling tool in patients with persistently thin endometrium who insist on autologous transfer.

Thus it can be surmised from the available data that a lining thickness >8 mm is ideal and that >7 mm is acceptable. Review of lining morphology and thickness during ovarian stimulation may reveal that supraphysiologic levels of E2 are needed to achieve a sufficient endometrial lining; thus dosing of E2 can be increased or extended if needed. However, care must be taken with this as markedly elevated levels of E2 (E2 levels >700 pg/mL) were implicated in decreased live birth rates [32]. Despite adequate E2 levels and adequate duration of E2 exposure, an endometrial lining that is persistently <7 mm is sometimes encountered and can be a clinically challenging situation. Options for these patients include what could be called "experimental" adjuvant treatments. Protocols such as intrauterine infusion of granulocyte-stimulating factor (G-CSF), co-treatment with sildenafil (Viagra™, Pfizer), and infusion of autologous platelet-rich plasma have been used in the setting of refractory thin endometrium [33–37]. There have even been pilot studies using bone marrow-derived stem cells (BMDSCs) in attempts to improve endometrial thickness in patients with refractory thin endometrial lining [38]. These approaches have yet to be validated in large well-designed studies.

In patients with persistently thin endometrium, issues such as prior surgical history causing Asherman's syndrome or chronic endometritis must be ruled out as potential causes of this phenomenon and corrected where possible. Specifically with chronic endometritis, improvements in implantation rate have been observed following treatment in patients with recurrent implantation failure [39]. Hysteroscopic lysis of adhesions may be indicated if intrauterine synechiae are suspected.

In addition to the endometrial thickness, the morphology and the characteristics of the endometrial lining merit close attention. Various publications have defined the phases of the endometrium in different ways. For the purposes of this chapter, the following nomenclature will be used: pattern 1 (late proliferative: hyperechoic endometrium measuring <50% of the endometrial thickness with a hypoechoic functionalis and a hyperechoic basalis), 2 (early secretory: hyperechoic basalis and functionalis extending >50% of the endometrial thickness, but not encompassing the entire endometrial cavity), and 3 (mid-late secretory: homogeneous hyperechoic functionalis extending all the way from the basalis to the lumen) [40]. Pattern 1 is considered the characteristic "trilaminar pattern" that is the hallmark of the mature proliferative endometrium. Overall, type 1 endometrial pattern ("trilaminar") is associated with improved pregnancy rates [41–44]. All these studies used embryo morphology as the criteria for embryo selection. A more recent study using preimplantation genetic testing for aneuploidy (PGT-A) confirmed euploid embryos (in theory removing to some extent chromosomal factors with the embryo) and found no statistically significant difference in implantation rate between pattern 1 and pattern 2 linings but showed decreased implantation rates for pattern 3 linings [45]. Given this, our clinical goal is the creation of a pattern 1 endometrial lining with at least 7 mm of thickness.

Lastly, during the endometrial lining assessment prior to progesterone administration, careful attention is also paid to the dynamic character of the endometrial stripe itself. Additionally, the presence and the extent of sub-endometrial contractions on 2D ultrasound are also carefully noted. Uterine contractility is a normal phenomenon during the menstrual cycle, reaching its peak in the late follicular/peri-ovulatory phase before subsiding greatly in the luteal phase [46]. Different studies assessed uterine contractility at various points in the cycle: the day of trigger in a fresh embryo transfer cycle [47], just prior to embryo transfer [48, 49], and at the time of embryo transfer [50, 51]. This has led to mixed results with some studies finding no correlation between sub-endometrial contractions and clinical outcomes [49], while others showed decreased pregnancy rates in those with the highest level of contractions [48, 50, 51]. In our practice, no ultrasonographic assessment of the lining is done after progesterone administration. If severe sub-endometrial contractions are seen at the time of lining assessment (contractions that resemble in character and speed the peristalsis of small bowel), then strong consideration is given toward cancelling that cycle. Anecdotally, such severe contractions are noted in patients who have had markedly fluctuating E2 levels during the endometrial preparation phase of their FET cycle, especially in cases that have had drastic falls in their serum E2 levels. If this was the case, alternative dosing strategies are sought in subsequent cycles to minimize changes in E2 levels.

21.2.3   Progesterone Supplementation/Luteal Phase Support

Similar to estrogen supplementation, the optimal progesterone supplement for luteal phase support in FET cycles has yet to be agreed upon. Various dosage forms have been developed and each has their own particular characteristics and potential drawbacks. Furthermore, owing to the heterogeneity between different approaches to FET, it can be hard to extrapolate from one study to another. Additionally, data from luteal phase support in IVF cycle cannot be extrapolated to artificial FET cycles as there is no formed or functioning corpus luteum; thus, all the progesterone needed to transform the endometrium and to maintain the early pregnancy is coming from an exogenous source.

Unfortunately, few studies directly examining luteal phase support in AC-FET cycles are available. Two small, randomized, prospective trials comparing vaginal progesterone with IM progesterone in donor oocyte recipients showed no difference in terms of ongoing pregnancy rates [52, 53]. Other retrospective studies examining donor oocyte recipients [54] and a study looking at both recipients of donor and autologous frozen blastocysts [55] also showed no differences in implantation, clinical pregnancy, or live birth rates. In contrast, two other showed decreased live birth rates in patients receiving vaginal progesterone (22.8% vs 34.5%) [56] and (24.4% vs 39.1%) [57]. Thus the best available data is not entirely clear on which form is superior.

A few issues should be discussed in regard to the benefits of IM progesterone despite some clear drawback. As discussed previously, estrogen is known to increase uterine contractility and progesterone antagonizes this action, thus reducing the extent of sub-endometrial contraction activity. Progesterone, when given vaginally, achieves higher endometrial concentrations then intramuscular progesterone despite lower serum level [58]. While vaginal progesterone does mature the endometrium at a faster rate than IM progesterone, the short half-life of vaginal administration necessitates more frequent dosing. It is possible that the intermittent peaks and troughs of progesterone result in less uterine quiescence than the progesterone in oil depot effect giving longer sustained tissue levels that promote a more evenly "relaxed" uterine environment that may give rise to higher implantation rates. Additionally long gaps in time do not occur with IM administration as they do with the overnight gap between the evening and morning vaginal progesterone administrations. When assessing the ability to reduce sub-endometrial contractility, a small randomized trial ($n = 34$) showed no difference between vaginal and IM progesterone in reducing endometrial contractility at the time of ET so this matter is still up for the debate [51]. A 2010 Cochrane review, with a total of four trials satisfying criteria for analysis, found no statistically significant difference in regard to live birth, clinical pregnancy, or miscarriage rates between vaginal and IM progesterone [59]. Still the authors acknowledge that further study concerning the optimal route of progesterone delivery is still needed. One recent trial that is worth mentioning examined the use of vaginal-only progesterone (Endometrin 200 mg BID; Ferring Pharmaceuticals), vaginal progesterone (Endometrin), and IM progestin every 3rd day or daily IM progesterone. The results of their interim analysis concluded that relative to IM progesterone and combination vaginal-IM progesterone, vaginal-only progesterone resulted in a decreased ongoing pregnancy rate due to a higher miscarriage rate in the vaginal-only treatment group [60]. The biggest takeaway from this study may be the equivalent outcome of combination therapy of progesterone which may allow some mitigation of the side effects of vaginal and IM administration. Further study is still needed to validate this approach.

Nonetheless, both IM and vaginal progesterone have their drawbacks when it comes to patient experience and patient satisfaction. IM progesterone can be painful, especially for long durations of use, and can cause sterile intramuscular abscesses. Vaginal progesterone may cause vaginal irritation in some women. The drawbacks of these methods have led some to explore oral dosing of progesterone to achieve the same ART success as other methods while limiting the side effects that are common with the other dosage forms. Oral preparations of progesterone have generally been avoided due to lower bioavailability and worse ART outcomes [61–63]. That said, dydrogesterone, a retroprogesterone with excellent oral bioavailability [64], currently not available in the United States, has been well researched in regard to luteal phase support after fresh cycle IVF and has shown equivalent outcomes [65–69]. Unfortunately, only limited data exists in its use for FET cycles. Two small studies examined the oral dydrogesterone as the sole source of progesterone in a FET cycle with one study finding comparable results to vaginal progesterone [70], while the other study reported lower pregnancy rates [71]. As with many issues concerning frozen cycles, further study is needed to define the feasibility of an oral-only approach, and if so, what is the optimal dose needed to achieve at least equivalent outcomes to more tried and true methods.

21.3   Natural Cycle

Next, we move on to the so-called "natural cycle" FET approaches. As with minimal/mild stimulation and ovarian stimulation approaches, no consistent definition of what exactly constitutes "natural" is agreed upon. The International Society for Mild Approaches in Assisted Reproduction (ISMAAR) proposed the following definition as it relates to IVF cycles: natural cycle IVF connotes unstimulated, spontaneous IVF cycles; modified natural cycle IVF connotes "semi-natural," controlled natural cycle IVF with hCG-only antagonist and FSH or HMG add-back [72]. We will extend the use of these terms to FET. Therefore, natural cycle FET (NC-FET) denotes no exogenous medications used during the endometrial growth phase and the corpus luteum is the sole source or progesterone. In modified natural cycle (mNC-FET), estrogen, progesterone, and even hCG can be added to support the underlying natural physiologic process.

The benefits of natural/modified natural cycle FET are numerous. These include using a more physiologic means of preparing the endometrium for implantation.

This means little to no medication is needed resulting in less medication cost to the patient. Additionally, avoiding the time and medication needed to suppress the hypothalamic pituitary axis via OCPs and GnRH agonist once again reduces medication cost and side effects and allows a shorter time to begin the FET cycle. Finally, as some patients express discomfort with both vaginal and IM administration of progesterone, avoiding luteal phase support can increase patient satisfaction as well as reduce cost. Unfortunately, natural/modified natural cycle techniques are not suited to patients with irregular cycles. This can especially be an issue for patients with ARA and/or DOR as they are prone to suffer the menstrual cycle characteristics typical of diminishing ovarian reserve, namely, short follicular phases, erratic follicular development (with accompanying erratic E2 levels), impaired corpus luteum development/function, and luteal phase insufficiency. To ensure these conditions are not present, intense laboratory monitoring with often daily lab draws is needed around the time of ovulation, and thus patients with limited access or unwillingness to attend intense monitoring would not be good candidates for this approach. The heightened demands of natural approaches may also burden the fertility clinic schedules as well. The unpredictability of cycle starts and timing of the FET can be stressful from a planning and staffing standpoint as the day of transfer can often fall on a weekend and occasionally on holidays.

A randomized controlled, non-inferiority trial (ANTARCTICA trial) compared artificial cycle with modified natural cycle. The study was conducted between February 2009 and April 2014 and it included an analysis of a total of 959 (n = 959) cycles and looked at 495 modified natural cycles and 464 artificial cycles. Using live birth as the primary outcome, modified natural cycle was shown to be non-inferior to artificial (LBR 11.5% for mNC-FET vs 8.8% AC-FET, 2.7% in favor of mNC-FET (95% confidence interval (CI) −0.065–0.012; P = 0.171) [23]. Similarly, there was no significant difference in clinical pregnancy rate or ongoing pregnancy rate observed. Interestingly, the cancellation rate for AC-FET was significantly higher than for mNC-FET (26.7% vs 20.4%, OR 1.4 95% CI 1.1–1.9 P value 0.02).

One question encountered during clinical practice is whether there needs to be a delay or an interval of time between the ovarian stimulation and the FET. Several retrospective studies examined this issue and have shown no difference between a delay of treatment and immediate start of post-ovarian stimulation and oocyte retrieval [73–76]; thus FET preparation can begin without delay with the first menses following oocyte retrieval.

21.3.1 Monitoring During NC

Integral to the success of a NC-FET is careful monitoring of the hormonal and ultrasonographic parameters as the cycle progresses. While a strict protocol for natural cycles is a contradiction in terms (i.e., a natural cycle varies for each patient and cannot necessarily be made to follow a strict set of rules), at our institution, we generally have a few principles which guide our efforts.

In a patient with regular menstrual cycles, they are instructed to contact the clinic with the onset of full flow of menstrual bleeding. This is considered cycle day 1 (CD1). They are then brought back on cycle day 10 for estradiol (E2), luteinizing hormone (LH), and progesterone (P4) levels. Based on the early values, they are then brought back for only blood work on a daily or every other day basis until their E2 level reaches ~200 pg/mL. At this time, they are brought in for ultrasound to assess the growth of the dominant follicle and the endometrial lining thickness. The goal lining thickness is at least 7 mm with trilaminar morphology. If the desired lining thickness is not achieved on the initial ultrasound, they can be brought back in the coming days as long as the E2 level is still rising and the P4 level is <1 ng/mL. Once the endometrial lining is at least 7 mm in thickness, the patient will come in for daily blood work to confirm ovulation (LH surge >15 IU/L, drop of E2 concentration, a rise in serum progesterone level). Some centers confirm collapse of the known follicle, but this is something we do not routinely do unless indicated by abnormalities in the hormone levels. As the progesterone rises to >1.5 ng/mL, it is our practice to begin progesterone in oil (PIO 50 mg/mL) at a dose of 1 mL IM injection. Additionally, micronized estradiol 2 mg (Estrace®, Teva Pharmaceuticals, Sellersville, PA) is started as well. Both of these medications function to "support" the underlying physiologic process. At the initiation of estrogen and progesterone, adjuvant medications like antibiotics and corticosteroids are also begun. As far as timing of the transfer, closely following the LH levels allows us to see the day of LH surge and thus we can calculate the date of the theoretical oocyte retrieval/pick up (tOPU). From this, we then transfer at the cleavage stage or blastocyst stage depending on the patient's frozen embryo status.

21.3.2 Modified Natural Cycle

To counter some of the unpredictability as well as to augment or shore up any lacking hormonal parameters, some centers have explored adding in various preparation to either support or augment the underlying physiologic processes that make up NC-FETs. This has given rise to the modified natural cycles (mNC-FET). One strategy explored has been the addition of an HCG trigger to the cycle rather than relying on spontaneous ovulation. Proponents of this technique cite several benefits to its use. Firstly, it allows some control and flexibility over the timing of ovulation so that there is some element of control over the timing of embryo warming and transfer. Secondly, it may be possible to decrease the number of monitoring/lab visits as spontaneous ovulation is not being awaited passively [77, 78]. Lastly, the addition of HCG may play a "support" role toward the corpus luteum thus potentially treating possible luteal dysfunction if it exists [79]. Negatives would include the increased cost of the medication and discomfort/inconvenience associated with injections and potential negative impacts on the endometrium which will be discussed below [80, 81].

One early prospective randomized controlled trial from 2010 directly compared outcomes for FET between spontaneous ovulation and induced ovulation via HCG trigger. This study notably did not give luteal support and an LH surge detected at the time HCG trigger was not an exclusion criteria. These factors may explain why this study was stopped prematurely as they noted a substantial decrease in ongoing pregnancy rate in the HCG group vs the pure natural cycle (14.3% vs 31.3%; $p = 0.025$) [80]. Another study by Montagut et al. also found the addition of HCG trigger to natural cycle decreased the pregnancy rates [81]. The authors of these studies suggested a possible negative impact of HCG on the endometrium via alterations of the luteinizing hormone/choriogonadotropin receptor (LHCGR) localization after exposure to exogenous HCG relative to changes that occur via endogenous LH exposure [80, 81].

In contrasts, two studies by Weissman et al. also compared the clinical outcome of pure NC-FET versus the addition of HCG trigger. The criteria for administration of HCG was the following: (i) existence of a dominant follicle at least 17 mm visualized by transvaginal ultrasound, (ii) serum progesterone <1 ng/mL, and (iii) serum E2 >150 pg/mL. An endometrial thickness of at least 7 mm was required prior to moving forward with the embryo transfer. As noted previously, luteal support was given in these studies. Both studies showed no statistically significant difference in implantation rate, clinical pregnancy, or live birth rate per transfer. Only the reduced number of monitoring visits was statistically significant in favor of the HCG trigger group [77, 78].

An important issue to consider regarding the use of HCG trigger relates to the interruption of the careful feedback between the developing follicle, the pituitary, and the developing endometrium. As has been noted many times previously [82], ovulation does not occur at a fixed dominant follicle size nor an exact E2 level. Allowing the body to decide on the optimal ovulatory time may maximize endometrial development and perhaps increase receptivity.

Lastly, the need for luteal phase support (LPS) has been questioned in regard to NC-FET. There have been a few studies published regarding this matter, and the results have been conflicting. In a retrospective analysis, Kyrou et al. showed no benefit for the inclusion of LPS with mNC-FET, while in contrast Bjuresten et al. showed higher live birth rates when LPS was added to true natural cycles [83, 84]. Still, others showed no difference in NC-FET with addition of LPS [85]. Furthermore, the exact route and dosage of LPS has not been universally agreed upon adding further confusion. Given these discrepancies, at this time there is a paucity of evidence in regard to recommending luteal phase support in NC-FET; thus this may be left up to provider/clinic preferences. As previously mentioned, our standard practice is to add low-dose estrogen and progesterone to our natural cycle patients once ovulation has been confirmed especially in women with DOR and ARA.

21.4 Additional Medications

In this next section, we will discuss some of the other medications that are sometimes used during an FET cycle apart from the main hormonal medications previously described in this chapter. Additionally, we will highlight the additional medications used in FET cycles performed at our center.

At the time of embryo transfer (ET), a catheter is placed through the cervical os to access the uterine cavity. Due to theoretical concerns of tracking upper genital tract microbes from the vagina into the uterus via the catheter, antibiotic administration prior to ET has been proposed as a way of improving pregnancy rates. Cochrane database analysis of this issue found that the use of amoxicillin and clavulanic acid prior ET reduced upper genital tract microbial contamination but did not alter clinical pregnancy rates [86]. This same finding was supported in another study [87], and thus according to most sources, the routine use of antibiotics prior to ET is not indicated [86, 88]. That said, it is our practice that all patients (fresh and frozen) receive 3 days of antibiotics (azithromycin 250 mg daily for 3 days) initiated at the start of progesterone initiation in fresh and frozen cycles.

Another medication often used as an adjuvant in ART is aspirin. Aspirin has been employed during FET cycles due to the potential for enhanced uterine perfusion and thus enhanced endometrial receptivity [89, 90]. The use of aspirin has shown mixed results when used in fresh transfer IVF cycles [90–93]. Data looking exclusively at frozen cycle outcomes is more limited. One early study found improved pregnancy rates by using high doses of aspirin 150–300 mg/day [94], but later small study found no improvements in pregnancy rate [95]. However, a more recent larger pilot randomized, double-blind placebo-controlled trial showed significant improvements in implantation rate, clinical pregnancy rate, and most importantly live birth with daily low-dose aspirin [96]. Importantly, this study used the standard and readily available dosing of 81 mg ("baby aspirin"). Given this, it is our standard practice to include aspirin in all of our frozen-thaw cycles (both natural and medicated). We continue baby aspirin through the first pregnancy test and subsequent ultrasounds. We do have a low threshold for stopping aspirin if any first trimester bleeding occurs.

Lastly, we will address the use of peri-implantation corticosteroids to embryo implantation. The theory behind this intervention is that the use of steroids will modulate uterine natural killer (NK) cells, improve the cytokine/growth factor milieu in the endometrium, and suppress endometrial inflammations in the hopes of improving receptivity [97, 98]. The most recent Cochrane review of 14 trials found no effect on clinical pregnancy or live birth rate in the general IVF/ICSI fresh transfer population [97]. Two nonrandomized trials revealed a benefit in patients with recurrent implantation failure [99, 100]. A large randomized controlled trial involving the use of corticosteroids alone or in combination with aspirin in frozen transfer cycles is lacking at this time. Furthermore, a trial examining the use of corticosteroids in cleavage state transfer in patients with advanced reproductive age and diminished ovarian reserve (reflective of our practice's patient population) needs to be performed. Given this, we prescribe 16 mg of methylprednisolone for 3 days starting at the time of progesterone initiation.

21.5   Adjunct Procedures

If an adequate trilaminar lining is achieved and there are no pregnancy results after the transfer of a high-grade embryo, one of the thoughts/suspicions is the failure of synchronization between the endometrium and the embryo resulting in failure to implant. Couples with an unsuccessful embryo transfer may feel desperate and inquire as to additional procedures or interventions that could be performed to increase their chances in subsequent cycles. Two of the most commonly asked for adjunct procedures among our patients are endometrial receptivity testing and endometrial scratch.

During the menstrual cycle, there is thought to be a "window of implantation" when the endometrium is receptive to the embryo [79]. One of the theories behind the lack of implantation of a "high-quality" embryo is since there is a mismatch between the "timing" of the endometrium and the "timing" of the embryo. By performing a mock cycle and obtaining a biopsy, an endometrial receptivity array (ERA) can be performed to guide the physician with transferring the embryo in a subsequent cycle. Our center has yet to adopt this in our patients. One of the central assumptions of ERA testing is that by repeating the same medication protocol, the same endometrial development and biopsy findings should always be the same over repetitive cycles. Therefore the transfer day should be indicated by the results of the ERA test as determined by the prior mock cycle. However, in our close observation of medicated cycles, we often observe quite dramatic fluctuations in serum levels of estradiol regardless of the dosage form (hence our strategy of frequent lab testing). Just as we feel there are variations from cycle to cycle in terms of ovarian response, we similarly feel there is cycle-to-cycle variation in endometrial preparation. As more research become available in the future, this issue may be revisited.

Local endometrial injury results in an inflammatory response that favors implantation. Specifically, this intervention was sought out by patients with recurrent implantation failure (RIF) as means of improving their chances of having a successful outcome. Some evidence exists in smaller studies; thus on occasion we have performed this upon request from patients (usually at the time of cavity assessment prior to an FET cycle). Additionally, by performing the endometrial scratch via an endometrial biopsy pipelle, a sample of tissue can be sent to test for chronic endometritis which has been shown to be more prevalent among patients with RIF. However, as a result of a recent large, well-designed, randomized controlled trial, there will likely be a decreased use of this technique in the future. The Pipelle for Pregnancy (PIP) trial investigated whether endometrial scratch via endometrial biopsy increased the probability of live birth. Endometrial scratching did not result in higher rates of live births in patients undergoing either their initial transfer or in those who had previously failed transfer [101]. It is interesting to note that this large study did not observe benefit in those with previous implantation failure given that this is the exact population that was purported to benefit the most from endometrial scratch.

Lastly, we can briefly mention that all our embryo transfers are performed under pelvic ultrasound guidance by using Wallace® Sure-Pro® embryo replacement with obturator (Cooper Surgical, Trumbull, CT). The cervix is gently irrigated by using 10 mL of sterile media to minimize mucus and debris. After passing the cervical internal os with the outer catheter very gently, the advancement is halted and the embryologist is notified. The inner catheter loaded with the embryo(s) is introduced into the outer catheter and the inner catheter is advanced toward the uterine fundus under ultrasonographic guidance. The inner catheter tip's advancement is stalled once the distance between the distal fundal end of the cavity and the catheter tip is between 1.5 cm and 2 cm. Then the plunger of the embryo transfer syringe was pushed to complete the embryo transfer. The air bubble density can be observed at the distal fundal portion of the cavity. Right after transfer, the inner catheter is gently withdrawn while still pressing the plunger and turning the inner catheter around its axis while withdrawing. When the level of outer catheter is reached, both catheters are removed out of the cervix and returned back to the embryologist. Once the embryologist indicates the absence of any stuck embryo, embryo transfer is completed by removing the speculum and repositioning the patient to the dorsal supine position. Although studies showed no benefit of prolonged or even short rest after the embryo transfer [102–106], we keep patients lying down in mild Trendelenburg position for 10 minutes or less while reviewing post-transfer recommendations and answering all their questions. Then the patient gets up and walks to the bathroom to empty the bladder and gets dressed. We recently stopped using oral anxiolytics like diazepam 5 mg tablet before the FET. Therefore, patients can just walk out of the clinic without needing assistance. Regular daily activities are allowed after the transfer.

21.6   Conclusion

There is a growing body of evidence that in high responders and patients with PCOS [107], FET cycles have a significantly higher or comparable clinical pregnancy rates compared to fresh transfers [1, 108–110] and that FET is at least equivalent in normal responders. The choice of which FET cycle to use for a patient can sometimes be a difficult one. Patient factors such as compliance, comorbidities, and previous reproductive history must be considered along with clinic factors that relate to frequency of lab checks and what medications and protocols to follow. While sometimes taxing for a busy clinical practice, natural cycle embryo transfers are an attractive option for patients looking to minimize interventions, interested in a more "natural" approach, and looking to reduce cost on medications and avoid medication side effects. Medicated cycles, on the other hand, can be advantageous for those with irregular/unpredictable cycles and for high-volume practices that need precise timing of embryo thaw and transfer. We believe that consistency and the same careful attention paid during the ovarian stimulation phase is the key to maintaining high pregnancy rates in frozen-thaw cycles. This may be of even more importance for women with ARA and DOR as the margin of error for a successful outcome is likely to be much smaller than with good prognosis patients.

References

1. Shapiro BS, Daneshmand ST, Garner FC, Aguirre M, Hudson C. Clinical rationale for cryopreservation of entire embryo cohorts in lieu of fresh transfer. Fertil Steril. 2014;102(1):3–9.
2. Rezazadeh Valojerdi M, Eftekhari-Yazdi P, Karimian L, Hassani F, Movaghar B. Vitrification versus slow freezing gives excellent survival, post warming embryo morphology and pregnancy outcomes for human cleaved embryos. J Assist Reprod Genet. 2009;26(6):347–54.
3. Practice Committee of the American Society for Reproductive Medicine. Electronic address ASRM@asrm.org. Practice Committee of the Society for Assisted Reproductive Technology. Penzias A, Bendikson K, Butts S, Coutifaris C, Fossum G, Falcone T, et al. Guidance on the limits to the number of embryos to transfer: a committee opinion. Fertil Steril. 2017;107(4):901–3.
4. Maxwell SM, Grifo JA. Should every embryo undergo preimplantation genetic testing for aneuploidy? A review of the modern approach to in vitro fertilization. Best Pract Res Clin Obstet Gynaecol. 2018;53:38–47.
5. Healy M, Patounakis G, Zanelotti A, Devine K, DeCherney A, Levy M, et al. Does premature elevated progesterone on the day of trigger increase spontaneous abortion rates in fresh and subsequent frozen embryo transfers? Gynecol Endocrinol. 2017;33(6):472–5.
6. Ghobara T, Gelbaya TA, Ayeleke RO. Cycle regimens for frozen-thawed embryo transfer. Cochrane Database Syst Rev. 2017;(7):CD003414.
7. Wallach EE, Younis JS, Simon A, Laufer N. Endometrial preparation: lessons from oocyte donation. Fertil Steril. 1996;66(6):873–84.
8. Borini A, Prato LD, Bianchi L, Violini F, Cattoli M, Flamigni C. CLINICAL ASSISTED REPRODUCTION: effect of duration of estradiol replacement on the outcome of oocyte donation. J Assist Reprod Genet. 2001;18(4):187–92.
9. Sunkara SK, Seshadri S, El-Toukhy T. The impact of the duration of estrogen supplementation on the outcome of medicated frozen-thawed embryo transfer (FET) cycles. Fertil Steril. 2011;96(3):S43.
10. Dougherty MP, Morin SJ, Juneau CR, Neal SA, Scott RT. Fewer than 9 days of estrogen exposure prior to progesterone initiation results in lower pregnancy rates in programmed frozen embryo transfer cycles. Fertil Steril. 2017;107(3):e11–2.
11. Fraser HM, Kelly RW, Jabbour HN, Critchley HOD. Endocrine regulation of menstruation. Endocr Rev. 2006;27(1):17–46.
12. Fauser BCJM, Macklon NS, Stouffer RL, Giudice LC. The science behind 25 years of ovarian stimulation for in vitro fertilization. Endocr Rev. 2006;27(2):170–207.
13. Davar R, Janati S, Mohseni F, Khabazkhoob M, Asgari S. A comparison of the effects of transdermal estradiol and estradiol valerate on endometrial receptivity in frozen-thawed embryo transfer cycles: a randomized clinical trial. J Reprod Infertil. 2016;17(2):97–103.
14. Rodriguez A, Madero S, Vernaeve V, Vassena R. Endometrial preparation: effect of estrogen dose and administration route on reproductive outcomes in oocyte donation cycles with fresh embryo transfer. Hum Reprod. 2016;31(8):1755–64.
15. Kawamura T, Motoyama H, Yanaihara A, Yorimitsu T, Arichi A, Karasawa Y, et al. Clinical outcomes of two different endometrial preparation methods for cryopreserved-thawed embryo transfer in patients with a normal menstrual cycle. Reprod Med Biol. 2007;6(1):53–7.
16. Tomás C, Alsbjerg B, Martikainen H, Humaidan P. Pregnancy loss after frozen-embryo transfer—a comparison of three protocols. Fertil Steril. 2012;98(5):1165–9.
17. Kuhl H. Pharmacokinetics of oestrogens and progestogens. Maturitas. 1990;12(3):171–97.
18. Krasnow JS, Lessey BA, Naus G, Hall L-LH, Guzick DS, Berga SL. Comparison of transdermal versus oral estradiol on endometrial receptivity. Fertil Steril. 1996;65(2):332–6.
19. Harden CL, Pennell PB. Neuroendocrine considerations in the treatment of men and women with epilepsy. Lancet Neurol. 2013;12(1):72–83.
20. Prato LD, Borini A, Cattoli M, Bonu MA, Sciajno R, Flamigni C. Endometrial preparation for frozen-thawed embryo transfer with or without pretreatment with gonadotropin-releasing hormone agonist. Fertil Steril. 2002;77(5):956–60.

21. Seltman HJ, Queenan JT, Jr, Ramey JW, Eure L, Veeck LL, Muasher SJ. Transfer of cryopreserved-thawed pre-embryos in a cycle using exogenous steroids without prior gonadotrophin-releasing hormone agonist suppression yields favourable pregnancy results. Hum Reprod. 1997;12(6):1176–80.
22. Hurwitz A, Simon A, Zentner BS, Laufer N, Bdolah Y. Transfer of frozen-thawed embryos in artificially prepared cycles with and without prior gonadotrophin-releasing hormone agonist suppression: a prospective randomized study. Hum Reprod. 1998;13(10):2712–7.
23. Groenewoud ER, Cohlen BJ, Al-Oraiby A, Brinkhuis EA, Broekmans FJM, de Bruin JP et al. A randomized controlled, non-inferiority trial of modified natural versus artificial cycle for cryo-thawed embryo transfer. Hum Reprod. 2016;31(7):1483–92.
24. Al-Ghamdi A, Coskun S, Al-Hassan S, Al-Rejjal R, Awartani K. The correlation between endometrial thickness and outcome of in vitro fertilization and embryo transfer (IVF-ET) outcome. Reprod Biol Endocrinol. 2008;6:37.
25. El-Toukhy T, Coomarasamy A, Khairy M, Sunkara K, Seed P, Khalaf Y, et al. The relationship between endometrial thickness and outcome of medicated frozen embryo replacement cycles. Fertil Steril. 2008;89(4):832–9.
26. Shufaro Y, Simon A, Laufer N, Fatum M. Thin unresponsive endometrium--a possible complication of surgical curettage compromising ART outcome. J Assist Reprod Genet. 2008;25(8):421–5.
27. Aydin T, Kara M, Nurettin T. Relationship between endometrial thickness and in vitro fertilization-intracytoplasmic sperm injection outcome. Int J Fertil Steril. 2013;7(1):29–34.
28. Wu Y, Gao X, Lu X, Xi J, Jiang S, Sun Y, et al. Endometrial thickness affects the outcome of in vitro fertilization and embryo transfer in normal responders after GnRH antagonist administration. Reprod Biol Endocrinol. 2014;12:96.
29. Bu Z, Sun Y. The impact of endometrial thickness on the day of human chorionic gonadotrophin (hCG) administration on ongoing pregnancy rate in patients with different ovarian response. PLoS One. 2015;10(12):e0145703.
30. Mahajan N, Sharma S. The endometrium in assisted reproductive technology: how thin is thin? J Hum Reprod Sci. 2016;9(1):3–8.
31. Liu KE, Hartman M, Hartman A, Luo ZC, Mahutte N. The impact of a thin endometrial lining on fresh and frozen-thaw IVF outcomes: an analysis of over 40 000 embryo transfers. Hum Reprod. 2018;33(10):1883–8.
32. Fritz R, Jindal S, Feil H, Buyuk E. Elevated serum estradiol levels in artificial autologous frozen embryo transfer cycles negatively impact ongoing pregnancy and live birth rates. J Assist Reprod Genet. 2017;34(12):1633–8.
33. Li Y, Pan P, Chen X, Li L, Li Y, Yang D. Granulocyte colony-stimulating factor administration for infertile women with thin endometrium in frozen embryo transfer program. Reprod Sci. 2014;21(3):381–5.
34. Kunicki M, Łukaszuk K, Woclawek-Potocka I, Liss J, Kulwikowska P, Szczyptańska J. Evaluation of granulocyte colony-stimulating factor effects on treatment-resistant thin endometrium in women undergoing in vitro fertilization. Biomed Res Int. 2014;2014:913235.
35. Kim A, Shohat-Tal A, Barad DH, Lazzaroni E, Lee H-J, Michaeli T, et al. A pilot cohort study of granulocyte colony-stimulating factor in the treatment of unresponsive thin endometrium resistant to standard therapies. Hum Reprod. 2012;28(1):172–7.
36. Lebovitz O, Orvieto R. Treating patients with "thin" endometrium – an ongoing challenge. Gynecol Endocrinol. 2014;30(6):409–14.
37. Kim H, Shin JE, Koo HS, Kwon H, Choi DH, Kim JH. Effect of autologous platelet-rich plasma treatment on refractory thin endometrium during the frozen embryo transfer cycle: a pilot study. Front Endocrinol. 2019;10:61.
38. Santamaria X, Mas A, Simon C, Cervelló I, Taylor H. Uterine stem cells: from basic research to advanced cell therapies. Hum Reprod Update. 2018;24(6):673–93.
39. Vitagliano A, Saccardi C, Noventa M, Di Spiezio Sardo A, Saccone G, Cicinelli E, et al. Effects of chronic endometritis therapy on in vitro fertilization outcome in women with repeated implantation failure: a systematic review and meta-analysis. Fertil Steril. 2018;110(1):103–112.e1.

40. Grunfeld L, Walker B, Bergh PA, Sandler B, Hofmann G, Navot D. High-resolution endovaginal ultrasonography of the endometrium: a noninvasive test for endometrial adequacy. Obstet Gynecol. 1991;78(2):200.
41. Järvelä IY, Sladkevicius P, Kelly S, Ojha K, Campbell S, Nargund G. Evaluation of endometrial receptivity during in-vitro fertilization using three-dimensional power Doppler ultrasound. Ultrasound Obstet Gynecol. 2005;26(7):765–9.
42. Zhao J, Zhang Q, Wang Y, Li Y. Endometrial pattern, thickness and growth in predicting pregnancy outcome following 3319 IVF cycle. Reprod Biomed Online. 2014;29(3):291–8.
43. Hock DL, Bohrer MK, Ananth CV, Kemmann E. Sonographic assessment of endometrial pattern and thickness in patients treated with clomiphene citrate, human menopausal gonadotropins, and intrauterine insemination. Fertil Steril. 1997;68(2):242–5.
44. Bohrer MK, Hock DL, Rhoads GG, Kemmann E. Sonographic assessment of endometrial pattern and thickness in patients treated with human menopausal gonadotropins**Presented in part in the 25th Annual Meeting of the American Society for Reproductive Medicine, San Antonio, Texas, November 5 to 10, 1994. Fertil Steril. 1996;66(2):244–7.
45. Gingold JA, Lee JA, Rodriguez-Purata J, Whitehouse MC, Sandler B, Grunfeld L, et al. Endometrial pattern, but not endometrial thickness, affects implantation rates in euploid embryo transfers. Fertil Steril. 2015;104(3):620–8.e5.
46. Bulletti C, de Ziegler D, Polli V, Diotallevi L, Ferro ED, Flamigni C. Uterine contractility during the menstrual cycle. Hum Reprod. 2000;15(suppl_1):81–9.
47. Vlaisavljevic V, Reljic M, Gavric–Lovrec V, Kovacic B . Subendometrial contractility is not predictive for in vitro fertilization (IVF) outcome. Ultrasound Obstet Gynecol. 2001;17(3):239–44.
48. Righini C, Olivennes F, Ayoubi J-M, Schönauer LM, Fanchin R, Frydman R. Uterine contractility decreases at the time of blastocyst transfers. Hum Reprod. 2001;16(6):1115–9.
49. Samara N, Casper RF, Bassil R, Shere M, Barzilay E, Orvieto R, et al. Sub-endometrial contractility or computer-enhanced 3-D modeling scoring of the endometrium before embryo transfer: are they better than measuring endometrial thickness? J Assist Reprod Genet. 2019;36(1):139–43.
50. Fanchin R, Righini C, Ayoubi JM, Olivennes F, de Ziegler D, Frydman R. Uterine contractions at the time of embryo transfer: a hindrance to implantation? Contracept Fertil Sex. 1998;26(7–8):498–505.
51. Hershko Klement A, Samara N, Weintraub A, Mitri F, Bentov Y, Chang P, et al. Intramuscular versus vaginal progesterone administration in medicated frozen embryo transfer cycles: a randomized clinical trial assessing sub-endometrial contractions. Gynecol Obstet Invest. 2018;83(1):40–4.
52. Gibbons WE, Toner JP, Hamacher P, Kolm P. Experience with a novel vaginal progesterone preparation in a donor oocyte program. Fertil Steril. 1998;69(1):96–101.
53. Jobanputra K, Toner JP, Denoncourt R, Gibbons WE. Crinone 8% (90 mg)**Crinone 8%, Serono Laboratories, Inc., Norwell, MA. given once daily for progesterone replacement therapy in donor egg cycles. Sponsored by Columbia Research Laboratories, Inc., Rockville Centre, New York. Fertil Steril. 1999;72(6):980–4.
54. Berger BM, Phillips JA. Pregnancy outcomes in oocyte donation recipients: vaginal gel versus intramuscular injection progesterone replacement. J Assist Reprod Genet. 2012;29(3): 237–42.
55. Shapiro DB, Pappadakis JA, Ellsworth NM, Hait HI, Nagy ZP. Progesterone replacement with vaginal gel versus i.m. injection: cycle and pregnancy outcomes in IVF patients receiving vitrified blastocysts. Hum Reprod. 2014;29(8):1706–11.
56. Haddad G, Saguan DA, Maxwell R, Thomas MA. Intramuscular route of progesterone administration increases pregnancy rates during non-downregulated frozen embryo transfer cycles. J Assist Reprod Genet. 2007;24(10):467–70.
57. Kaser DJ, Ginsburg ES, Missmer SA, Correia KF, Racowsky C. Intramuscular progesterone versus 8% Crinone vaginal gel for luteal phase support for day 3 cryopreserved embryo transfer. Fertil Steril. 2012;98(6):1464–9.

58. Cicinelli E, De Ziegler D, Bulletti C, Matteo MG, Schonauer LM, Galantino P. Direct transport of progesterone from vagina to uterus. Obstet Gynecol. 2000;95(3):403–6.
59. Glujovsky D, Pesce R, Fiszbajn G, Sueldo C, Hart RJ, Ciapponi A. Endometrial preparation for women undergoing embryo transfer with frozen embryos or embryos derived from donor oocytes. Cochrane Database Syst Rev. 2010;(1):CD006359.
60. Devine K, Richter KS, Widra EA, McKeeby JL. Vitrified blastocyst transfer cycles with the use of only vaginal progesterone replacement with Endometrin have inferior ongoing pregnancy rates: results from the planned interim analysis of a three-arm randomized controlled noninferiority trial. Fertil Steril. 2018;109(2):266–75.
61. Nahoul K, Dehennin L, Jondet M, Roger M. Profiles of plasma estrogens, progesterone and their metabolites after oral or vaginal administration of estradiol or progesterone. Maturitas. 1993;16(3):185–202.
62. Licciardi FL, Kwiatkowski A, Noyes NL, Berkeley AS, Krey LL, Grifo JA. Oral versus intramuscular progesterone for in vitro fertilization: a prospective randomized study. Fertil Steril. 1999;71(4):614–8.
63. Simon JA, Robinson DE, Andrews MC, Hildebrand JR, Rocci ML, Blake RE, et al. The absorption of oral micronized progesterone: the effect of food, dose proportionality, and comparison with intramuscular progesterone∗†∗Supported in part by a grant from Besins-Iscovesco, Paris, France.†Presented in part at the 35th Annual Meeting of the Society for Gynecologic Investigation, Baltimore, Maryland, March 17 to 20, 1988. Fertil Steril. 1993;60(1):26–33.
64. Griesinger G, Tournaye H, Macklon N, Petraglia F, Arck P, Blockeel C, et al. Dydrogesterone: pharmacological profile and mechanism of action as luteal phase support in assisted reproduction. Reprod Biomed Online. 2019;38(2):249–59.
65. Ganesh A, Chakravorty N, Mukherjee R, Goswami S, Chaudhury K, Chakravarty B. Comparison of oral dydrogestrone with progesterone gel and micronized progesterone for luteal support in 1,373 women undergoing in vitro fertilization: a randomized clinical study. Fertil Steril. 2011;95(6):1961–5.
66. Tomic V, Tomic J, Klaic DZ, Kasum M, Kuna K. Oral dydrogesterone versus vaginal progesterone gel in the luteal phase support: randomized controlled trial. Eur J Obstet Gynecol Reprod Biol. 2015;186:49–53.
67. Barbosa MWP, Silva LR, Navarro PA, Ferriani RA, Nastri CO, Martins WP. Dydrogesterone vs progesterone for luteal-phase support: systematic review and meta-analysis of randomized controlled trials. Ultrasound Obstet Gynecol. 2016;48(2):161–70.
68. Saharkhiz N, Zamaniyan M, Salehpour S, Zadehmodarres S, Hoseini S, Cheraghi L, et al. A comparative study of dydrogesterone and micronized progesterone for luteal phase support during in vitro fertilization (IVF) cycles. Gynecol Endocrinol. 2016;32(3):213–7.
69. Griesinger G, Blockeel C, Sukhikh GT, Patki A, Dhorepatil B, Yang D-Z, et al. Oral dydrogesterone versus intravaginal micronized progesterone gel for luteal phase support in IVF: a randomized clinical trial. Hum Reprod. 2018;33(12):2212–21.
70. Rashidi BH, Ghazizadeh M, Tehrani Nejad ES, Bagheri M, Gorginzadeh M. Oral dydrogesterone for luteal support in frozen-thawed embryo transfer artificial cycles: a pilot randomized controlled trial. Asian Pac J Reprod. 2016;5(6):490–4.
71. Zarei A, Sohail P, Parsanezhad ME, Alborzi S, Samsami A, Azizi M. Comparison of four protocols for luteal phase support in frozen-thawed Embryo transfer cycles: a randomized clinical trial. Arch Gynecol Obstet. 2017;295(1):239–46.
72. Nargund G. ISMAAR: The International Society for mild approaches in Assisted Reproduction. Facts Views Vis Obgyn. 2011;3(1):5–7.
73. Santos-Ribeiro S, Siffain J, Polyzos NP, van de Vijver A, van Landuyt L, Stoop D, et al. To delay or not to delay a frozen embryo transfer after a failed fresh embryo transfer attempt? Fertil Steril. 2016;105(5):1202–1207.e1.
74. Tournaye H, Siffain J, Van Landuyt L, Mackens S, Santos-Ribeiro S, Polyzos NP, et al. The effect of an immediate frozen embryo transfer following a freeze-all protocol: a retrospective analysis from two centres. Hum Reprod. 2016;31(11):2541–8.

75. Maas KH, Baker VL, Westphal LM, Lathi RB. Optimal timing of frozen embryo transfer after failed IVF attempt. Fertil Steril. 2008;90:S285.
76. Lattes K, Checa MA, Vassena R, Brassesco M, Vernaeve V. There is no evidence that the time from egg retrieval to embryo transfer affects live birth rates in a freeze-all strategy. Hum Reprod. 2017;32(2):368–74.
77. Weissman A, Horowitz E, Ravhon A, Steinfeld Z, Mutzafi R, Golan A, et al. Spontaneous ovulation versus HCG triggering for timing natural-cycle frozen–thawed embryo transfer: a randomized study. Reprod Biomed Online. 2011;23(4):484–9.
78. Weissman A, Levin D, Ravhon A, Eran H, Golan A, Levran D. What is the preferred method for timing natural cycle frozen–thawed embryo transfer? Reprod Biomed Online. 2009;19(1):66–71.
79. Casper RF, Yanushpolsky EH. Optimal endometrial preparation for frozen embryo transfer cycles: window of implantation and progesterone support. Fertil Steril. 2016;105(4):867–72.
80. Fatemi HM, Kyrou D, Bourgain C, Van den Abbeel E, Griesinger G, Devroey P. Cryopreserved-thawed human embryo transfer: spontaneous natural cycle is superior to human chorionic gonadotropin–induced natural cycle. Fertil Steril. 2010;94(6):2054–8.
81. Montagut M, van de Vijver A, Verheyen G, Tournaye H, van Landuyt L, De Vos M, et al. Frozen–thawed embryo transfers in natural cycles with spontaneous or induced ovulation: the search for the best protocol continues. Hum Reprod. 2016;31(12):2803–10.
82. Hackelöer BJ, Fleming R, Robinson HP, Adam AH, Coutts JR. Correlation of ultrasonic and endocrinologic assessment of human follicular development. Am J Obstet Gynecol. 1979;135(1):122–8.
83. Kyrou D, Fatemi HM, Popovic-Todorovic B, Van den Abbeel E, Camus M, Devroey P. Vaginal progesterone supplementation has no effect on ongoing pregnancy rate in hCG-induced natural frozen–thawed embryo transfer cycles. Eur J Obstet Gynecol Reprod Biol. 2010;150(2):175–9.
84. Bjuresten K, Landgren B-M, Hovatta O, Stavreus-Evers A. Luteal phase progesterone increases live birth rate after frozen embryo transfer. Fertil Steril. 2011;95(2):534–7.
85. Lee VCY, Li RHW, Ng EHY, Yeung WSB, Ho PC. Luteal phase support does not improve the clinical pregnancy rate of natural cycle frozen-thawed embryo transfer: a retrospective analysis. Eur J Obstet Gynecol Reprod Biol. 2013;169(1):50–3.
86. Kroon B, Hart RJ, Wong BMS, Ford E, Yazdani A. Antibiotics prior to embryo transfer in ART. Cochrane Database of Syst Rev. 2012;(3):CD008995.
87. Coomarasamy A, Brook N, Khalaf Y, Braude P, Edgeworth J. A randomized controlled trial of prophylactic antibiotics (co-amoxiclav) prior to embryo transfer. Hum Reprod. 2006;21(11):2911–5.
88. Pereira N, Hutchinson AP, Lekovich JP, Hobeika E, Elias RT. Antibiotic prophylaxis for gynecologic procedures prior to and during the utilization of assisted reproductive technologies: a systematic review. J Pathog. 2016;2016:4698314.
89. Merien A, Gerris J, Galajdova L, Dhont M, Cabri P, De Sutter P, et al. Does low-dose aspirin improve pregnancy rate in IVF/ICSI? A randomized double-blind placebo controlled trial. Hum Reprod. 2009;24(4):856–60.
90. Dentali F, Ageno W, Rezoagli E, Rancan E, Squizzato A, Middeldorp S, et al. Low-dose aspirin for in vitro fertilization or intracytoplasmic sperm injection: a systematic review and a meta-analysis of the literature. J Thromb Haemost. 2012;10(10):2075–85.
91. Siristatidis CS, Basios G, Pergialiotis V, Vogiatzi P. Aspirin for in vitro fertilisation. Cochrane Database Syst Rev. 2016;(11):CD004832.
92. Ruopp MD, Collins TC, Whitcomb BW, Schisterman EF. Evidence of absence or absence of evidence? A reanalysis of the effects of low-dose aspirin in in vitro fertilization. Fertil Steril. 2008;90(1):71–6.
93. Gelbaya TA, Kyrgiou M, Li TC, Stern C, Nardo LG. Low-dose aspirin for in vitro fertilization: a systematic review and meta-analysis. Hum Reprod Update. 2007;13(4):357–64.
94. Wada I, Hsu CC, Williams G, Macnamee MC, Brinsden PR. Pregnancy: the benefits of low-dose aspirin therapy in women with impaired uterine perfusion during assisted conception. Hum Reprod. 1994;9(10):1954–7.

95. Check JH, Dietterich C, Lurie D, Nazari A, Chuong J. A matched study to determine whether low-dose aspirin without heparin improves pregnancy rates following frozen embryo transfer and/or affects endometrial sonographic parameters. J Assist Reprod Genet. 1998;15(10):579–82.
96. Madani T, Ahmadi F, Jahangiri N, Bahmanabadi A, Bagheri Lankarani N. Does low-dose aspirin improve pregnancy rate in women undergoing frozen-thawed embryo transfer cycle? A pilot double-blind, randomized placebo-controlled trial. J Obstet Gynaecol Res. 2019;45(1):156–63.
97. Boomsma CM, Keay SD, Macklon NS. Peri-implantation glucocorticoid administration for assisted reproductive technology cycles. Cochrane Database Syst Rev. 2012;(6):CD005996.
98. Datta AK, Campbell S, Deval B, Nargund G. Add-ons in IVF programme – Hype or Hope? Facts Views Vis Obgyn. 2015;7(4):241–50.
99. Siristatidis C, Chrelias C, Creatsa M, Varounis C, Vrachnis N, Iliodromiti Z, et al. Addition of prednisolone and heparin in patients with failed IVF/ICSI cycles: a preliminary report of a clinical trial. Hum Fertil. 2013;16(3):207–10.
100. Fawzy M, El-Refaeey AA. Does combined prednisolone and low molecular weight heparin have a role in unexplained implantation failure? Arch Gynecol Obstet. 2014;289(3):677–80.
101. Lensen S, Osavlyuk D, Armstrong S, Stadelmann C, Hennes A, Napier E, et al. A randomized trial of endometrial scratching before in vitro fertilization. N Engl J Med. 2019;380(4):325–34.
102. Gaikwad S, Garrido N, Cobo A, Pellicer A, Remohi J. Bed rest after embryo transfer negatively affects in vitro fertilization: a randomized controlled clinical trial. Fertil Steril. 2013;100(3):729–735.e2.
103. Lambers MJ, Lambalk CB, Schats R, Hompes PGA. Ultrasonographic evidence that bedrest after embryo transfer is useless. Gynecol Obstet Invest. 2009;68(2):122–6.
104. Sharif K, Afnan M, Lashen H, Elgendy M, Morgan C, Sinclair L. Is bed rest following embryo transfer necessary? Fertil Steril. 1998;69(3):478–81.
105. Purcell KJ, Schembri M, Telles TL, Fujimoto VY, Cedars MI. Bed rest after embryo transfer: a randomized controlled trial. Fertil Steril. 2007;87(6):1322–6.
106. Practice Committee of the American Society for Reproductive Medicine. Electronic address: ASRM@asrm.org, Practice Committee of the American Society for Reproductive Medicine. Performing the embryo transfer: a guideline. Fertil Steril. 2017;107(4):882–96.
107. Chen Z-J, Shi Y, Sun Y, Zhang B, Liang X, Cao Y, et al. Fresh versus frozen embryos for infertility in the polycystic ovary syndrome. N Engl J Med. 2016;375(6):523–33.
108. Shapiro BS, Daneshmand ST, Garner FC, Aguirre M, Hudson C, Thomas S. Evidence of impaired endometrial receptivity after ovarian stimulation for in vitro fertilization: a prospective randomized trial comparing fresh and frozen–thawed embryo transfer in normal responders. Fertil Steril. 2011;96(2):344–8.
109. Shapiro BS, Daneshmand ST, Restrepo H, Garner FC, Aguirre M, Hudson C. Matched-cohort comparison of single-embryo transfers in fresh and frozen-thawed embryo transfer cycles. Fertil Steril. 2013;99(2):389–92.
110. Ozgur K, Berkkanoglu M, Bulut H, Humaidan P, Coetzee K. Perinatal outcomes after fresh versus vitrified-warmed blastocyst transfer: retrospective analysis. Fertil Steril. 2015;104(4):899–907.e3.

Chapter 22
Minimal and Mild Stimulation IVF Results

David Prokai, John Wu, and Orhan Bukulmez

22.1 Introduction

We assessed our database over two time periods. The initial period between 2012 and 2015 encompasses a different assisted reproductive technologies (ART) laboratory team with earlier protocols. After this period, we had a different and more established ART laboratory team, patients showed more profound poor ovarian response (POR) and diminished ovarian reserve (DOR) characteristics, and protocol monitoring was intensified. We offered minimal and mild stimulation protocols as discussed in this book only for women with DOR and/or advanced reproductive age (ARA) and POR.

22.2 Results

22.2.1 Minimal and/or Mild Stimulation Cycle Outcomes

Our database from 2012 to 2015 suggests that 89 women underwent minimal or mild stimulation cycles. The number of started stimulation cycles was 206. Thirty-seven out of 206 (17.9%) cycles were canceled due to various factors. Ten out of 169 (5.9%) oocyte retrievals did not yield oocytes and 66 out of 159 (41.5%) cycles yielding oocytes did not result in frozen embryos. 22 out of 89 (24.7%) women did not have any frozen embryos.

D. Prokai (✉) · J. Wu · O. Bukulmez
Division of Reproductive Endocrinology & Infertility, Fertility and Advanced Reproductive Medicine Assisted Reproductive Technologies Program, Department of Obstetrics and Gynecology, University of Texas Southwestern Medical Center, Dallas, TX, USA
e-mail: David.Prokai@UTSouthwestern.edu; john.wu@utsouthwestern.edu

© Springer Nature Switzerland AG 2020   273
O. Bukulmez (ed.), *Diminished Ovarian Reserve and Assisted Reproductive Technologies*, https://doi.org/10.1007/978-3-030-23235-1_22

Our database from 2016 to 2018 suggests that 102 women underwent minimal or mild stimulation cycles. The number of started stimulation cycles was 305. Fifty-eight out of 305 (19%) were canceled due to various reasons including medication errors, concurrent illness, and poor response. The number of cycles canceled due to poor response was 50 out of 58 (86.2%). 12 out of 247 (4.8%) oocyte retrievals did not yield an oocyte. 111 out of 235 (47.2%) cycles yielding oocytes did not result in frozen embryos. 17 out of 102 (16.6%) women did not have any frozen embryos. At least a partial impression about the age and cycle characteristics of the patients who underwent minimal and/or mild stimulation can be attained from the data presented in Chap. 16.

In general, these numbers can be used to counsel the patients about the performance of such protocols in women with DOR and/or ARA or POR.

22.2.2 Frozen-Thawed Embryo Transfer (FET) Cycle Outcomes

The age distribution of women who underwent FET is provided in Fig. 22.1. As expected, majority of the patients were with ARA, >35 years of age. More than 2/3 of the women were over the age of 38 years. Table 22.1 shows the characteristics of 154 FET cycles. We report ongoing pregnancy since live birth rates were not completely available for 2018 cycles. The data from a large multicenter IVF-based study suggested that ongoing pregnancy rates after 10 weeks may be associated with live birth at a mean rate of 92% [1].

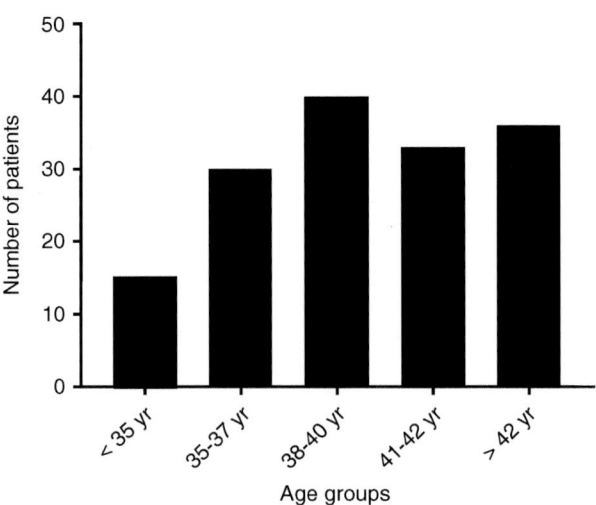

Fig. 22.1 The number of patients per age group who underwent frozen-thawed embryo transfer (FET)

Table 22.1 The characteristics of 154 FET cycles

Factors	Mean ± SD
Age (years) (range)	39.47 ± 3.6 (29–46)
Number of conventional cycles before (range)	0.81 ± 0.97 (0–5)
Number of minimal/mild stimulation cycles started per patient including canceled cycles (range)	3.21 ± 1.94 (1–11)
Number of frozen embryos accumulated per patient	3.72 ± 2.29 (1–13)
Number of FET cycles per patient (range)	1.37 ± 0.67 (1–4)
AMH (ng/mL) (range)	0.99 ± 0.86 (0.07–4.0)
Number of day-3 stage embryos transferred per FET	1.7 ± 0.53
Number of day-5 stage embryos transferred per FET	1.6 ± 0.63
Days to pregnancy from the first minimal/mild stimulation cycle (range)	324 ± 176 (93–877)
Ongoing pregnancy rate per FET cycle	46.8% (72/154)
Ongoing twin pregnancy rate per FET cycle	8.4% (13/154)

SD standard deviation

Table 22.2 FET cycle pregnancy outcomes in women who underwent minimal/mild stimulation per age groups

		Age group (years)				
		<35	35–37	38–40	41–42	>42
		Count	Count	Count	Count	Count
Outcome	Not pregnant	3	9	18	16	20
	Biochemical/SAB	2	3	3	2	6
	Ongoing pregnancy	10 (66%)	18 (60%)	19 (47.5%)	15 (45.5%)	10 (27.8%)

Ongoing pregnancy rate in parenthesis (%)
SAB spontaneous abortion

Ongoing pregnancy rate was 46.8% per FET cycle. The data also confirms that the process of minimal/mild stimulation cycles and then FET and achievement of pregnancy take time, ranging from 93 to 877 days. Therefore, this process requires considerable commitment from the patients with POR, DOR, and/or ARA. The mean number of cycles corresponds to our counseling that we recommend about three minimal and/or mild stimulation cycles for such patients to accumulate frozen embryos (Table 22.1). The range of stimulation cycles per each women shows a wide range of 1–11. We limit the number of embryos transferred in any age group. Recently, we have avoided transferring more than two embryos at any age. Our overall ongoing twin pregnancy rate is acceptably low at 8.4% (13/154). The pregnancy outcome data per age groups was provided and depicted in Table 22.2 and Fig. 22.2, respectively. Again as discussed, younger DOR patients achieve much higher ongoing pregnancies as compared to older women. Therefore, younger DOR women still show high pregnancy chances with each FET than older women.

Fig. 22.2 Ongoing
pregnancy rates per FET in
various female age groups

Ongoing pregnancy rates per FET cycle per female age

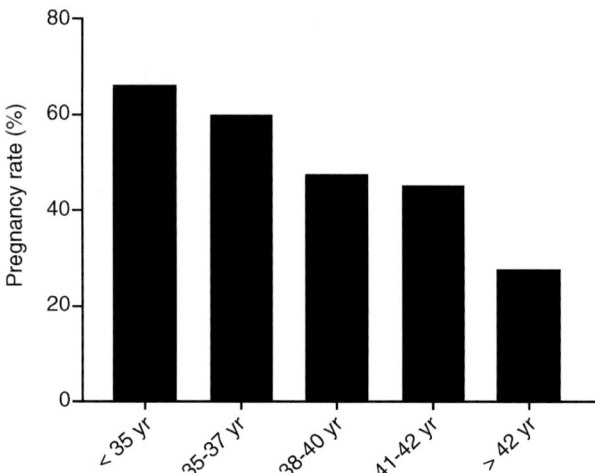

22.3 Conclusion

Our simple tally without any advanced statistics suggests that women with expected POR such as with DOR and/or ARA may achieve clinically meaningful ongoing pregnancy rates once they undergo FET. However, with minimal and mild stimulation, 16.6–24.7% of women may not have any frozen embryos for delayed FET after such stimulation cycles. We feel that with careful counseling and appropriate setting of expectations, this group may find such odds acceptable especially because many such women may have only been offered donor oocyte/donor embryo treatment by majority of the fertility clinics favoring conventional stimulation protocols for IVF. Minimal/mild stimulation approaches with embryo banking afford the best chance for autologous pregnancy for this special and deserving population and as such warrant further studies and validation in the future.

Reference

1. The European and Israeli Study Group on Highly Purified Menotropin versus Recombinant Follicle-Stimulating Hormone. Efficacy and safety of highly purified menotropin versus recombinant follicle-stimulating hormone in in vitro fertilization/intracytoplasmic sperm injection cycles: a randomized, comparative trial. Fertil Steril. 2002;78(3):520–8.

Part III
Utilization of Contemporary Technologies in Diminished Ovarian Reserve Patients

Chapter 23
Fresh Versus Frozen Embryo Transfer

Zexu Jiao

23.1 Introduction

The fresh embryo transfer has traditionally performed in vitro fertilization (IVF) since its successful introduction in 1978. To date, about 5 million IVF babies have been born around the world as the result of fresh embryo transfer. However, in spite of considerable advances in the optimization of ovarian stimulation protocols and new technologies for the assessment of embryo quality, the success rates for IVF in fresh transfer cycles are less than ideal. As IVF technology improved, embryo freezing was performed to allow subsequent transfer if the fresh cycle was unsuccessful. The first pregnancy following the transfer of a frozen-thawed human embryo was reported by Trounson et al. in 1983 [1]. Since then, the clinical value of embryo cryopreservation has steadily increased over the decades.

23.2 Cryopreservation of Human Embryos

Cryopreservation involves a series of complex and dynamic physiochemical processes of temperature and water transport between a cell and the surrounding medium. The basic goal of cryopreservation is to achieve intracellular vitrification while avoiding intracellular ice formation and membrane and organelle damage [2, 3]. Two major methods are used in the cryopreservation of human embryos: slow freezing and vitrification.

Z. Jiao (✉)
Division of Reproductive Endocrinology & Infertility, Fertility and Advanced Reproductive Medicine Assisted Reproductive Technologies Program, Department of Obstetrics and Gynecology, University of Texas Southwestern Medical Center, Dallas, TX, USA
e-mail: Zexu.Jiao@utsouthwestern.edu

© Springer Nature Switzerland AG 2020

O. Bukulmez (ed.), *Diminished Ovarian Reserve and Assisted Reproductive Technologies*, https://doi.org/10.1007/978-3-030-23235-1_23

23.2.1 Slow Freezing

Slow freezing attempts to maintain a delicate balance between cryoprotectants and the aqueous embryo compartment, in which the embryos are cooled at very slow rates after being treated with cryoprotectants at a relatively low concentration (1.0–1.5 M), thus limiting the toxic and osmotic damage. In this protocol, the dehydration of the cells and the diffusion of cryoprotectant agents into the cells take place very slowly during a long period. At the end, the procedure allows the equilibration of the extra- and intracellular fluids [4].

If we have to do slow freezing in a particular case, commercially prepared G-FreezeKit Blast from VitroLife is used in the University of Texas Southwestern Medical Center IVF laboratory, which contains:

- Blastocyst freezing solution 1 (BFS1) contains 100 mM of surcose and 5% glycerol.
- Blastocyst freezing solution 2 (BFS2) contains 200 mM of sucrose and 10% glycerol.
- Blastocyst thaw solution 1 (BTS1) contains 200 mM of sucrose and 10% glycerol.
- Blastocyst thaw solution 2 (BTS2) contains 100 mM of sucrose and 5% glycerol.
- Blastocyst thaw solution 3 (BTS3) contains 100 mM of sucrose.
- Blastocyst incubation medium (BIM) does not contain sucrose or glycerol.

23.2.1.1 Protocol for Embryo Slow Freezing

1. Preparation: supplement BIM, BFS1, and BFS2 with 20% SSS (synthetic serum substitute).
2. Remove the embryo(s) from the incubator and rinse in BIM + 20% SSS solution.
3. Transfer embryo(s) to the BFS1 + 20% SSS solution for 10 min.
4. Transfer embryo(s) to the BFS2 + 20% SSS solution for 7 min.
5. Load embryos into vials. Do not exceed 15 min in BFS2 + 20% SSS solution.
6. Cool the samples at a rate of 2 °C/min to −7 °C, and "hold" at this temperature to allow thermal equilibration before ice nucleation (seeding).
7. Following seeding, with initiation and growth of ice crystals, cool the samples at a slow rate, −0.3 °C/min down to −30 °C.
8. Cool the samples rapidly to liquid nitrogen temperatures, then plunge and store in liquid nitrogen.

23.2.1.2 Protocol for Embryo Thawing After Slow Freezing

1. Preparation: supplement BTS1, BTS 2, BTS3, and BIM with 20% SSS (synthetic serum substitute).
2. Hold vial(s) in air for 1 min.
3. Tighten vial top and immerse the vial(s) in a 30 °C water bath for 3 min.
4. Transfer the contents of the vial containing the embryo to Nunc plate to search for embryos and note embryo's appearance and grade.
5. Transfer the embryo(s) to BTS1 + 20% SSS solution for 1 min.

6. Transfer the embryo(s) to BTS2 + 20% SSS solution for 5 min.
7. Transfer the embryo(s) to BTS3 + 20% SSS solution for 5 min.
8. Transfer the embryo(s) to BIM + 20% SSS solution for 5 min.
9. Transfer the embryos to pre-equilibrated culture medium.
10. Assess post-thawed embryo(s) and document survival.

23.2.2   Vitrification

Vitrification is a process involving exposure of embryo to high concentration of cryoprotectants and ultrarapid cooling to solidify the cell into glass-like state without the formation of ice crystals. This technique requires critical process control. All samples must be handled and moved precisely, and there is zero tolerance to any changes/fluctuations.

Two different types of carrier, open or closed systems, named due to the necessity of contact with liquid nitrogen in the former, or not in the latter, are available for vitrification. The University of Texas Southwestern Medical Center IVF laboratory currently uses VitriGuard from Origio as a closed system.

Ready-to-use media for vitrification and warming of embryos are available from the majority of companies who supply the culture media. Individual methods and protocols vary slightly with the different reparations, and manufacturers' instructions should be followed for each. The University of Texas Southwestern Medical Center IVF laboratory currently uses vitrification and warming solution from Irvine Scientific.

23.2.2.1   Protocol for Embryo Vitrification

All procedures are performed at room temperature (22–27 °C).

1. Prepare a four-well dish with 1.0 mL equilibration solution (ES) and 1.0 mL vitrification solution (VS) in each well.
2. Transfer the embryos to ES for 6–10 min.
3. Transfer the embryos to VS for 1 min.
4. Load the embryo(s) onto the VitriGuard with a minimal volume within 80 s, not to exceed 110 s after initial exposure to VS.
5. Plunge the VitriGuard into liquid nitrogen.
6. Move the plunged VitriGuard to the liquid nitrogen tank for long-term storage.

23.2.2.2   Protocol for Embryo Warming

1. Identify the embryo(s) to be thawed.
2. Take the VitriGuard out of the liquid nitrogen and quickly transfer embryo(s) into thawing solution (TS) at 37 °C for 1 min.
3. Transfer the embryos into 1.0 mL dilution solution (DS) for 4 min at room temperature.

4. Transfer the embryos into 1.0 mL washing solution (WS) 1 then WS2 for 4 min each undisturbed at room temperature.
5. Transfer the warmed embryos into pre-equilibrated culture medium.
6. Assess post-thawed embryo(s) and document survival and grade.

23.2.3 The Implications of Cryopreservation

For the past two decades, slow freezing has been the method of choice for embryo cryopreservation. However, when the process is completed, the extracellular liquid crystallizes and intracellular ice formation cannot be avoided completely, which is one of the greatest shortcomings of this strategy. Intracellular ice formation is one of the causes responsible for the partial blastomere loss observed in a high proportion of embryos after slow freezing. It is well known that partial lysis in frozen-thawed embryos results in an impaired implantation potential [5].

Compared to slow freezing, vitrification involves a very high cooling rate and passages rapidly through the dangerous temperature zone between +15 °C and −5 °C, significantly decreasing chilling injury to the embryos [6]. The complete absence of crystallization achieved with vitrification leads to an extremely high proportion of fully intact embryos of 95% [7], which may explain the studies showing that vitrification has higher post-thaw survival rates and clinical pregnancy rates compared with slow freezing of embryos [8–10]. So vitrification has become more widely utilized in IVF centers currently (Figs. 23.1, 23.2, and 23.3).

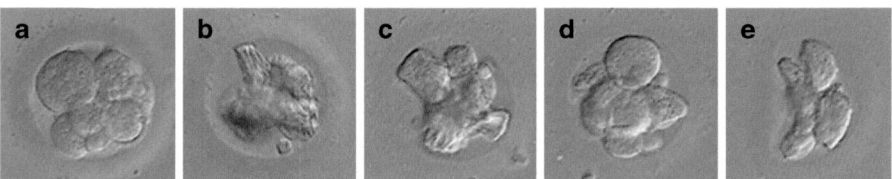

Fig. 23.1 Morphological change of the embryo during vitrifaction: (**a**) Day 3 embryo before vitrification; (**b**) dehydration immediately after the exposure to equilibration solution; (**c**) partial rehydration as cryoprotectants enter the embryo; (**d**) the embryo regaining original form with cryoprotectant filling; (**e**) further dehydration in vitrification solution

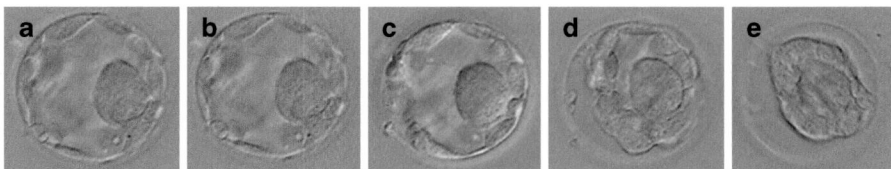

Fig. 23.2 Artificial collapsing of blastocysts: (**a**) prior to the artificial shrinkage; (**b**) a single laser pulse at a junction between two trophectoderm cells away from inner cell mass; (**c**) beginning of shrinkage 10 s after laser shot; (**d**) partial shrinkage 30 s after laser shot; (**e**) blastocyst is fully collapsed and ready to get vitrified

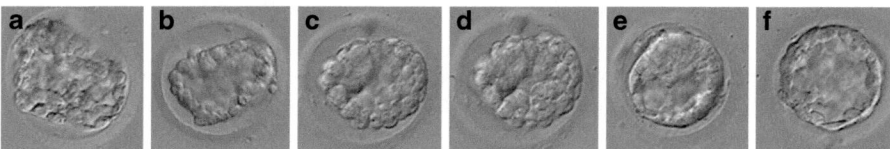

Fig. 23.3 Morphological changes of a human blastocyst during thawing: (**a**) blastocyst in thawing solution; (**b**) blastocyst in diluent solution; (**c**) blastocyst in washing solution 1; (**d**) blastocyst in washing solution 2; (**e**) the thawed blastocyst starts to re-expand within 1 h of incubation in culture media; (**f**) the thawed blastocyst shows 90% blastocoel re-expansion after 2 h of in vitro culture

23.3 Freeze-All Embryos in IVF

The availability of vitrification for embryo storage has also made possible the segmentation of IVF, leading to the so-called freeze-all strategy, which has gained much attention lately [11]. With this strategy, the entire cohort of embryos is cryopreserved following IVF with transfer of a thawed embryo in one or several subsequent cycles [12]. The rationale behind this hypothesis is that the transfer of an embryo into a more "physiologic environment" would result not only in higher pregnancy rates but potentially a decrease in both maternal and perinatal morbidity, when compared with a fresh embryo transfer [13, 14].

23.3.1 Indication of Freeze-All Embryos

The most common reasons for cryopreservation and delayed embryo transfer are the presence of risk factors for ovarian hyperstimulation syndrome (OHSS), the need for pre-implantation genetic diagnosis or testing for aneuploidy (PGD/PGT-A), or the presence of embryo/endometrial asynchrony. The other indications include altered endocrine and cardiovascular profile at the time of transfer (elevated progesterone, hypertension, etc.), inadequate uterine cavity for embryo transfer (i.e., fluid in cavity), and women with poor ovarian response, diminished ovarian reserve (DOR), or advanced reproductive age who seek a strategy to accumulate frozen oocytes or embryos. We still need the evidence to support routine use of the freeze-all policy [15]. However, frozen embryo transfer has become increasingly common and currently there is an accelerating trend toward the implementation for all patient categories [16, 17].

23.3.2 Perinatal and Obstetric Outcomes

First, there is a large body of evidence suggesting that freezing all embryos in a fresh IVF cycle followed by thawed frozen transfer in subsequent cycles (frozen embryo transfer, FET) might improve clinical and ongoing pregnancy rates [14, 18].

A population study suggest that there is a specific risk of blastogenesis birth defects arising very early in pregnancy after IVF or ICSI and that this risk may be lower with use of frozen-thawed embryo transfer [19]. Secondly, compared with embryo transfers following ovarian stimulation, large retrospective cohort studies [20, 21] have shown that frozen-thawed embryo transfers, both at cleavage and blastocyst stages, significantly reduce the rate of ectopic pregnancy. Third, a recent systematic review and meta-analysis suggested that pregnancies occurring after frozen embryo transfer are associated with fewer complications (e.g., lower rates of antepartum hemorrhage) and better neonatal outcomes, including higher birth weight and lower risk of perinatal death [18, 22–24]. These findings have led many to propose that the strategy should apply routinely in IVF. However, these evidences should be taken with caution, since some of the studies available have been criticized due to serious flaws in their design. So more research is still needed to prove the validity of the "freeze-all strategy."

23.4 Optimal Embryo Transfer Strategy in Diminished Ovarian Reserve Patient

Considering the available evidence that supports freeze-all strategy has great relevance for advances in assisted reproductive technology (ART). Comparisons made between fresh and frozen cycles are mainly based on studies including high responders [15, 18, 25, 26]. Therefore, extrapolating these data to the DOR population should be further investigated.

Several recent studies have explored to analyze the success rate of fresh ET versus FET cycle in cohorts of patients with varying number of oocyte retrieved. Dieamant et al. analyzed the outcomes based on the number of oocytes retrieved and found that the freeze-all strategy appeared beneficial when a high number of oocytes was collected, but that when the mean number of oocytes collected is <15, the freeze-all strategy does not appear to be advantageous [27]. Roque et al. found that when the group with 4–9 oocytes retrieved was analyzed separately, there was no statistically significant difference in pregnancy rates [28]. Recently, in a retrospective study published in 2018, Xue et al. examined 559 poor responders who met Bologna criteria, including 256 in the fresh embryo transfer group and 303 in the freeze-all group [29]. Their result showed similar live birth rate per cycle and per transfer between these two groups. They also found that maternal age at retrieval and number of good quality embryos transferred were significantly associated with the live birth rate. Another retrospective cohort study examined 433 poor responders, including 277 patients who underwent fresh ET and 156 who followed the freeze-all policy. They found the freeze-all strategy, compared with fresh ET, had no impact on IVF outcomes in poor responder patients. Maternal age and number of embryo transferred were the only independent variables associated with ongoing pregnancy rate [30].

Successful implantation of an embryo depends not only on embryo quality but also on endometrial receptivity and the microenvironment for embryo-maternal signaling within the uterine cavity during the peri-implantation period. The main pathophysiologic mechanism involved in the selection of the freeze-all strategy seems to be controlled ovarian stimulation and consequent impairment in endometrial receptivity [31, 32]. We retrospectively analyzed a cohort of 230 cycles in 119 poor ovarian response patients. The IVF cycles were studied in three groups: minimal stimulation cycles, mild stimulation cycles, and conventional high-dose gonadotropin-releasing hormone (GnRH) antagonist cycles. 33 minimal stimulation IVF patients had 41 FET cycles which allowed us to study whether the clomiphene citrate use in minimal stimulation effects were prolonged. We found that endometrial thickness in the minimal stimulation group was significantly lower than the mild and conventional stimulation groups. In patients who underwent minimal stimulation IVF followed by FET, significantly thicker endometrial thickness was achieved during their FET cycles as compared to their minimal stimulation cycles. We concluded that endometrial thickness is impacted during minimal stimulation IVF cycles. Since negative effects on endometrial thickness are not observed in the patients' subsequent FET cycle, a freeze-all approach is justified to mitigate adverse endometrial effects of clomiphene citrate in minimal stimulation IVF cycles [33].

Moreover, the applicability of vitrification of all embryos to the DOR population can only be a fact when laboratories acquire optimal vitrification systems. However, a consensus is currently lacking in this aspect, and, as a result, ART centers have developed their own freezing strategies based on their personal experiences and choices, which is an important drawback that limits our ability to effectively compare the freeze-all policy available in DOR population [34]. Furthermore, a cost-effectiveness analysis and cumulative pregnancy rates comparison between fresh and frozen embryo transfer is also necessary in order to assess if the potential effects of a freeze-all policy on perinatal outcomes justify the additional cost and extra workload of elective cryopreservation [35].

23.5 Conclusion

Taken together, several observations provide reassuring evidence that the abnormal hormonal milieu and the suboptimal endometrial development observed in conventional ovarian stimulation cycles may be the main risk factor for fresh embryo transfer. The physiological intrauterine conditions of FET may have a positive impact not only on endometrial receptivity but also on early implantation. Although confirmation of the clinical benefits of a freeze-all strategy through well-designed clinical trials is necessary, the freeze-all strategy is an acceptable treatment in DOR patients undergoing minimal and mild stimulation protocols as detailed in this book. In some cases, freezing all embryos might be suggested by physicians as an alternative to cycle cancelation when a fresh transfer would not be advantageous. At the same time, potential costs, delays in treatment, and potential risks associated with this strategy need to be discussed with the patients.

References

1. Trounson A, Mohr L. Human pregnancy following cryopreservation, thawing and transfer of an eight-cell embryo. Nature. 1983;305(5936):707–9.
2. Mazur P, Leibo SP, Chu EH. A two-factor hypothesis of freezing injury. Evidence from Chinese hamster tissue-culture cells. Exp Cell Res. 1972;71(2):345–55.
3. Ghetler Y, Yavin S, Shalgi R, Arav A. The effect of chilling on membrane lipid phase transition in human oocytes and zygotes. Hum Reprod. 2005;20(12):3385–9.
4. Schneider U. Cryobiological principles of embryo freezing. J In Vitro Fert Embryo Transf. 1986;3(1):3–9.
5. El-Toukhy T, Khalaf Y, Al-Darazi K, Andritsos V, Taylor A, Braude P. Effect of blastomere loss on the outcome of frozen embryo replacement cycles. Fertil Steril. 2003;79(5):1106–11.
6. Rall WF, Fahy GM. Ice-free cryopreservation of mouse embryos at −196 degrees C by vitrification. Nature. 1985;313(6003):573–5.
7. Cobo A, de los Santos MJ, Castello D, Gamiz P, Campos P, Remohi J. Outcomes of vitrified early cleavage-stage and blastocyst-stage embryos in a cryopreservation program: evaluation of 3,150 warming cycles. Fertil Steril. 2012;98(5):1138–46.e1.
8. AbdelHafez FF, Desai N, Abou-Setta AM, Falcone T, Goldfarb J. Slow freezing, vitrification and ultra-rapid freezing of human embryos: a systematic review and meta-analysis. Reprod Biomed Online. 2010;20(2):209–22.
9. Loutradi KE, Kolibianakis EM, Venetis CA, Papanikolaou EG, Pados G, Bontis I, et al. Cryopreservation of human embryos by vitrification or slow freezing: a systematic review and meta-analysis. Fertil Steril. 2008;90(1):186–93.
10. Vajta G, Nagy ZP. Are programmable freezers still needed in the embryo laboratory? Review on vitrification. Reprod Biomed Online. 2006;12(6):779–96.
11. Doody KJ. Cryopreservation and delayed embryo transfer-assisted reproductive technology registry and reporting implications. Fertil Steril. 2014;102(1):27–31.
12. Devroey P, Polyzos NP, Blockeel C. An OHSS-Free Clinic by segmentation of IVF treatment. Hum Reprod. 2011;26(10):2593–7.
13. Melo MA, Meseguer M, Garrido N, Bosch E, Pellicer A, Remohi J. The significance of premature luteinization in an oocyte-donation programme. Hum Reprod. 2006;21(6):1503–7.
14. Roque M, Lattes K, Serra S, Sola I, Geber S, Carreras R, et al. Fresh embryo transfer versus frozen embryo transfer in *in vitro* fertilization cycles: a systematic review and meta-analysis. Fertil Steril. 2013;99(1):156–62.
15. Basile N, Garcia-Velasco JA. The state of "freeze-for-all" in human ARTs. J Assist Reprod Genet. 2016;33(12):1543–50.
16. Weinerman R, Mainigi M. Why we should transfer frozen instead of fresh embryos: the translational rationale. Fertil Steril. 2014;102(1):10–8.
17. Roque M, Valle M, Kostolias A, Sampaio M, Geber S. Freeze-all cycle in reproductive medicine: current perspectives. JBRA Assist Reprod. 2017;21(1):49–53.
18. Chen ZJ, Shi Y, Sun Y, Zhang B, Liang X, Cao Y, et al. Fresh versus frozen embryos for infertility in the polycystic ovary syndrome. N Engl J Med. 2016;375(6):523–33.
19. Halliday JL, Ukoumunne OC, Baker HW, Breheny S, Jaques AM, Garrett C, et al. Increased risk of blastogenesis birth defects, arising in the first 4 weeks of pregnancy, after assisted reproductive technologies. Hum Reprod. 2010;25(1):59–65.
20. Huang B, Hu D, Qian K, Ai J, Li Y, Jin L, et al. Is frozen embryo transfer cycle associated with a significantly lower incidence of ectopic pregnancy? An analysis of more than 30,000 cycles. Fertil Steril. 2014;102(5):1345–9.

21. Londra L, Moreau C, Strobino D, Garcia J, Zacur H, Zhao Y. Ectopic pregnancy after *in vitro* fertilization: differences between fresh and frozen-thawed cycles. Fertil Steril. 2015;104(1):110–8.
22. Maheshwari A, Pandey S, Shetty A, Hamilton M, Bhattacharya S. Obstetric and perinatal outcomes in singleton pregnancies resulting from the transfer of frozen thawed versus fresh embryos generated through *in vitro* fertilization treatment: a systematic review and meta-analysis. Fertil Steril. 2012;98(2):368–77.e1–9.
23. Roy TK, Bradley CK, Bowman MC, McArthur SJ. Single-embryo transfer of vitrified-warmed blastocysts yields equivalent live-birth rates and improved neonatal outcomes compared with fresh transfers. Fertil Steril. 2014;101(5):1294–301.
24. Zhu Q, Chen Q, Wang L, Lu X, Lyu Q, Wang Y, et al. Live birth rates in the first complete IVF cycle among 20 687 women using a freeze-all strategy. Hum Reprod. 2018;33(5):924–9.
25. Shi Y, Sun Y, Hao C, Zhang H, Wei D, Zhang Y, et al. Transfer of fresh versus frozen embryos in ovulatory women. N Engl J Med. 2018;378(2):126–36.
26. Wang A, Santistevan A, Hunter Cohn K, Copperman A, Nulsen J, Miller BT, et al. Freeze-only versus fresh embryo transfer in a multicenter matched cohort study: contribution of progesterone and maternal age to success rates. Fertil Steril. 2017;108(2):254–61.e4.
27. Dieamant FC, Petersen CG, Mauri AL, Comar V, Mattila M, Vagnini LD, et al. Fresh embryos versus freeze-all embryos - transfer strategies: nuances of a meta-analysis. JBRA Assist Reprod. 2017;21(3):260–72.
28. Roque M, Valle M, Guimaraes F, Sampaio M, Geber S. Freeze-all cycle for all normal responders? J Assist Reprod Genet. 2017;34(2):179–85.
29. Xue Y, Tong X, Zhu H, Li K, Zhang S. Freeze-all embryo strategy in poor ovarian responders undergoing ovarian stimulation for *in vitro* fertilization. Gynecol Endocrinol. 2018;34(8):680–3.
30. Roque M, Valle M, Sampaio M, Geber S. Does freeze-all policy affect IVF outcome in poor ovarian responders? Ultrasound Obstet Gynecol. 2018;52(4):530–4.
31. Shapiro BS, Daneshmand ST, Garner FC, Aguirre M, Hudson C, Thomas S. Evidence of impaired endometrial receptivity after ovarian stimulation for *in vitro* fertilization: a prospective randomized trial comparing fresh and frozen-thawed embryo transfer in normal responders. Fertil Steril. 2011;96(2):344–8.
32. Venetis CA, Kolibianakis EM, Bosdou JK, Tarlatzis BC. Progesterone elevation and probability of pregnancy after IVF: a systematic review and meta-analysis of over 60 000 cycles. Hum Reprod Update. 2013;19(5):433–57.
33. Reed BG, Wu JL, Nemer LB, Carr BR, Bukulmez O. Use of Clomiphene Citrate in minimal stimulation *in vitro* fertilization negatively impacts endometrial thickness: an argument for a freeze-all approach. JBRA Assist Reprod. 2018;22:355–62.
34. Groenewoud ER, Cantineau AE, Kollen BJ, Macklon NS, Cohlen BJ. What is the optimal means of preparing the endometrium in frozen-thawed embryo transfer cycles? A systematic review and meta-analysis. Hum Reprod Update. 2013;19(5):458–70.
35. Blockeel C, Drakopoulos P, Santos-Ribeiro S, Polyzos NP, Tournaye H. A fresh look at the freeze-all protocol: a SWOT analysis. Hum Reprod. 2016;31(3):491–7.

Chapter 24
Comprehensive Chromosome Analysis in Diminished Ovarian Reserve Patients

Zexu Jiao and Orhan Bukulmez

24.1 Brief History

Chromosomal aneuploidy is the most common genetic abnormality and the leading cause of implantation failure, miscarriage, and congenital abnormalities in humans, with an incidence at birth of less than 0.3%. Comprehensive chromosome analysis, now termed preimplantation genetic testing for aneuploidy (PGT-A), involves in vitro fertilization (IVF), embryo biopsy, diagnosis, and selective chromosomally normal embryo transfer in order to increase the live birth rates per embryo transferred and to prevent abnormal pregnancies.

Initially, preimplantation genetic diagnosis (PGD) is applicable for monogenic disorder where the mutation is identifiable by molecular techniques. The first instance of PGD was reported in 1990 for gender determination to avoid an X-linked disease [1]. Since then, various approaches have been applied for single-gene disorders [2]. To date, PGD has been licensed for over 400 different conditions including late-onset disorders, mitochondrial disorders, rare disorders, and HLA typing and has resulted in the birth of thousands of healthy children [3].

More recently, the indications for PGD have expanded for the assessment of aneuploidies. From the 1990s to 2010s, thousands of IVF patients have had their embryos screened for aneuploidy using fluorescence in situ hybridization (FISH), which was limited by its inability to simultaneously evaluate all 24 chromosomes [4]. In the early to mid-2000s, several laboratories began developing new technologies offering the ability to test all 24 chromosomes for aneuploidy, simultaneously testing for structural chromosome aberrations [5]. The development of techniques for whole genome amplification (WGA) led to a number of platforms with the abil-

Z. Jiao (✉) · O. Bukulmez
Division of Reproductive Endocrinology & Infertility, Fertility and Advanced Reproductive Medicine Assisted Reproductive Technologies Program, Department of Obstetrics and Gynecology, University of Texas Southwestern Medical Center, Dallas, TX, USA
e-mail: Zexu.Jiao@utsouthwestern.edu

© Springer Nature Switzerland AG 2020
O. Bukulmez (ed.), *Diminished Ovarian Reserve and Assisted Reproductive Technologies*, https://doi.org/10.1007/978-3-030-23235-1_24

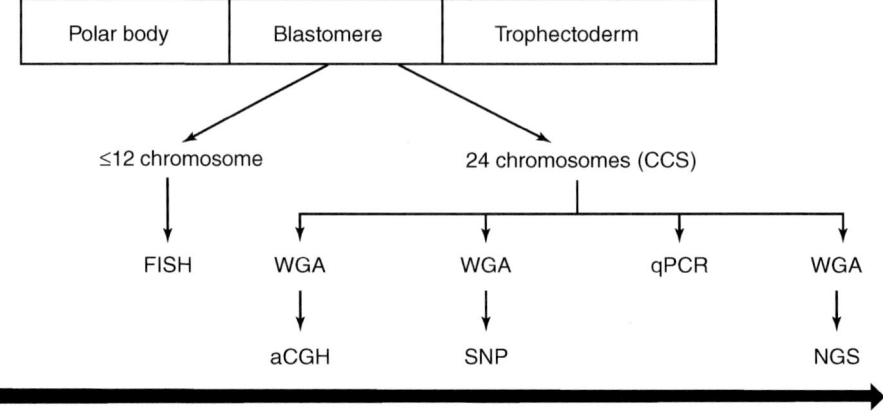

Fig. 24.1 Preimplantation genetic testing for aneuploidy

ity to perform comprehensive chromosome screening, including array comparative genomic hybridization (aCGH) [6], single nucleotide polymorphism (SNP) arrays, and shortly thereafter, quantitative real-time (RT) polymerase chain reaction (qPCR). The most recent development in this area is next-generation sequencing (NGS) (Fig. 24.1).

The evolution of aneuploidy screening techniques has provided more reliable and faster results about genetic status of the embryos. It has been estimated that approximately 100,000 PGD cycles have been performed worldwide over the past 23 years and nearly 80% of these cycles have been PGT-A [7]. Currently, PGT-A constitutes the majority of PGD cycles performed globally. PGT-A is also controversial in terms of the effectiveness of comprehensive techniques used in different patient groups and using different cell types for biopsy.

24.2   Biopsy

24.2.1   The Source of Sample

There are currently three sources of cellular materials that can be used for PGT-A. Polar body (PB) is usually retrieved from oocytes and zygotes. This approach restricts detection of chromosome abnormalities to the female. Blastomere biopsy involves the removal of a single cell from a day 3 stage embryo. This approach allows identification of both maternal and paternal contributions. Embryo transfer can be performed 2 days later, on day 5 of development. However, this approach cannot detect mosaicism and may damage the embryo viability.

Improvements in embryo culture conditions as well as in vitrification systems have paved the way for the current trend of trophectoderm (TE) biopsies. TE biopsy is performed at the blastocyst stage, on day 5, day 6, or sometimes day 7. At this stage, embryos have undergone their first cellular differentiation, resulting in two cell lineages: the inner cell mass (ICM) and TE cells. Biopsy of TE cells does not adversely affect embryo development. With TE biopsy, multiple cells can be sampled from each embryo, which can improve accuracy in the genetics laboratory. Current most PGT-A research focuses on genome-wide aneuploidy screening of biopsies from the TE, which may better represent the ultimate genetic constitution of the embryo. More recently, new types of sample, like blastocentesis and analysis of spent embryo culture medium, have also been proposed. However, further results are needed to ensure reliability of the results before widespread clinical application [8, 9].

24.2.2 Sampling Method

For each biopsy approach, the zona pellucida (ZP) must be perforated. This can be accomplished by several methods, including mechanically cutting through the ZP with a micropipette, chemically dissolving the ZP with a weak acid solution (acid Tyrode's), or laser via the optical system of a microscope. The laser approach is most commonly used because it is faster, safer, and more reproducible among technicians.

Currently, two methods are used for TE biopsy. The first method requires a hole in the ZP on day 3, and then the embryo is cultured up to the blastocyst stage [10]. A hatching of TE cells makes the blastocyst biopsy relatively easy. However, the risk that the blastocyst will hatch starting from the ICM also exists. The second method, which is used at the University of Texas Southwestern Medical Center, leaves the embryo undisturbed up to blastocyst stage and then ZP drilling and TE biopsy are performed at the same time [11]. The advantage of this method is that no extra stress at the cleavage stage is required, allowing a more physiological embryo growth to the blastocyst stage, as well as no additional operations in the laboratory (Fig. 24.2).

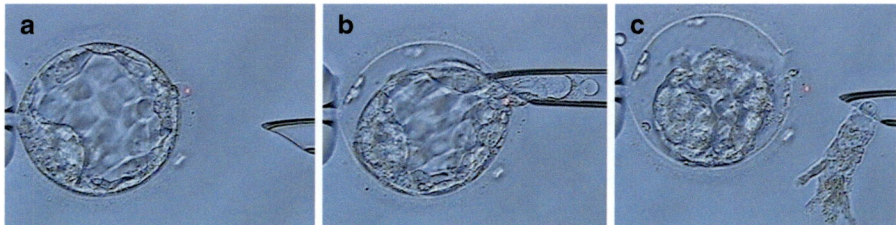

Fig. 24.2 Blastocyst biopsy is performed by simultaneous zona pellucida opening and trophectoderm biopsy. (**a**) Laser-assisted hatching on day 5 blastocyst, (**b**) 5–10 trophectoderm cells were sucked into the biopsy pipette and then targeted with few laser pulses, (**c**) trophectoderm cells are dissected from the blastocyst by gentle suction during the laser firing

24.3 Diagnostic Technologies

24.3.1 FISH

FISH with chromosome-specific DNA probes can be applied to polar body, blastomere, or TE cell that had been fixed on slides and gives detectable signals in interphase nuclei as well as on metaphase chromosomes. However, The FISH technique is limited by having relatively few discrete colors available, and typically up to five chromosomes can be tested at the same time. The same nucleus can be retested (reprobed), and in this way, 12 chromosomes have been tested in clinical practice. In addition, FISH requires high technical skills and scoring FISH signals in a single nucleus is inherently subjective and prone to errors.

24.3.2 aCGH

aCGH is the first technology to be widely available for reliable, accurate, and relatively fast 24-chromosome copy number analysis. In this method, the biopsied cells are amplified using a WGA technique. Amplified sample DNA and control DNA are differentially labeled with fluorophores and then competitively hybridized on the array platform at the same time. Chromosome loss or gain is revealed by the color of each spot after hybridization. This is because the technique involves the competitive hybridization of differentially labeled test and reference euploid DNA samples. Fluorescence intensity is detected using a laser scanner and data processing software, which can analyze whole chromosome aneuploidy and sub-chromosomal structural imbalances. aCGH is now used extensively around the world despite the relatively high cost of testing multiple samples [12].

24.3.3 SNP Array

Single nucleotide polymorphism (SNP) is a DNA sequence variant in which, at a particular position or locus, one of two or more nucleotides may be present on different chromosomes within a population. SNP arrays involves tracking the inheritance of polymorphisms from the parents to their embryos. Each of the parental chromosomes has a unique combination of SNP alleles providing a means of confirming whether a particular chromosome is present or absent from a sample. The process of SNP array involves WGA, fluorescent labeling of the amplified embryo DNA, and ascertainment of SNP genotypes using a microarray. The results from embryos are compared with data obtained from the mother and father and ploidy status can be inferred and assigned to each embryo. A significant advantage of SNP array is that the simultaneous analysis of thousands of polymorphisms scattered throughout the genome produces a unique DNA fingerprint for each embryo tested. The DNA fingerprint allows parental origin to be confirmed, reducing the risk that a laboratory error could lead to embryos being transferred to the wrong patient. The main drawbacks of SNP array are that the test is more expensive and takes longer to perform than aCGH or qPCR [13].

24.3.4   qPCR

qPCR technique is a robust, rapid, accurate, and cost-effective comprehensive chromosome screening method. Briefly, a preamplification step involving the multiplex amplification of 96 loci is performed with the use of TaqMan copy number assays. The preamplified products are then quantified using RT-qPCR in a 384-well plate, and whole chromosome aneuploidies are determined. The whole procedure lasts about 4 h and can also be combined with mutation detection. In this approach, PCR is performed directly on the sample, without WGA, which demonstrates the biggest advantage of this technique. However, the main drawbacks of this system are the facts that it is unable to detect segmental abnormalities and has yet to be validated for the detection of mosaicism [7, 14].

24.3.5   NGS

Most recently, next-generation sequencing (NGS) has been applied to PGT-A as a potentially more efficient and affordable technique. NGS is based upon the ability to massively parallel sequence small DNA fragments until the required depth of coverage is attained. Succeeding WGA, a barcoding step follows to allow the identification of embryo-specific sequences after which the amplified product is broken down into small sequence-ready fragments. Those fragments are then subjected to massively parallel sequencing with low coverage for the purpose of aneuploidy screening. The number of reads per chromosome ("binning") is proportional to the copy number of each chromosome and serves as a basis for aneuploidy calls [15]. The most important benefit of NGS is that it has the power of simultaneous assessment of aneuploidy, translocations, single-gene disorders, small copy number variations, and low-level mosaicism (<25%) from the same biopsy sample using the same platform technology [16]. Another benefit is, with NGS, a large number of samples can be simultaneously tested which results in reducing the cost and workload.

24.4   Clinical Outcome of PGT-A

Currently, multiple reports including meta-analysis and systematic reviews have demonstrated an improvement on implantation, clinical pregnancy, ongoing pregnancy, and live birth rates while reducing miscarriage rates and multiple pregnancy rates through the use of PGT-A [17, 18]. A randomized controlled trial (RCT) comparing blastocyst-stage single embryo fresh transfer with and without aCGH in good prognosis patients showed a significantly higher clinical pregnancy rate in the PGT-A group (70.9% vs. 45.8%). PGT-A group yielded a lower miscarriage rate than those without PGT-A [19]. A combination of the findings of 19 articles were summarized including 3 RCTs and 16 observational studies which revealed that in both young and advanced maternal age (AMA) patient populations, PGT-A results in a higher delivery rate per embryo transferred compared to the traditional method of morphology-based selection of embryos [20]. However, the data on patients of AMA, recurrent miscarriage, and implantation failure were from matched cohort studies, limiting their validity to make decisive conclusions. Similarly, in a meta-analysis where four RCTs and seven cohort studies were assessed for the effectiveness of PGT-A over traditional morphological methods, according to that, the transfer of euploid embryos can improve the implantation rate [21].

24.5   The Implementation Dilemma on Diminished Ovarian Reserve Patients

Despite the large and rapidly growing weight of evidence in support of PGT-A, some clinicians continue to have reservations about the clinical utility of this technique, particularly on diminished ovarian reserve (DOR) patients [22].

So why is PGT-A so controversial in DOR patients? One of the main reasons is that DOR patients have a reduced potential to produce an adequate number of oocytes and hence embryos, which may not allow PGT-A to be applied. Actually, many DOR patients who undergo IVF-PGT-A do not reach embryo transfer owing to the culmination of low embryo numbers and high aneuploidy rate in tested blastocyst-stage embryos. Shahine et al. found that the risk of not having a euploid blastocyst available for transfer in an IVF-PGT-A cycle was 13% in the normal ovarian reserve group and 25% in the DOR group. After including the eight patients with DOR who did not even make it to retrieval, the risk of no transfer for DOR patients was at least 37% [23]. It is important to note that the average number of oocytes retrieved was eight, and the mean number of blastocysts biopsied was 3.6 in this study, which still is a reasonable number to proceed with IVF-PGT-A. Some patients with severe DOR will have even fewer oocytes, blastocysts, and higher likelihood of no blastocyst formation. So when counseling DOR patients about the success rates with IVF-PGT-A, it is important to quote not only the success rates per transfer but also the likelihood of having an euploid blastocyst available for transfer

[24]. There are two studies that provided data comparing PGT-A with standard morphology assessment among anticipated poor responders. The authors reported that although more poor responders in the PGT-A arm had no transfer performed because of no euploid embryos being available, the PGT-A arm had a higher delivery rate per randomized patient (36 versus 21.9%, $P < 0.05$). This improvement was because of a significantly higher pregnancy rate per transfer (52.9 versus 24.2%, $P < 0.001$) and a significant reduction in miscarriage (2.7 versus 39%, $P < 0.001$) in the PGT-A arm [25]. Indeed, many patients randomized to PGT-A in such a study will have no embryos available to transfer if the only clinically usable embryos are found to be aneuploid. The true benefit in such patients may be the result of avoiding futile transfers and expeditiously moving into either another stimulation cycle or egg/embryo donation. Thus, time to pregnancy may be a better metric with miscarriage rate being a useful secondary measure [26].

Another reason for the controversy is the accuracy of the PGT-A's diagnostic results. The importance of avoiding a false diagnosis of euploidy and eliminating the chance of an aneuploid ongoing gestation is obvious. However, given the small number of embryos available for transfer in DOR patients, the avoidance of a false diagnosis of aneuploidy is very important in this patient population. Indeed, discarding an embryo because of incorrectly labeling it as abnormal may eliminate a patient's only chance at transfer. The chance of misdiagnosis results from both technical and biological limitations. Technical error can arise with any screening platform and occurs because of DNA contamination, allele dropout, human error, failed amplification, or a variety of other causes [27]. Even when technical aspects of the platform run flawlessly, biologic errors can still occur. One source of biologic error is related to the presence of chromosomal mosaicism within the developing embryo, which is characterized by the presence of a mixture of diploid and aneuploid cell lines. Mosaic embryos may not transferred usually because they are deemed abnormal. However, single TE biopsy cannot reliably reflect the whole TE and ICM [28]. Moreover, the ability of aCGH to detect mosaicism is dependent on the percentage of aneuploid cells in the TE biopsy. NGS now has the ability to detect mosaicism molecularly. The higher rates of reporting mosaicism by NGS compared with aCGH have called into question the validity of a diagnosis of mosaicism [29]. So if some viable embryos are discarded either because of false positives or mosaicism, then for DOR patients, where the number of available oocytes and embryos is strictly limited, treatment may be compromised [30].

Furthermore, the implementation of expensive technologies in healthcare, even when shown to offer an incremental improvement to outcomes, requires careful consideration of their relative cost-effectiveness. Currently, the cost of PGT-A remains high, making it unaffordable in many patients if not paid for by health insurance. In addition, it is difficult to quantify the intangible costs of failed implantation, miscarriage, all obstetric, neonatal, and ongoing costs of disease/aneuploidy. More research is needed to help patients, clinicians, and insurers in their decision regarding whether to utilize and pay for this technology [22].

Recently after reviewing the data, the American Society of Reproductive Medicine (ASRM) concluded that studies on use of PGT-A have limitations, and there are concerns about appropriate patient selections and testing platforms. For instance, patients in RCTs are mostly good responders and some started randomization on the day of blastulation rather than on the day of commencing stimulation. The questions about false-positive testing, potential embryonic damage with biopsy, loss of potential euploid embryos between day 3 and day 5, and blastocyst formation are not addressed. As we also discussed in Chap. 19, ASRM also agrees that not all the embryos survive in culture to develop into blastocyst stage for biopsy, although potentially they may have resulted in live birth if transferred in the cleavage stage [22]. Debates continue on the pros and cons of PGT-A [31].

24.6 Conclusion

The techniques of PGT-A, blastocyst culture, and biopsy as well as freeze-all approaches have the potential to reduce time to ongoing pregnancy and decrease miscarriages and ongoing aneuploid gestations in DOR patients. A complete assessment of the efficacy in this population will require more information regarding genetic variations, the biological ovarian aging, and multiple phenotypes of DOR. At present, however, there is insufficient evidence to recommend the routine use of blastocyst biopsy for aneuploidy testing in DOR patients. Therefore, taking into consideration each patient's unique circumstance, extensive counseling based on the pros and cons of the PGT-A procedure should be provided to best take care of this challenging patient population.

References

1. Handyside AH, Kontogianni EH, Hardy K, Winston RM. Pregnancies from biopsied human preimplantation embryos sexed by Y-specific DNA amplification. Nature. 1990;344(6268):768–70.
2. Handyside AH, Lesko JG, Tarin JJ, Winston RM, Hughes MR. Birth of a normal girl after in vitro fertilization and preimplantation diagnostic testing for cystic fibrosis. N Engl J Med. 1992;327(13):905–9.
3. Harper JC, Sengupta SB. Preimplantation genetic diagnosis: state of the art 2011. Hum Genet. 2012;131(2):175–86.
4. Griffin DK, Wilton LJ, Handyside AH, Winston RM, Delhanty JD. Dual fluorescent in situ hybridisation for simultaneous detection of X and Y chromosome-specific probes for the sexing of human preimplantation embryonic nuclei. Hum Genet. 1992;89(1):18–22.
5. Munne S, Sandalinas M, Escudero T, Velilla E, Walmsley R, Sadowy S, et al. Improved implantation after preimplantation genetic diagnosis of aneuploidy. Reprod Biomed Online. 2003;7(1):91–7.
6. Wells D, Delhanty JD. Comprehensive chromosomal analysis of human preimplantation embryos using whole genome amplification and single cell comparative genomic hybridization. Mol Hum Reprod. 2000;6(11):1055–62.
7. Griffin DK, Ogur C. Chromosomal analysis in IVF: just how useful is it? Reproduction. 2018;156(1):F29–50.

8. Gianaroli L, Magli MC, Pomante A, Crivello AM, Cafueri G, Valerio M, et al. Blastocentesis: a source of DNA for preimplantation genetic testing. Results from a pilot study. Fertil Steril. 2014;102(6):1692–9.e6.
9. Liu W, Liu J, Du H, Ling J, Sun X, Chen D. Non-invasive pre-implantation aneuploidy screening and diagnosis of beta thalassemia IVSII654 mutation using spent embryo culture medium. Ann Med. 2017;49(4):319–28.
10. McArthur SJ, Leigh D, Marshall JT, de Boer KA, Jansen RP. Pregnancies and live births after trophectoderm biopsy and preimplantation genetic testing of human blastocysts. Fertil Steril. 2005;84(6):1628–36.
11. Capalbo A, Rienzi L, Cimadomo D, Maggiulli R, Elliott T, Wright G, et al. Correlation between standard blastocyst morphology, euploidy and implantation: an observational study in two centers involving 956 screened blastocysts. Hum Reprod. 2014;29(6):1173–81.
12. Treff NR, Su J, Tao X, Levy B, Scott RT Jr. Accurate single cell 24 chromosome aneuploidy screening using whole genome amplification and single nucleotide polymorphism microarrays. Fertil Steril. 2010;94(6):2017–21.
13. Wells D, Alfarawati S, Fragouli E. Use of comprehensive chromosomal screening for embryo assessment: microarrays and CGH. Mol Hum Reprod. 2008;14(12):703–10.
14. Treff NR, Tao X, Ferry KM, Su J, Taylor D, Scott RT Jr. Development and validation of an accurate quantitative real-time polymerase chain reaction-based assay for human blastocyst comprehensive chromosomal aneuploidy screening. Fertil Steril. 2012;97(4):819–24.
15. Knapp M, Stiller M, Meyer M. Generating barcoded libraries for multiplex high-throughput sequencing. Methods Mol Biol. 2012;840:155–70.
16. Yan L, Huang L, Xu L, Huang J, Ma F, Zhu X, et al. Live births after simultaneous avoidance of monogenic diseases and chromosome abnormality by next-generation sequencing with linkage analyses. Proc Natl Acad Sci U S A. 2015;112(52):15964–9.
17. Brezina PR, Kutteh WH. Clinical applications of preimplantation genetic testing. BMJ. 2015;350:g7611.
18. Scott RT Jr, Ferry K, Su J, Tao X, Scott K, Treff NR. Comprehensive chromosome screening is highly predictive of the reproductive potential of human embryos: a prospective, blinded, nonselection study. Fertil Steril. 2012;97(4):870–5.
19. Yang Z, Liu J, Collins GS, Salem SA, Liu X, Lyle SS, et al. Selection of single blastocysts for fresh transfer via standard morphology assessment alone and with array CGH for good prognosis IVF patients: results from a randomized pilot study. Mol Cytogenet. 2012;5(1):24.
20. Lee E, Illingworth P, Wilton L, Chambers GM. The clinical effectiveness of preimplantation genetic diagnosis for aneuploidy in all 24 chromosomes (PGD-A): systematic review. Hum Reprod. 2015;30(2):473–83.
21. Chen M, Wei S, Hu J, Quan S. Can comprehensive chromosome screening technology improve IVF/ICSI outcomes? A meta-analysis. PLoS One. 2015;10(10):e0140779.
22. Practice Committees of the American Society for Reproductive Medicine, the Society for Assisted Reproductive Technology. Electronic address: ASRM@asrm.org, Practice Committees of the American Society for Reproductive Medicine, the Society for Assisted Reproductive Technology. The use of preimplantation genetic testing for aneuploidy (PGT-A): a committee opinion. Fertil Steril. 2018;109(3):429–36.
23. Shahine LK, Marshall L, Lamb JD, Hickok LR. Higher rates of aneuploidy in blastocysts and higher risk of no embryo transfer in recurrent pregnancy loss patients with diminished ovarian reserve undergoing in vitro fertilization. Fertil Steril. 2016;106(5):1124–8.
24. Lathi RB, Kort JD. Caution: counseling patients with diminished ovarian reserve and recurrent pregnancy loss about in vitro fertilization with preimplantation genetic screening. Fertil Steril. 2016;106(5):1041–2.
25. Rubio C, Bellver J, Rodrigo L, Castillon G, Guillen A, Vidal C, et al. In vitro fertilization with preimplantation genetic diagnosis for aneuploidies in advanced maternal age: a randomized, controlled study. Fertil Steril. 2017;107(5):1122–9.

26. Morin SJ, Kaser DJ, Franasiak JM. The dilemma of aneuploidy screening on low responders. Curr Opin Obstet Gynecol. 2018;30(3):179–84.
27. Brezina PR, Kutteh WH, Bailey AP, Ke RW. Preimplantation genetic screening (PGS) is an excellent tool, but not perfect: a guide to counseling patients considering PGS. Fertil Steril. 2016;105(1):49–50.
28. Gleicher N, Orvieto R. Is the hypothesis of preimplantation genetic screening (PGS) still supportable? A review. J Ovarian Res. 2017;10(1):21.
29. Munne S, Grifo J, Wells D. Mosaicism: "survival of the fittest" versus "no embryo left behind". Fertil Steril. 2016;105(5):1146–9.
30. Rosenwaks Z, Handyside AH. Is preimplantation genetic testing for aneuploidy an essential tool for embryo selection or a costly 'add-on' of no clinical benefit? Fertil Steril. 2018;110(3):351–2.
31. Rosenwaks Z, Handyside AH, Fiorentino F, Gleicher N, Paulson RJ, Schattman GL, et al. The pros and cons of preimplantation genetic testing for aneuploidy: clinical and laboratory perspectives. Fertil Steril. 2018;110(3):353–61.

Part IV
Future Prospects

Chapter 25
Artificial Oocyte and Artificial Ovary Development

Kotaro Sasaki

25.1 Introduction

The last several decades has witnessed the rapid progression of developmental engineering and stem cell biology, including reproductive cloning and the establishment of pluripotent stem cells from various mammalian species, including humans. Notably, pluripotent stem cells, including embryonic stem cells (ESCs) and inducible pluripotent stem cells (iPSCs) obtained from preimplantation embryos or any somatic cells, respectively, have the potential to differentiate into any cell type in the human body, thereby providing an unprecedented opportunity for tissue regeneration for therapeutic purposes [1]. Do these cells also have the potential to differentiate into germ cells such as oocytes or spermatozoa in vitro? If successful in humans, such technology will not only provide a highly valuable platform to understand the molecular mechanisms of mammalian germ cell formation but also the novel treatment modality against infertility caused by the loss or functional defect of gametes. On the other hand, such technology enables the creation of the "life" from "nonliving" somatic cells, thereby necessitating careful scrutiny of its safety and ethicolegal considerations. Due to its broad impact on science and medicine, the concept of "in vitro gametogenesis" has attracted many scientists for over several centuries. Nonetheless, the paucity of information on how mammalian germ cells develop in vivo, a prerequisite for in vitro reconstitution, has hindered the development of such technology until very recently [2]. Accumulation of such knowledge on germ cell development, especially the mechanisms of the early segregation of germ cell lineage from somatic lineages in mice over the last 20 years, gradually enables the reconstitution of germline in vitro. In this chapter, the progress in understanding the mechanisms of early mouse germ cell development and its successful reconstitution

K. Sasaki (✉)
Department of Biomedical Sciences, University of Pennsylvania School of Veterinary Medicine, Philadelphia, PA, USA
e-mail: ksasaki@vet.upenn.edu

© Springer Nature Switzerland AG 2020
O. Bukulmez (ed.), *Diminished Ovarian Reserve and Assisted Reproductive Technologies*, https://doi.org/10.1007/978-3-030-23235-1_25

in vitro will be reviewed, followed by recent groundbreaking discoveries in human germ cell development and attempts for in vitro human gametogenesis.

25.2 Mechanisms of Early Germ Cell Development in Mice

Primordial germ cells (PGCs), a transient entity only present in the embryonic/fetal period, are the common precursors for both oocytes and spermatozoa [2]. The development of mammalian PGCs has been studied mostly using mice as a model organism. Mouse zygotes form the epiblast, a pluripotent cell lineage at the peri-implantation period, from which the entire fetus forms. The gastrulation starts within the posterior aspect of the epiblast to generate three germ layers (ectoderm, mesoderm, and endoderm) at around E6.5 [3]. This is about the time when a small number of founder mouse PGCs (mPGCs) are first specified within the posterior and proximal epiblast, which subsequently expand to establish a cluster of about 30 PGCs within the extraembryonic mesoderm (ExM) at around E7.0 (Fig. 25.1) [4, 5]. Based on transplantation experiments recombining the different parts of epiblasts ex vivo, peri-gastrulating epiblasts were shown to possess the competency to generate mPGCs regardless of their position in vivo, suggesting that extraembryonic signals dictate the fate of the epiblast to become either germline or somatic lineages

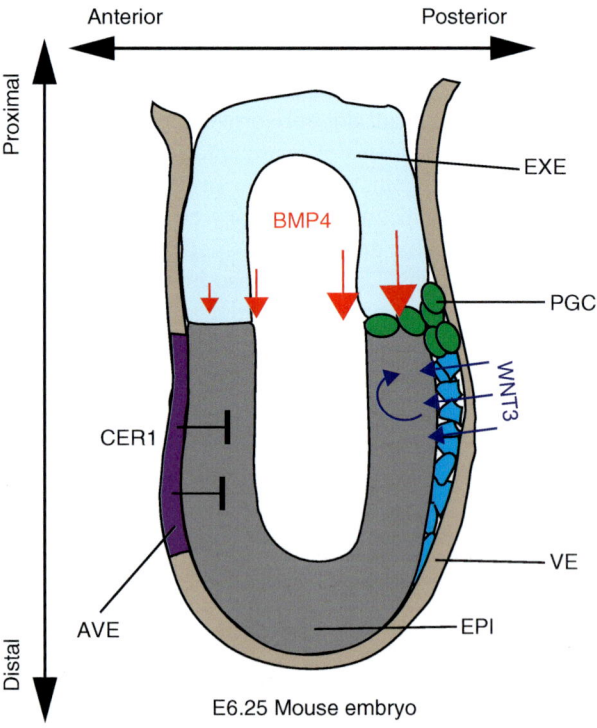

Fig. 25.1 The PGC specification in mouse embryos. Mouse PGCs are specified at the posterior and proximal end of the epiblast (EPI) by receiving BMP4 from extraembryonic ectoderm (EXE), a trophectoderm lineage, which later contributes to the placenta, and WNT3 from visceral endoderm (VE) and/or EPI. CER1, an antagonistic factor for BMP4 produced by anterior visceral endoderm (AVE), inhibits the formation of PGCs at the anterior EPI

[6]. Subsequent studies using mouse genetics demonstrated that BMP4 and WNT3, secreted from the extraembryonic ectoderm (EXE) or visceral endoderm (VE), respectively, play an essential role for mPGC specification within the epiblast and that the inhibitory factors for such signals (CER1, DKK1) secreted from the anterior visceral endoderm (AVE) inhibit the mPGC specification at the anterior epiblast [7, 8]. Together, these studies showed that mice, and perhaps most other mammalian germline, are specified within the pluripotent epiblast by receiving extrinsic inductive signals through "epigenesis" in contrast to other metazoan species (e.g., *Drosophila*, *Xenopus*) where germ cells are specified by the maternally inherited determinants through "preformation." These studies also suggest that the mammalian germline can be reconstituted in vitro from pluripotent stem cells. In early 2000, key transcription factors and marker genes for the specification stage of mPGCs, including *Stella*, *Blimp1*, *Tfap2c*, and *Prdm14*, were identified by several laboratories [4, 9–11]. Identification of these factors has not only provided critical insight into the mechanisms of mouse germ cell specification but also enables the visualization of nascent PGCs both in vivo and in vitro. Through a series of elegant studies using mouse genetics, Saitou and colleagues demonstrated that inducing *Blimp1* and *Prdm14* within the epiblast through BMP4 signaling triggers the expression of PGC specific genes such as *Nanos3*, *Tdrd5*, *Dnd1*, and *Stella* and pluripotency-associated genes, such as *Pou5f1*, *Nanog*, and *Sox2*, while suppressing the genes expressed in somatic lineages. Both *Blimp1* and *Prdm14* also play a critical role in the genome-wide epigenetic reprogramming processes such as global DNA demethylation [12].

25.2.1 In Vitro Gametogenesis in Mice

PGCs are a scarce and transient entity, present only at the embryonic period thereby precluding the detailed biochemical analysis requiring a large number of cells. Induction of PGCs from pluripotent cells, such as mouse ESCs (mESCs) or iPSCs (miPSCs), therefore, have been awaited to overcome such hurdles. Many of such attempts have been done since early 2000, but none of them have successfully demonstrated the contribution to functional gametes or healthy offspring, likely due to the poor induction efficiency and/or the lack of appropriate markers to isolate and characterize the in vitro derivatives [13–16]. Notably, these studies utilized markers that have poor PGC specificity or are expressed only at a late stage, thereby failing to recapitulate the early PGC development and thus the following developmental trajectories leading to mature gametes. To reconstitute the perplexed and protracted germ cell developmental processes in vitro, faithful reconstitution of such processes in a stepwise manner is of paramount importance. By using epiblast cells harboring *Blimp1-mVenus* (BV), *Stella-Ecfp* (SC) reporters to visualize the formation of early PGCs, Ohinata et al. successfully induced the BVSC (+) PGC-like state from pregastrulating epiblast cells in a dish by adding BMP4 and other growth factors (SCF, EGF, LIF, BMP8b) (Fig. 25.2) [8]. These cells closely resembled PGCs in vivo in

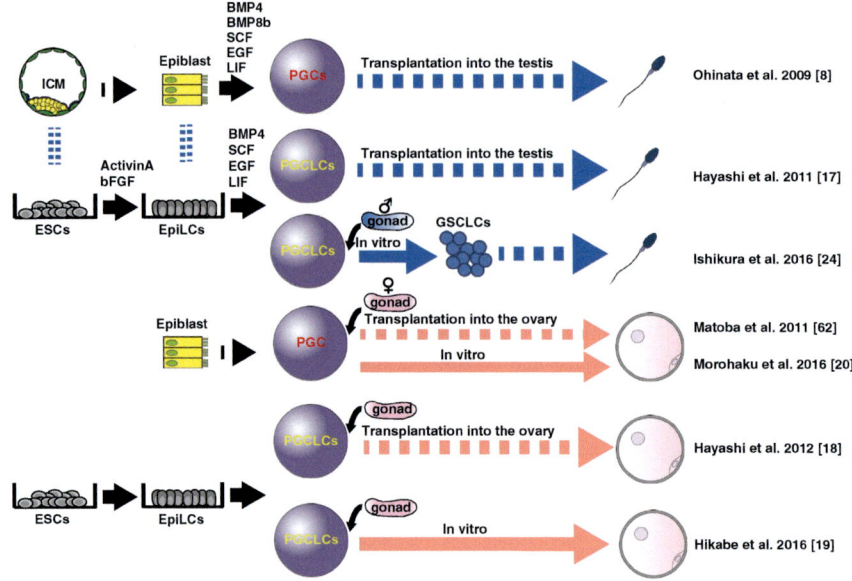

Fig. 25.2 Functionally validated in vitro gametogenesis in mice. First successful demonstration of the reconstitution of mouse PGC development dates back to 2009, when Ohinata et al. showed that epiblasts at E6.0 can be induced ex vivo into PGC-like cells (PGCLCs) by culturing in the presence of BMP4, BMP8b, SCF, EGF, and LIF, which matured into functional sperm upon transplantation into the neonatal testis [8]. In subsequent studies, ESCs were used as a starting material to induce epiblast-like cells (EpiLCs) through the monolayer culture in the presence of Activin-A and bFGF, which were in turn induced into PGCLCs [17]. PGCLCs similarly contribute to functional spermatogenesis upon transplantation. In 2011, Matoba et al. developed a method in which PGCs were induced ex vivo into mature oocytes through ectopic transplantation into kidney capsules [62]. With minor modification of this method, Hayashi et al. successfully induced fertile oocytes derived from PGCLCs [18]. More recently, the latter oogenesis processes were recapitulated in vitro first using PGCs ex vivo [20] then PGCLCs induced from mESCs [19]. These studies used the "reconstituted ovary" by which germ cells were cultured together with gonadal somatic cells obtained from E12.5 ovaries. Male spermatogenesis has also been partially reconstituted; germline stem cell-like cells (GSCLCs) were induced from PGCLCs through reconstituted testis, which, upon transplantation into recipient testis, contributed to the fertile spermatozoa [24]

both gene expression and epigenome pattern. Upon transplantation into the seminiferous tubules of *c-Kit* mutant (W/Wv) mice depleted of endogenous germ cells, they differentiated into functional sperm and successfully contributed to the healthy offspring after intracytoplasmic sperm injection (ICSI). In the following study, Hayashi et al. successfully induced mouse primordial germ cell-like cells (mPGCLCs) in vitro from BVSC (+) naïve mESCs or miPSCs maintained in the presence of 2i (CHIR99021, PD0325901) + LIF [17]. In this study, they first cultivated naïve mESCs or miPSCs for 2 days in the presence of Activin-A and bFGF to induce epiblast-like cells (EpiLCs), which closely resemble germline competent E 5.75 pre-gastrulating epiblast. EpiLCs were further induced into mPGCLCs by BMP4-based cytokine cocktails as above used by Ohinata et al. Notably, mPGCLCs exhibit highly similar transcriptome and epigenome profiles with in vivo PGCs at ~E9.0 and contribute to the functional spermatogenesis upon transplantation into W/Wv mice. Again, healthy pups were generated through intracytoplasmic sperm injection (ICSI) of the mPG-CLC-derived sperms and transferring the resultant zygotes to foster mothers.

In a subsequent study, Hayashi et al. similarly induced female mESCs into mPG-CLCs in vitro (Fig. 25.2) [18]. By culturing with somatic cells obtained from embryonic ovaries ("reconstituted ovary" method), mPGCLCs further differentiated into the oocytes that were in prophase of the first meiotic division. Upon transplantation into ovaries of immune-deficient mice, mPGCLC-derived oocytes matured into fully grown oocytes, which, through in vitro maturation (IVM) and in vitro fertilization (IVF), became zygotes and contributed to fertile offspring [18]. Together, these studies for the first time provided convincing evidence that the mouse germline can be reconstituted in vitro by using pluripotent stem cells.

Notably, all of the above attempts of mouse in vitro gametogenesis relied on host niche environment for terminal maturation into oocytes or spermatozoa through the transplantation of mPGCLCs into recipient mice (Fig. 25.2) [8, 17, 18]. More recently, however, several groups have reported the successful reconstitution of the latter half of oogenesis in vitro. In these studies, authors divided the culture into three steps – in vitro differentiation (IVD), in vitro growth (IVG), and IVM according to the in vivo oogenesis pathway. By careful validation of each step using the reconstituted ovaries, authors successfully reconstituted the entire process of oogenesis in vitro and generated healthy offspring by IVF of the in vitro reconstituted eggs [19–21]. These studies provide a valuable platform for analyzing the mechanisms of oogenesis in vitro and will serve as a guide for future in vitro gametogenesis in humans.

In male testes, the presence of spermatogonial stem cells with self-renewal capabilities allow for production of terminally differentiated spermatozoa for a prolonged period of time [21]. In mice, long-term culture of cells with robust spermatogonial potential, named germline stem cells (GSCs), can be established from both neonatal and adult testes [22, 23]. Recently, Ishikura et al. successfully induced GSC-like cells (GSCLCs) from male mPGCLCs by culturing with gonadal somatic cells obtained from E12.5 male embryos (Fig. 25.2) [24]. Upon transplantation, GSCLCs were capable of colonizing in the adult testis and generated functional sperm, features characteristic of GSCs. Previously, Ogawa and colleagues successfully induced sperm from GSCs through organ culture of neonatal testes into which GSCs were transplanted before culture [25]. Combining these methods together, reconstitution of the entire process of spermatogenesis in vitro will be technically feasible and achieved in the near future.

25.3 The Development of Germline in Humans and Nonhuman Primates

Precise understanding of how human germline develops in vivo is the prerequisite information for human in vitro gametogenesis. However, until very recently, human germ cell development has been poorly understood due to ethical and technical constraints in analyzing a scarce population which is only present in embryos and fetuses. To date, our knowledge of human germ cell development has been mostly attributed to the morphologic description conducted in the early to mid-twentieth century.

One of such earliest descriptions dates back to nearly a century ago, when Fuss identified the cluster of cells with unique morphologic features suggestive of human PGCs (hPGCs) at the posterior aspect of the yolk sac at ~4 weeks post conception (wpc) of human embryos [26, 27]. Subsequent series of histological and ultrastructural evaluation provided further evidence that PGCs emigrate from the yolk sac endoderm and further migrate through the hindgut endoderm and dorsal mesentery until they reach the gonads at ~5 wpc [28–30]. Recently, several groups reported transcriptome and immunohistochemical profiles of hPGCs within the gonads [31–34]. Gonadal hPGCs show expression of germ cell markers (e.g., *BLIMP1, TFAP2C, NANOS3, DND1, DDX4, DAZL*) and pluripotency-associated genes (e.g., *POU5F1, NANOG, SALL4, LIN28A, PRDM14*) similar to mPGCs. Notable divergence, however, does exist between hPGCs and mPGCs. *SOX2*, a core transcription factor for pluripotency and critical for germ cell development in mPGCs, is not expressed in hPGCs, which instead shows strong and persistent expression of *SOX17*, previously known as an endodermal marker [32, 35]. *SOX17*, on the other hand, is only transiently expressed in early mPGCs but not in gonadal mPGCs [36]. Epigenetic features of hPGCs in particular genome-wide methylation has also been investigated over the last few years, which showed that global demethylation occurs in hPGCs at the migratory and early gonadal stage with their genome-wide 5-methylcytosine (5mC) levels reaching ~5% at 9 wpc, similar to mPGCs [31–33].

Although the above recent studies provide some insight into the biologic properties of gonadal hPGCs in vivo from 5 wpc and onward, how hPGCs develop and are specified in earlier phases is still a mystery due to our inaccessibility of such specimens. Of note, there are striking differences in the anatomical structures in pre-gastrulating embryos between mice and primates that include humans [37]. For example, EXE, a source of BMP4, which also plays an essential role in mPGC specification, is not present in early postimplantation primate embryos. On the other hand, the nascent amnion which emerges in early pre-gastrulating primate embryos dorsal to the epiblastic disc is not present at the pre-gastrulating mouse embryos (Figs. 25.1 and 25.3). Therefore, direct extrapolation of the signaling principles in the formation of mice pre-gastrulating embryos to those of primates is not possible. To overcome this hurdle, Sasaki et al. recently used cynomolgus monkey embryos as a surrogate model, which exhibit very similar early developmental processes to human embryos [38, 39]. By series of immunohistochemical evaluation in cynomolgus embryos at various stages, they found that the origin of cynomolgus PGCs (cyPGCs) are traced back to clusters of ~10 cells at the dorsal aspect of the nascent amnion in the pre-gastrulating embryos at E11, which thereafter move toward the posterior end and further into the yolk sac (visceral) endoderm by E17 (Fig. 25.3) [38]. These early cyPGCs express germ cell markers (BLIMP1, TFAP2C, and SOX17) and pluripotency-associated markers (POU5F1, NANOG, and

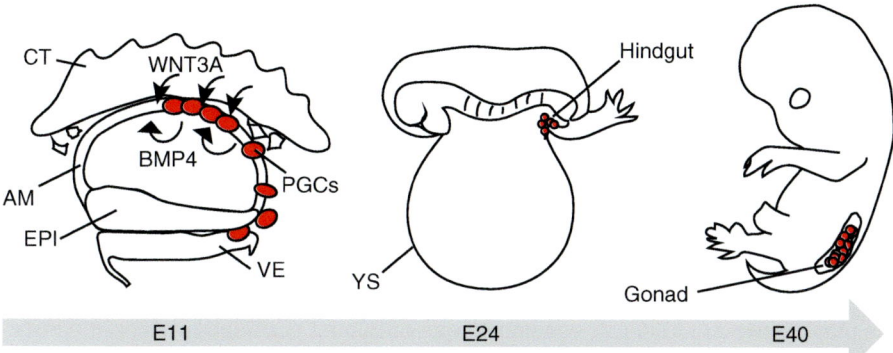

Fig. 25.3 Primate germ cell development in vivo. Cynomolgus PGCs (cyPGCs) first appear at the dorsal aspect of the nascent amnion at E11. BMP4 and WNT3A, critical specifiers of germ cell fate, are expressed in the nascent amnion (AM) and cytotrophoblast (CT), respectively. cyPGCs subsequently move into the visceral endoderm (VE) through the posterior AM. Note that cyPGCs are not identified within the epiblast (EPI). cyPGCs thereafter form the loose cluster at the posterior end of the yolk sac endoderm (YS) (a derivative of VE), which is incorporated into the hindgut endoderm upon folding of the embryo at ~E24. cyPGCs further migrate into the bilateral gonads through the dorsal mesentery by ~E40

PRDM14) but lack SOX2, similar to gonadal hPGCs. Interestingly, cyPGCs before E17 do not express DDX4 or DAZL, suggesting that these markers serve as a late (gonadal) PGC marker in both mice and primates. In situ hybridization on histologic sections further demonstrated the specific localization of *BMP4*, a key determinant of mPGC specification, and their downstream target genes, *ID2* and *MSX2* in the nascent amnion, suggesting that cyPGCs may be specified within the nascent amnion through the autocrine action of BMP4 signaling [38]. This surprising finding is at odds with the mode of mPGC specification, where mPGCs are originated from the posterior epiblast by receiving BMP4 signaling from EXE (Fig.25.1) and highlights the mechanistic divergence of PGC specification among species [7, 8]. Nonetheless, the study is based on static observation and therefore awaits further validation, such as the tracing of cyPGCs using a reporter system ex vivo. This will prove to be challenging even with the current developmental engineering technologies.

25.3.1   Induction of Human PGC-Like Cells in Humans

Reconstitution of the human germline in vitro using hESCs or hiPSCs has a tremendous impact on both basic research and clinical perspectives. Since human embryos before 4 wpc, which is when specification of hPGCs occurs, are inaccessible due to ethical reasons, human PGC-like cells (hPGCLCs) induced in vitro from pluripotent stem cells provide the indispensable tool in understanding the molecular mechanisms of hPGC specification. Additionally, the reconstitution of the human germline in vitro will also enable the molecular dissection of the critical events during the subsequent germline development including epigenetic reprogramming, genomic imprinting, X-chromosome reactivation, or meiosis through gain- or loss-of-function analysis which, in turn, provides critical insight into causes of infertility or birth defects as a consequence of abnormal germ cell development [2]. Moreover, creation of fertile eggs or sperms in a dish provides new opportunities for infertile couples possessing defective gametes. Despite such significance, human in vitro gametogenesis has several hurdles to be overcome, making it more challenging than its mouse counterpart. First, our knowledge of human germline in vivo, in particular, that of before 4 wpc is very limited, which makes it difficult to assure that hPG-CLCs recapitulate hPGC development in vivo. Second, species specific differences exist in the property of ESCs/iPSCs between mice and humans. hESCs/hiPSCs exhibit "primed" pluripotency, resembling peri-gastrulating epiblasts in vivo, while mESCs/miPSCs show "naïve" pluripotency recapitulating the features characteristic of inner cell mass (ICM) [37]. Although mESCs/miPSCs are known to be germline competent, it has yet to be known whether hESCs/hiPSCs have such competency. Third, an appropriate assay system to test the functionality of germ cells is lacking in humans. Although with ethical and legal constraints, fertilization using hPGCLC-derived gametes and observing the successive embryo development may provide clues that such germ cells have a potential to create the embryonic and extraembryonic tissues, a hallmark of germline [2].

Despite such technical and ethical constraints, many laboratories have attempted the induction of human germline from pluripotent stem cells over the last two decades. These studies used various methods including random differentiation [40, 41], directed differentiation using BMP4 [42–44] or retinoic acids [45], or overexpression of DAZ gene family [43]. These studies however suffer from either low induction efficiency due to the failure to recapitulate hPGC development in vivo or inappropriately gauge the induction using markers that is not specific to or only detectable at the late stage of human germ cells (e.g., DDX4, DAZL, or meiotic markers).

More recently, Sasaki et al. employed a stepwise approach to reconstitute the first step of human PGC development (Fig. 25.4) [39]. To recapitulate early PGC development, they generated dual reporter hiPSCs harboring tdTomato or EGFP reporter genes under the promoter of *BLIMP1* and *AP2γ* (also known as *TFAP2C*), respectively [*BLIMP1-tdTomato* (BT); *AP2γ-EGFP* (AG)], the earliest known markers in both mPGCs and cyPGCs [10, 38, 46] as well as in gonadal hPGCs in vivo [32, 47]. BTAG hiPSCs were maintained in feeder-free, defined conditions through multiple passages with stable karyotypes and a gene expression pattern consistent with "primed pluripotency." Authors demonstrated that BTAG hiPSCs first differentiated into incipient mesoderm-like cells (iMeLCs) by WNT agonist, CHIR99021, and Activin-A could be further induced robustly into hPGCLCs by culturing in the presence of BMP4, SCF, EGF, and LIF, the similar growth factors used for mPGCLC induction [17, 39]. These cells strongly express both BT and AG

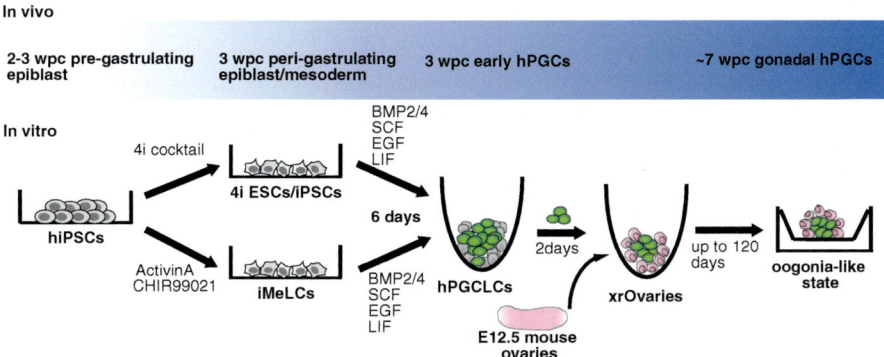

Fig. 25.4 In vitro gametogenesis in humans. Feeder free hiPSCs or ESCs were first cultured in monolayer in the presence of Activin-A and CHIR99021 for the induction of iMeLCs as demonstrated by Sasaki et al. [39, 52]. In the alternative method proposed by Irie et al. [35], hiPSCs or ESCs were cultured on feeders in the presence of 4i cocktail containing inhibitors for GSK3, p38, JNK, and MAPK together with LIF, bFGF, and TGF-β1 to induce 4i ESCs/iPSCs [48]. 4i ESCs/iPSCs or iMeLCs were further induced into hPGCLCs by BMP2/4, SCF, EGF, and LIF in 3D aggregates similar to mPGCLC induction. hPGCLCs mixed with somatic cells from E12.5 mouse ovaries were cultured for 2 days to form the xenogeneic reconstituted ovaries, which, upon air-liquid interface culture on nitrocellulose membranes for up to 120 days, generate cells with oogonia-like state expressing later germ cell markers (e.g., DDX4 and DAZL) and with global DNA demethylation

fluorescence proteins with efficiency reaching 60% and exhibit a gene expression pattern similar to that of cyPGCs and hPGCs in vivo. Notably, however, in contrast to gonadal PGCs, hPGCLCs lack late germ cell markers such as DDX4 or DAZL that are only expressed after they migrate into the gonads. Further comparison of hPGCLCs with early cyPGCs (obtained from E13–E21 embryos) versus gonadal cyPGCs confirmed that hPGCLCs do in fact resemble early cyPGCs more than gonadal cyPGCs they have yet to undergo overt epigenetic reprogramming such as global demethylation [38, 39]. Sasaki et al. also identified highly specific cell surface markers, ITGA6 and EpCAM, which, when used in combination, enables isolation of hPGCLCs with nearly 99% accuracy from hPGCLC-induction culture using various hiPSCs, which do not harbor fluorescence reporter genes [39].

Around the same time this study was published, Surani and colleagues also induced hPGCLCs from hESCs and hiPSCs maintained in "4i condition," consisting of the inhibitors for four kinases (MAPK, GSK3, p38, and c-Jun N-terminal kinase [JNK]), which has been used for inducing naïve human pluripotency [35, 48]. Authors demonstrated that the 4i-conditioned hESCs/hiPSCs were successfully induced into hPGCLCs through the similar protocol used for mPGCLC induction with the efficiency of ~50%, while conventional "primed" state hESCs/hiPSCs failed to generate hPGCLCs, in contrast to the study by Sasaki et al. (Fig. 25.4) [39]. Later studies resolved the discrepancy by showing that 4i-conditioned hESCs/hiP-SCs do not possess the naïve pluripotency despite their intention and rather show early mesodermal differentiation similar to iMeLCs in the induction method by

Sasaki et al. [39, 49]. These seminal studies laid the foundation for the mechanistic dissection of human germline development and downstream in vitro gametogenesis. By using the method by Sasaki et al., several studies identified the critical determinant in human germline specification [50–52]. Accordingly, *EOMES*, a target gene of WNT3 signaling, induces *SOX17*. *EOMES*, in concert with *TFAP2C*, which is downstream in the BMP4 signaling pathway, instates the transcription program for hPGCLC induction including the upregulation of *BLIMP1*, which in turn suppresses the somatic and neuronal programs and further reinforces the germline transcriptional circuit [51].

Despite similarity in gene expression with PGCs in vivo, whether hPGCLCs represent bona fide hPGCs awaits future studies that validate its functionality, ultimately to create mature gametes and offspring. Such stringent functionality testing has numerous technical and ethical barriers; therefore, the stepwise comparison in transcriptome or epigenome with in vivo hPGCs or cyPGCs at different stages will serve as a valuable surrogate to move this technology forward.

25.4 Further Differentiation of hPGCLCs and the Future of In Vitro Gametogenesis

Recently, by xenogeneic ovary reconstitution, Yamashiro et al. successfully induced oogonia-like cells from hPGCLCs (Fig. 25.4) [53]. In this study, they first induced hiPSCs into hPGCLCs through iMeLCs, which subsequently reaggregated with mouse gonadal somatic cells from E12.5 embryonic ovaries to create xenogeneic reconstituted ovaries (xrOvaries). After a long-term organ culture (up to 120 days), a small portion of the hPGCLCs upregulated late germ cell markers, such as DDX4 and DAZL, and acquired oogonia-like gene expression profiles. Importantly, these cells showed evidence of partial imprint erasure, X chromosome reactivation, and progressive DNA demethylation with their global DNA methylation reaching to ~13% after the 120-day culture, suggesting that this system recapitulates epigenetic reprogramming processes in vivo. Nonetheless, these cells failed to enter meiotic prophase even after 4 months of induction, by the time at least some of the human oogonia at the corresponding stage would have initiated meiotic recombination in vivo. Moreover, induction efficiency is generally very low (~4%), suggesting that the xenogeneic niche environment fails to provide the appropriate supportive signaling for the survival and maturation of hPGCLCs. Utilization of human or monkey embryonic gonads may provide more physiological niche signaling, thereby helping to enhance their survival and maturation, including entry into meiosis.

Alternatively, using this platform, screening and validation of various factors such as BMP2 or retinoic acid [54] may be worthwhile in order to identify the critical determinants of meiotic entry of human oogonia. Once established, such reconstitution system will provide the essential tools to understand the mechanistic details of human meiosis responsible for the evolution of species as well as the congenital anomalies that result from aberrant meiotic recombination.

Whether or not spermatogenesis can also be reconstituted using hPGCLCs awaits further investigation. Notably, the culture methods for GSCs has not been established in humans, adding another layer of challenges in the reconstitution of male pathways. Characterization of human spermatogonia and their niche environment by single cell studies [55–57] may provide important clues in developing an effective strategy for culturing human GSCs.

25.5 Conclusion

Given the rapid advances of mammalian germ cell research both on mice and humans, it is not surprising that the in vitro derived mature human gametes with certain functionalities will be generated in the near future. However, rigorous validation of efficacy and safety will be mandatory before translating such technology into a clinical trial, such as infertility treatment. Specifically, there must be careful scrutinization of the genome and epigenome of such gametes as surrogate markers for their functionality, validation of developmental potential during preimplantation cultures, and of the normality of offspring derived from in vitro derived gametes across several generations using monkeys as a surrogate. Somatic cells, from which hiPSCs are derived, have already accumulated a significant number of mutations, while such mutations are suppressed to a minimal degree in the germline [58]. Therefore, creating germ cells using somatic cells has the potential risk to introduce deleterious mutations into the next generation. It is therefore essential to quality control the genome of the in vitro derived gametes through high-resolution whole-genome sequencing to rule out the presence of such mutations. If such mutations are inevitable, the correction of the deleterious mutations using genome-editing technologies such as CRISPR/Cas9 might be an option but has the potential to create additional "off-target" mutations [59]. Moreover, given the difficulty in strictly distinguishing mutations versus polymorphisms, referring to the patient's decision of which genes to correct might create room for "designing" babies. Importantly, fertilization of in vitro derived gametes is under certain regulations in some countries [60, 61]. Future use of such technology for clinical application needs to be carefully discussed from ethical and legal standpoints.

Acknowledgment KS thanks Ms. Karen Makar for the discussion of the study, careful review, and editing of the manuscript.

References

1. Shi Y, Inoue H, Wu JC, Yamanaka S. Induced pluripotent stem cell technology: a decade of progress. Nat Rev Drug Discov. 2016;16:245.
2. Saitou M, Miyauchi H. Gametogenesis from pluripotent stem cells. Cell Stem Cell. 2016;18:721–35.

3. Takaoka K, Hamada H. Cell fate decisions and axis determination in the early mouse embryo. Development. 2012;139:3–14.

4. Saitou M, Barton SC, Surani AM. A molecular programme for the specification of germ cell fate in mice. Nature. 2002;418:293.

5. Lawson K, Hage W. Clonal analysis of the origin of primordial germ cells in the mouse. Ciba Found Symp. 1994;182:68–84; discussion 84–91.

6. Tam P, Zhou SX. The allocation of epiblast cells to ectodermal and germ-line lineages is influenced by the position of the cells in the gastrulating mouse embryo. Dev Biol. 1996;178:124–32.

7. Lawson KA, Dunn RN, Roelen B, Zeinstra LM, Davis AM, Wright C, Korving J, Hogan B. Bmp4 is required for the generation of primordial germ cells in the mouse embryo. Genes Dev. 1999;13:424–36.

8. Ohinata Y, Ohta H, Shigeta M, Yamanaka K, Wakayama T, Saitou M. A signaling principle for the specification of the germ cell lineage in mice. Cell. 2009;137:571–84.

9. Yamaji M, Seki Y, Kurimoto K, Yabuta Y, Yuasa M, Shigeta M, Yamanaka K, Ohinata Y, Saitou M. Critical function of Prdm14 for the establishment of the germ cell lineage in mice. Nat Genet. 2008;40:186.

10. Ohinata Y, Payer B, O'Carroll D, et al. Blimp1 is a critical determinant of the germ cell lineage in mice. Nature. 2005;436:207.

11. Pauls K, Jäger R, Weber S, Wardelmann E, Koch A, Büttner R, Schorle H. Transcription factor AP-2γ, a novel marker of gonocytes and seminomatous germ cell tumors. Int J Cancer. 2005;115:470–7.

12. Saitou M, Yamaji M. Primordial germ cells in mice. Cold Spring Harb Perspect Biol. 2012;4:a008375.

13. Nayernia K, Nolte J, Michelmann HW, et al. In vitro-differentiated embryonic stem cells give rise to male gametes that can generate offspring mice. Dev Cell. 2006;11:125–32.

14. Hübner K, Fuhrmann G, Christenson LK, Kehler J, Reinbold R, Fuente R, Wood J, Strauss JF, Boiani M, Schöler HR. Derivation of oocytes from mouse embryonic stem cells. Science. 2003;300:1251–6.

15. Geijsen N, Horoschak M, Kim K, Gribnau J, Eggan K, Daley GQ. Derivation of embryonic germ cells and male gametes from embryonic stem cells. Nature. 2003;427:148.

16. Lacham-Kaplan O, Chy H, Trounson A. Testicular cell conditioned medium supports differentiation of embryonic stem cells into ovarian structures containing oocytes. Stem Cells. 2006;24:266–73.

17. Hayashi K, Ohta H, Kurimoto K, Aramaki S, Saitou M. Reconstitution of the mouse germ cell specification pathway in culture by pluripotent stem cells. Cell. 2011;146:519–32.

18. Hayashi K, Ogushi S, Kurimoto K, Shimamoto S, Ohta H, Saitou M. Offspring from oocytes derived from in vitro primordial germ cell–like cells in mice. Science. 2012;338:971–5.

19. Hikabe O, Hamazaki N, Nagamatsu G, et al. Reconstitution in vitro of the entire cycle of the mouse female germ line. Nature. 2016;539:299–303.

20. Morohaku K, Tanimoto R, Sasaki K, Kawahara-Miki R, Kono T, Hayashi K, Hirao Y, Obata Y. Complete in vitro generation of fertile oocytes from mouse primordial germ cells. Proc Natl Acad Sci U S A. 2016;113:9021–6.

21. Kubota H, Brinster RL. Spermatogonial stem cells. Biol Reprod. 2018;99:52. https://doi.org/10.1093/biolre/ioy077.

22. Kubota H, Avarbock MR, Brinster RL. Growth factors essential for self-renewal and expansion of mouse spermatogonial stem cells. Proc Natl Acad Sci U S A. 2004;101:16489–94.

23. Kanatsu-Shinohara M, Ogonuki N, Inoue K, Miki H, Ogura A, Toyokuni S, Shinohara T. Long-term proliferation in culture and germline transmission of mouse male germline stem cells. Biol Reprod. 2003;69:612–6.

24. Ishikura Y, Yabuta Y, Ohta H, et al. In vitro derivation and propagation of spermatogonial stem cell activity from mouse pluripotent stem cells. Cell Rep. 2016;17:2789–804.

25. Sato T, Katagiri K, Gohbara A, Inoue K, Ogonuki N, Ogura A, Kubota Y, Ogawa T. In vitro production of functional sperm in cultured neonatal mouse testes. Nature. 2011;471:504.

26. Fuss A. Über die Geschlechtszellen des Menschen und der Säugetiere. Arch Mikrosk Anat. 1912;81:a1–23.
27. Fuss A. Uber extraregionare Geschlechtszellen bei einem menschlichen Embryo von 4 Wochen. Anat Am. 1911;39:407–9.
28. Witschi E. Migration of the germ cells of human embryos from the yolk sac to the primitive gonadal folds: with 24 plates. Contrib Embryol Carnegie Inst. 1948;32:67–80.
29. Politzer G. Über einen menschlichen Embryo mit sieben Urwirbelpaaren. Z Anat Entwicklungsgesch. 1930;93:386–428.
30. Politzer G. Die Keimbahn des Menschen. Z Anat Entwicklungsgesch. 1933;100:331–61.
31. Gkountela S, Zhang KX, Shafiq TA, Liao W-W, Hargan-Calvopiña J, Chen P-Y, Clark AT. DNA demethylation dynamics in the human prenatal germline. Cell. 2015;161:1425–36.
32. Tang W, Dietmann S, Irie N, Leitch HG, Floros VI, Bradshaw CR, Hackett JA, Chinnery PF, Surani AM. A unique gene regulatory network resets the human germline epigenome for development. Cell. 2015;161:1453–67.
33. Guo F, Yan L, Guo H, et al. The transcriptome and DNA methylome landscapes of human primordial germ cells. Cell. 2015;161:1437–52.
34. Li L, Dong J, Yan L, et al. Single-cell RNA-seq analysis maps development of human germline cells and gonadal niche interactions. Cell Stem Cell. 2017;20:858–873.e4.
35. Irie N, Weinberger L, Tang WW, Kobayashi T, Viukov S, Manor YS, Dietmann S, Hanna JH, Surani AM. SOX17 is a critical specifier of human primordial germ cell fate. Cell. 2015;160:253.
36. Kurimoto K, Yabuta Y, Ohinata Y, Shigeta M, Yamanaka K, Saitou M. Complex genome-wide transcription dynamics orchestrated by Blimp1 for the specification of the germ cell lineage in mice. Genes Dev. 2008;22:1617–35.
37. Boroviak T, Nichols J. Primate embryogenesis predicts the hallmarks of human naïve pluripotency. Development. 2017;144:175–86.
38. Sasaki K, Nakamura T, Okamoto I, et al. The germ cell fate of cynomolgus monkeys is specified in the nascent amnion. Dev Cell. 2016;39:169–85.
39. Sasaki K, Yokobayashi S, Nakamura T, et al. Robust in vitro induction of human germ cell fate from pluripotent stem cells. Cell Stem Cell. 2015;17:178–94.
40. Clark AT, Bodnar MS, Fox M, Rodriquez RT, Abeyta MJ, Firpo MT, Pera RA. Spontaneous differentiation of germ cells from human embryonic stem cells in vitro. Hum Mol Genet. 2004;13:727–39.
41. Chen H-F, Kuo H-C, Chien C-L, Shun C-T, Yao Y-L, Ip P-L, Chuang C-Y, Wang C-C, Yang Y-S, Ho H-N. Derivation, characterization and differentiation of human embryonic stem cells: comparing serum-containing versus serum-free media and evidence of germ cell differentiation. Hum Reprod. 2007;22:567–77.
42. West FD, Roche-Rios MI, Abraham S, Rao RR, Natrajan MS, Bacanamwo M, Stice SL. KIT ligand and bone morphogenetic protein signaling enhances human embryonic stem cell to germ-like cell differentiation. Hum Reprod. 2010;25:168–78.
43. Kee K, Angeles VT, Flores M, Nguyen H, Pera RA. Human DAZL, DAZ and BOULE genes modulate primordial germ-cell and haploid gamete formation. Nature. 2009;462:222.
44. Kee K, Gonsalves JM, Clark AT, Pera RA. Bone morphogenetic proteins induce germ cell differentiation from human embryonic stem cells. Stem Cells Dev. 2006;15:831–7.
45. Eguizabal C, Montserrat N, Vassena R, Barragan M, Garreta E, Garcia-Quevedo L, Vidal F, Giorgetti A, Veiga A, Belmonte IJ. Complete meiosis from human induced pluripotent stem cells. Stem Cells. 2011;29:1186–95.
46. Weber S, Eckert D, Nettersheim D, et al. Critical function of AP-2gamma/TCFAP2C in mouse embryonic germ cell maintenance. Biol Reprod. 2010;82:214–23.
47. Schäfer S, Anschlag J, Nettersheim D, Haas N, Pawig L, Schorle H. The role of BLIMP1 and its putative downstream target TFAP2C in germ cell development and germ cell tumours. Int J Androl. 2011;34:e152–9.

48. Gafni O, Weinberger L, Mansour A, et al. Derivation of novel human ground state naive pluripotent stem cells. Nature. 2013;504:282.

49. Kobayashi T, Zhang H, Tang WW, et al. Principles of early human development and germ cell program from conserved model systems. Nature. 2017;546:416.

50. Yokobayashi S, Okita K, Nakagawa M, Nakamura T, Yabuta Y, Yamamoto T, Saitou M. Clonal variation of human induced pluripotent stem cells for induction into the germ cell fate. Biol Reprod. 2017;96:1154. https://doi.org/10.1093/biolre/iox038.

51. Kojima Y, Sasaki K, Yokobayashi S, et al. Evolutionarily distinctive transcriptional and signaling programs drive human germ cell lineage specification from pluripotent stem cells. Cell Stem Cell. 2017;21:517–532.e5.

52. Chen D, Liu W, Lukianchikov A, et al. Germline competency of human embryonic stem cells depends on eomesodermin. Biol Reprod. 2017;97:850. https://doi.org/10.1093/biolre/iox138.

53. Yamashiro C, Sasaki K, Yabuta Y, et al. Generation of human oogonia from induced pluripotent stem cells in vitro. Science. 2018;362:eaat1674.

54. Miyauchi H, Ohta H, Nagaoka S, Nakaki F, Sasaki K, Hayashi K, Yabuta Y, Nakamura T, Yamamoto T, Saitou M. Bone morphogenetic protein and retinoic acid synergistically specify female germ-cell fate in mice. EMBO J. 2017;36:3100–19.

55. Guo J, Grow EJ, Yi C, et al. Chromatin and single-cell RNA-seq profiling reveal dynamic signaling and metabolic transitions during human spermatogonial stem cell development. Cell Stem Cell. 2017;21:533–546.e6.

56. Hermann BP, Cheng K, Singh A, et al. The mammalian spermatogenesis single-cell transcriptome, from spermatogonial stem cells to spermatids. Cell Rep. 2018;25:1650–1667.e8.

57. Wang M, Liu X, Chang G, et al. Single-cell RNA sequencing analysis reveals sequential cell fate transition during human spermatogenesis. Cell Stem Cell. 2018;23:599–614.e4.

58. Milholland B, Dong X, Zhang L, Hao X, Suh Y, Vijg J. Differences between germline and somatic mutation rates in humans and mice. Nat Commun. 2017;8:ncomms15183.

59. Adli M. The CRISPR tool kit for genome editing and beyond. Nat Commun. 2018;9:1911.

60. Ishii T, Saitou M. Promoting in vitro gametogenesis research with a social understanding. Trends Mol Med. 2017;23:985. https://doi.org/10.1016/j.molmed.2017.09.006.

61. Ishii T, Pera R, Greely HT. Ethical and legal issues arising in research on inducing human germ cells from pluripotent stem cells. Cell Stem Cell. 2013;13:145–8.

62. Matoba S, Ogura A. Generation of functional oocytes and spermatids from fetal primordial germ cells after ectopic transplantation in adult mice. Biol Reprod. 2011;84:631–8.

Chapter 26
Activation of Ovarian Cortex

Orhan Bukulmez

26.1 Ovarian Autotransplantation

Ovarian cortical tissue freezing before life-saving treatment in young females has found worldwide acceptance as an important fertility preservation option and currently; it is the sole option for prepubertal female children. The main intention of ovarian cortical tissue freezing is to perform the autotransplantation of such tissues for induction of puberty and to restore fertility [1–4].

Accidental autografting of ovarian tissue to the laparoscopic umbilical incision site was reported after removing the ovarian endometrioma specimen out of the pelvis by using the umbilical port site [5]. Ovarian tissue could regain its function with neovascularization without requiring a vascular pedicle. Although this was reported to be the first case and quoted by many articles concerning ovarian autotransplantation, the history of ovarian autotransplantation itself goes back to the early twentieth century.

The autotransplantation procedure used to be performed during hysterectomy and bilateral salpingo-oopherectomy. Transplantation of parts of one or both ovaries was performed into the abdominal wall. The postmenopausal (as described as "ablation") symptoms since the performed operation were observed to be substantially relieved during the period that the grafts showed activity in three women. Ovarian autotransplantation was also performed into the wall of the uterus if hysterectomy was not performed, to preserve menstruation [6]. It was eloquently described that the ovaries were completely removed and wrapped in gauze and placed in a vessel containing normal salt solution at about 100 °F. Then a peritoneal pocket was created by blunt dissection between the peritoneum and the undersurface of the rectus muscle. The visually healthy looking ovarian tissue was used for grafting. The ova-

O. Bukulmez (✉)
Division of Reproductive Endocrinology and Infertility, Fertility and Advanced Reproductive Medicine Assisted Reproductive Technologies Program, Department of Obstetrics and Gynecology, University of Texas Southwestern Medical Center, Dallas, TX, USA
e-mail: Orhan.Bukulmez@UTSouthwestern.edu

ries were cut into 2 by 2.5 cm discoid pieces, and two to three pieces were transplanted into those peritoneal pockets without requiring any sutures to keep the grafts in their locations. The authors believed that grafting ovarian tissue in multiple small tissue pieces provides better results since a larger surface area would assure a better blood supply [6]. It was reported that the average age of such women undergoing ovarian tissue autografting was 30.5 years, the youngest being 20 years and the oldest being 41 years. Graft functioning was observed anywhere from 5 weeks to 6 months after the surgery. Indeed, there is a lot to learn from the history of medicine, as now older publications can become reachable electronically. Let us now review the present state of ovarian autotransplantation with the intention to activate ovarian cortex in women with premature ovarian insufficiency.

26.1.1 Applications of Lessons from History

In its landmark article, Pincus pointed out his observations in rabbits. He reported that removal of oocytes from the follicle itself resulted in maturation regardless of the presence or absence of pituitary hormones or of thyroxin in the culture medium. Therefore the maturation of the oocyte could be achieved simply by isolating it from its normal follicular environment which also leads to normal fertilization when exposed to sperm [7]. As mentioned above, it has already been shown that the ovarian tissue when autotransplanted in small pieces within a peritoneal pocket gets activated with follicle development, leading to diminished symptoms of menopause. In oncofertility studies, the activity of the frozen ovarian tissue could be restored more than 93% of the time after thawing and autotransplantation in small fragments and by repeating the autotransplantation procedure ovarian activity could be extended for over 11 years [8, 9].

Silber observed that even the vitrified ovarian tissue autotransplantation was performed in large cortical strips, extended graft survival can be achieved. Contrary to the common belief and to the older models of ovarian aging, increased primordial follicle loss with follicle growth leads to lower oocyte reserve but with eventual slower gradual decline of the ovarian reserve which may lead to extended functioning of the autotransplanted thin but unfragmented strip of the ovarian cortex. This may well be related to the relief of ovarian stromal and medullary pressure to the ovarian cortex, which is achieved through autotransplantation. Hence, such an extended graft survival can even be helpful to physiologically postpone the menopause in females [10, 11].

26.1.2 Relevance to Diminished Ovarian Reserve and/or Premature Ovarian Insufficiency-Associated Gonadotropin Increase

Some clinical data suggest that DOR is not only associated with disturbed ovarian – pituitary and hypothalamic axis – but also with increased gonadotropin levels, which results in some changes in the ovary itself resulting in a forward feedback loop of further deterioration of ovarian function. Hypergonadotropic levels of FSH, mostly above 20 IU/L, may be associated with abnormal follicle growth dynamics, while desensitization of the G protein-coupled receptors may also ensue. Hence, the prolonged suppression of FSH may decrease the forced early follicle selection and may restore the responsiveness of follicles to FSH when needed, perhaps through mitigation of desensitization [12, 13]. Therefore, suppression of FSH in the luteal phase before ovarian stimulation and following ovarian autotransplantation while waiting for ovarian function return was attempted with exogenous estrogen [14]. However, now the effects of chronically elevated LH levels on the ovarian stroma are also under scrutiny.

Ovarian stromal fibrosis can be seen in women with advanced reproductive age (ARA) with increased basal LH levels [15]. Increased risk of ovarian cancer was also associated with increased LH levels in women with polycystic ovary syndrome [16]. Increased stromal androgens with LH increase may result in ovarian stromal hyperplasia and fibrosis [17, 18]. In mice, unexpected accumulation of cells in the ovarian stroma with increased expressions of CYP17A1 (17OHlase/17–20 desmolase for glucocorticoid, androgen, and eventual estrogen production), CYP19A1 (aromatase for estrogen production from androgens), and LH/HCG receptors was noted to be due to increased LH levels [19, 20]. The ovarian stromal fibrosis in mice induced by both elevated LH and androgens was shown to be reversed by prolonged GnRH antagonist treatment [20]. It was also suggested that ovarian stromal fibrosis may impede secondary follicle or pre-antral follicle development, and this can be mitigated by prolonged GnRH antagonist treatment [20]. This aspect is important since there are proposed noninvasive methods to assess ovarian tissue rigidity associated with ovarian fibrosis [21] and treatment protocols can be refined accordingly. As reviewed in mild stimulation section, our prolonged GnRH agonist suppression protocol with estradiol priming until antral follicles are observed before mild stimulation as recommended in patients with profound DOR showing increased gonadotropins may reflect the mitigating factors achieved by prolonged suppression of FSH and LH.

Therefore, actually relieving the mechanical stress within the ovary via medical or surgical means may result in secondary follicle growth possibly through inhibition of the Hippo pathway via decreased phosphorylation of Yes-associated protein (YAP). This can be achieved surgically by cutting the ovary into fragments in vitro or in vivo via autotransplantation of the ovarian cortex [10, 11, 22].

26.1.3 How to Fit In Vitro Activation into This Paradigm

Hippo(potamus) pathway, although not well defined, controls the organ size by regulating cell proliferation, apoptosis, and stem cell self-renewal [23, 24]. It is involved in cell contact inhibition regulated by cytoskeleton and protein ubiquitination. It has been observed that protein kinase Hippo mutations, namely, MST-1/2, lead to organ overgrowth. Furthermore, dysregulation of Hippo pathway may result in cancer development. Hence Hippo signaling is considered as a tumor suppressor cascade

[25]. Actually, some members of Hippo pathway like YAP (Yes-associated protein tyrosine kinase)/TAZ are considered as oncogenes, since they play roles in the programming of cancer stem cells with increased proliferation and inhibition of apoptosis. YAP/TAZ (transcriptional co-activator with PDZ binding motif) phosphorylation results in their inactivation by keeping them in the cytoplasm. Disrupted Hippo pathway leads to YAP/TAZ de-phosphorylation leading to their nuclear entry, acting on organ growth, cell proliferation, inhibition of apoptosis, and oncogenesis.

Mechanical stress created in the ovarian cortex may suppress follicle growth by inhibition of YAP/TAZ as part of the mechano-induction system in granulosa cells. With the same rationale, cutting ovarian cortex in pieces in vitro disrupts Hippo signaling. Polymerization of globular actin to filamentous actin was shown to result in Hippo signaling disruption. Fragmentation of ovarian tissue induces actin polymerization, which in turn is associated with nuclear localization of YAP in granulosa cells of primary and secondary follicles in mice [22]. As phosphorylated YAP decreases, nuclear levels for YAP increase. This leads to their interaction with transcription factors TAED, which leads to extracellular matrix enhancement of CCN growth factors that include cysteine-rich angiogenic protein 6 CCN1, connective tissue growth factor CCN2, nephroblastoma overexpressed gene CCN3, and 3 Wnt-induced secreted proteins. CCN growth factors stimulate cell growth and proliferation and inhibit apoptosis [26]. Therefore, the stimulation of secondary follicle growth in the ovary may be achieved through these mechanisms following the fragmentation of ovarian cortex or with decreased pressure to the ovarian cortex from stromal components.

26.2 Ovarian Cortical In Vitro Activation and Autotransplantation

It was observed that anovulation associated with polycystic ovary syndrome (PCOS) responds to surgically induced controlled ovarian injury via wedge resection or ovarian drilling [27, 28]. Although PCOS is associated with high rather than diminished ovarian reserve (DOR), the FSH sensitivity is restored in antral follicles leading to follicle growth and eventual ovulation after such ovarian tissue disruptive procedures.

It is widely believed that primary germ cell proliferation stops at around midgestation in the fetus and then germ cells arrested at prophase I of meiosis are surrounded by a layer of somatic granulosa cells to form primordial follicles. The number of primordial follicles may be between 1.5 and 2 million at birth but with follicle atresia decreases to about 400,000 at puberty, and there may be about 1000 primordial follicles still remaining at menopause [29]. In diminished ovarian reserve cases, primordial follicle pool is decreased, and more profound decrease is expected in the presence of premature ovarian insufficiency (POI). In POI cases, primordial follicles still exist as evidenced by the observation that 50% of POI cases may show intermittent ovarian function and 5–10% may conceive [30]. The women with POI may show a resumption of ovulatory function mostly within the first year of diagnosis. The offspring conceived from women who later develop POI or who were diagnosed with POI are reported to be healthy. Even, it was reported that the reproductive capacity of young women with POI (early 20s to early 30s) might be comparable to the women of the SAME age range [31, 32]. Therefore, primordial follicle can be activated to support follicle growth and ovulation leading to competent oocytes and to healthy offspring.

The stimulation of primordial follicle may be through another oncogenic pathway. It has been shown in mice that oocyte-specific deletion of phosphatase and tensin homolog deleted from chromosome 10 (PTEN) causes premature activation of primordial follicles leading to depletion of ovarian reserve and to an eventual premature ovarian failure [33]. PTEN is a major suppressor of phosphatidylinositol 3-kinase (PI3K) and PI3K induces eventual activation of Akt (acute transforming retrovirus thymoma protein kinase), a serine/threonine kinase also known as protein kinase B. Akt signaling, in general was found to be important in the growth of primordial follicles. PI3K activation in granulosa cells of mice by selective PTEN disruption was also shown to increase ovulated follicles while increasing the life span of corpora lutea [34]. Akt signaling stimulation has been shown to stimulate secondary follicle growth as well [22].

In mice, PTEN inhibitor bpV(HOPIC) was used transiently to activate primordial follicles to generate mature oocytes which were then subjected to IVF to achieve progeny mice [35]. Therefore, from mouse studies, it was suggested that ovarian cortical activation can be achieved in women with POI. Then the technique was translated into human ovaries.

Human ovarian tissue was obtained from women with POI via laparoscopy for in vitro activation based on Hippo signaling pathway disruption and Akt signaling stimulation, aided by autotransplantation followed by in vitro fertilization (IVF) [22]. Ovaries were removed by laparoscopy and then ovarian cortical tissue strips, which were 1–2 mm thick and measuring 1x1 cm, were frozen with vitrification. Then ovarian cortical strips were thawed and further fragmented into smaller sized (1–2 mm) pieces. Then these tissues were cultured with reversible inhibitor of PTEN bisperoxovanadium or bpV (dipotassium bisperoxo meaning 5-hydroxypyridine-2-carboxyl, oxovanadate, HOPIC) and Akt stimulator 740YP (Tocris) for 24 hours and then only with 740YP for another 24 hours followed by a final wash. Then 40 to 80 such pieces were autotransplanted beneath the fallopian tube serosa into a created peritoneal pouch via laparoscopy, and sutures were used to keep these fragments in place. Patients were followed by weekly or biweekly transvaginal ultrasound and serum estradiol and FSH levels. Out of 27 patients, 13 patients showed histological evidence of residual follicles, and 8 patients showed follicular activity. All eight patients showed histological presence of residual follicles in their tissue samples before autografting. All such women developed pre-ovulatory follicles (of about 20 mm in size) in less than 6 months of autotransplantation, and even some patients developed pre-ovulatory follicles in 3 weeks. Hence, secondary follicle development may be the reason for shorter follicle growth times since per common knowledge primordial follicle to pre-ovulatory follicle development phase may require at least 6 months [36]. When follicles reached >5 mm in diameters, FSH treatment was started and HCG trigger was used with the follicular size >16 mm. Oocyte retrieval was scheduled 36 hours after the HCG administration. Mature oocytes could be obtained from 5 women, which were fertilized with intracytoplasmic sperm injection. Three patients underwent embryo transfers. One did not get pregnant, the other one showed only elevated HCG level, and the last one, who was a 29-year-old patient at the time of ovarian removal with POI diagnosed at the age of 25, got pregnant with a singleton pregnancy and delivered a healthy baby at 37 weeks and 2 days with a birth weight of 3254 grams [22].

The same group had a follow-up report about the outcome of in vitro activation and autotransplantation [14]. They described 37 women with POI who underwent the process, 54% (n: 20) of which showed histological evidence of residual follicles before autotransplantation. Then among these 20 women with evidence of residual follicles, 9 showed follicle growth in autografts (45%). Oocyte retrieval was possible in 6 women with a total of 24 oocytes obtained. IVF with embryo transfer was possible in four women. Three had a positive pregnancy test but two had live birth. Hence, the live birth rate among women with histological evidence of residual follicles was 10% (2/20). Much lower rates would be calculated if the denominator were 37 women. The authors initially included the women with POI with a history of amenorrhea for more than 1 year and elevated serum FSH levels of >40 mIU/mL (n = 31). Then the last 6 women were included if they had a history of amenorrhea >4 months, and serum FSH levels of >35 mIU/mL (n = 6) to include POI patients with a shorter history of amenorrhea. Although more studies are required, the reported rates of ovarian activity and pregnancy rates are reminiscent of those reported in POI patients in general as discussed above (50% of POI cases may show intermittent ovarian function and 5–10% may conceive naturally).

26.2.1 Safety Concerns for In Vitro Activation

Since the report of live births with this technique, some arguments followed. It is not clear if the sole fragmentation of the ovarian tissue followed by autotransplantation can be adequate to activate the follicle growth across the board. It seems that Hippo signaling disruption is more relevant to activation of secondary to antral follicles as discussed above. For primordial follicle activation, the in vitro activation focused also on blocking PTEN action while enhancing Akt signaling, and it is not clear whether this step is really necessary due to the concerns about application of potentially oncogenic chemicals.

The data from ovarian cortical tissue autotransplantation after life-saving treatments suggest the primordial follicle growth follows autografting without needing in vitro activation [37, 38]. The main criticism about in vitro activation studies is that they did not include a control group solely with autotransplantation without in vitro activation [39].

There are also some concerns that in vitro activation before autotransplantation may actually decrease the graft longevity since generalized activation of resting follicle pool may result in follicle burnout. Another concern is about keeping the size of the autografted fragments very small in in vitro activation studies. It was suggested that the strips of thawed ovarian cortex resumes function better than the small fragments injected into the ovary [40]. As discussed above, it was observed that vitrification, thawing, and autotransplantation of long strips of ovarian cortical tissue resulted in extended graft survival and function [10, 11, 41]. Extended endocrine function of the graft is also important to mitigate health issues and consequences of early menopause. Naturally, the recruitment rate of follicles may be reduced when the ovarian reserve is decreased. However, with in vitro activation, follicle burnout seems to be accelerated. Hence, the patients undergoing in vitro activation before ovarian cortical tissue autotransplantation should look into immediate, short-term outcomes for follicle activation and pregnancy [39].

The researchers working on in vitro activation before autotransplantation in patients with POI also acknowledge that ovarian cortical tissue cryopreservation for fertility preservation is different than in vitro activation which is in fact for infertility treatment. They even recommend in vitro activation of the fresh ovarian cortex without vitrification and thawing, but just autotransplanting the ovarian cortical tissue fragments after 2 days of treatment [42]. Certainly, this approach may raise some other safety concerns that the growing follicles already exposed to these potentially toxic chemicals may result in a pregnancy. Then the authors stated that in vitro drug treatment could also be omitted and immediate autotransplantation could be undertaken if the tissues still show residual secondary and early antral follicles. Hence, the terms cryopreservation-free in vitro activation and drug- and cryopreservation-free in vitro activation were introduced quoting an ongoing pregnancy in China with the former. The latter method involving just ovarian cortical tissue procurement and autografting back in fragments was performed in women with poor ovarian response (POR) per Bologna criteria with the observation of an increased number of oocytes retrieved [42].

In terms of chemicals used for in vitro activation, the authors defend that ovarian cubes exposed to these chemicals for 2 days are rinsed extensively before grafting and no abnormal growth in the graft sites was observed under ultrasound. In addition, the patients getting their repeat autografting did not show any abnormalities in the past autografting sites as observed by laparoscopy [42]. Certainly, any long-term observational data is lacking to address such safety concerns at this time. However, there is a tendency to promote such approaches for women with DOR and POR and to those who underwent cryopreserved ovarian cortical tissue before their life-saving treatment [43].

On the other hand, human ovarian tissue fragments cultured with 1 μM of bpV (HOPIC) or control medium for 24 hours followed by culture only in control medium for both groups for another 5 days demonstrated that the follicle activation occurred in both treatment groups but with significantly more secondary follicles developed in the group treated with HOPIC. This increased activation with HOPIC was associated with increased Akt phosphorylation and increased nuclear localization of forkhead box O3 (FOXO3) as expected from PTEN inhibition. Nevertheless, isolated and cultured such follicles showed restricted growth and decreased survival if the ovarian tissue was exposed to HOPIC as compared to control tissues not exposed to the chemical. Therefore, PTEN inhibition promotes follicle activation toward the secondary stage but then severely compromises the survival of secondary follicles [44].

In summary, time will show if these surgical approaches with or without chemical treatment will, in fact, become widely accepted approaches for women with POI or profound DOR.

26.3 Platelet-Rich Plasma to Activate Ovarian Cortex

Platelet-rich plasma (PRP) concentrates have found some new uses in regenerative medicine. Platelets, in addition to playing role in hemostasis, secrete various products playing role in cell migration, proliferation, and differentiation and in angiogenesis and tissue repair [45, 46]. Therefore, PRP has been used to support tissue repair and regeneration in various clinical scenarios such as androgenic alopecia [47]. One such attempt was made on four DOR patients older than 35 years of age, with infertility and at least one failed or canceled IVF cycle or amenorrhea for at least 3 months. The authors prepared the PRP from 8 mL of blood collected from patients through a regular venipuncture followed by centrifugation for platelet separation; platelets were then activated by using calcium gluconate. Then PRP was injected into the ovary by using a 17 G, 35 cm single lumen needle while paying attention that about 1 ml of PRP sample was deposited just under the ovarian capsule. The procedure was applied to both ovaries. The patients did not require any sedation or anesthesia. All patients were then started with monitoring every 2 weeks. Especially cycle day 2 or 3, FSH and E2 testing were obtained after the procedure. When increased AMH and/or decreased FSH is noted, the patients were subjected to IVF. All four patients showed decreased FSH levels as compared to the levels before PRP injection. Also, three out of four patients showed an AMH level increase shortly after PRP injection. IVF resulted in at least one day five blastocysts in all four patients which were frozen for banking purposes in three patients. One patient underwent embryo transfer and had an ongoing pregnancy [48].

Since the anti-aging industry has thrived with similar statements, some of the fertility practices, worldwide, advertise for "ovarian rejuvenation" directed toward women with POI and those with DOR. The PRP applications along with ovarian autotransplantation methods as discussed above and stem cell approaches are involved with such promotions. We will then briefly mention about stem cells in relevance to the ovary.

26.4 Activation of Ovaries with Stem Cells and Other Proposed Stem Cell Involved Treatments

The presence of ovarian stem cells postulated by Jonathan Tilly's group was briefly introduced at the beginning of this book. Oogonial stem cells (OSCs) have been defined in mice as mitotically active cells leading to oocyte renewal, which are also putatively present in the bone marrow and the peripheral blood of adult mice [49,

50]. Although its relevance to humans has been debated, OSCs were isolated from both murine and human ovarian cortex. The current lack of gene promoter exclusively expressed in OSCs but not in differentiating pre-meiotic germ cells or oocytes has been found concerning to definitely prove the presence of OSCs. It seems that OSCs in the ovarian cortex are found in very small numbers. It was estimated that OSCs can be 0.014% of all cells in mouse ovaries, and their numbers decline with chronologic aging. In addition, the introduction of the human OSCs, engineered to express green fluorescent protein (GFP), into human ovarian cortical tissue leads to the formation of follicles containing GFP-positive oocytes about 2 weeks after xenotransplantation into immune-deficient female mice [51].

In order to isolate OSCs from neonatal mice, two-step enzymatic digestion of ovarian tissue was followed by immunomagnetic separation based on DEAD box polypeptide 4 protein (DDX4/VAS, MVH in mice) expression as the membrane marker with cytoplasmic tail common to cells of germ cell lineage in both sexes since it is also expressed in spermatogonia. These cells, also called female germline stem cells, could be cultured more than 15 months with more than 68 passages, unexpected from any somatic cell. The similar isolation could also be made from adult mice. After transfection to express GFP, injection of these cells into the ovaries of mice sterilized with chemotherapy, resulted in GFP and DDX4 expressing oocytes [52]. The use of a membrane marker with cytoplasmic tail produced some concerns. DDX4 is expressed in the cytoplasm of oocytes but it has been claimed that DDX4 has a transmembrane component in OSCs which can be used for cell sorting [53]. In addition, it was shown that GFP by itself causes mitosis since, without GFP, mitosis of putative OSCs did not occur. Some groups developed a different fluorescent mouse model for tracking of DDX4 expressing OSCs and could not detect fluorescence in the ovaries with a conclusion that OSCs do not enter mitosis and hence do not contribute to egg renewal [54].

Small OSC like cells producing oocyte-like cells in culture were also isolated from human ovarian cortical cell cultures by using a strict membrane marker, stage-specific embryonic antigen-4 (SSEA-4) [55, 56]. Some other researchers used other stem cell markers to detect and define OSCs, but in one study, only Fragilis worked [57]. It is agreed that the cells with characteristics of OSCs exist in the ovary of many species including humans. Literature is still undecided about their best method of detection. It is also not clear if these cells contribute to ovarian follicle development in women [58].

One of the proposed applications of OSCs in humans has been some sort of autologous cytoplasmic transfer to improve oocyte quality in women undergoing treatment with assisted reproductive technologies (ART). This technique is called autologous germline mitochondrial energy transfer (AUGMENT) which still requires more studies [59, 60]. One recent prospective randomized trial though did not show any clinically significant benefit of AUGMENT in women with a history of poor embryo quality [61].

Most proposed ovarian stem cell-based therapies have been directed to women with POI or profound DOR. These approaches are usually explored under the basic title of ovarian rejuvenation. One of such protocols is based on the bone marrow-derived stem cell therapy. This protocol is entitled as rejuvenation of premature ovarian failure with stem cells (ROSE-1) (ClinicalTrials.gov identifier:

NCT02696889). The study is based on bone marrow aspiration with separation of bone marrow mesenchymal stem cells (MSCs). Then autologous MSCs are injected into the biopsied right ovary. The first abstract on this technique was presented in March of 2018. The authors presented two patients. Human autologous MSCs were isolated from the posterior iliac crest and injected into the ovary through a laparoscopic approach. The patients followed for up to 1 year after the procedure. Both patients resumed menses and had relief from their postmenopausal symptoms with increased estrogen levels. At the time of this review, the study was still open to enroll more subjects [62].

Autologous stem cell ovarian transplantation (ASCOT) was attempted in women with poor ovarian response. Bone marrow-derived stem cells were obtained from peripheral blood after mobilization of such cells with a 5-day course of granulocyte colony-stimulating factor. Then CD34+ cells were collected with apheresis. Then the samples were subjected to the separation of CD133+ cells, which were then infused into one of the ovaries through ovarian artery catheterization. Seventeen patients underwent the procedure. Within 2 weeks of infusion, antral follicle count increased in patients especially in the treated ovary. Some patients showed increased AMH level. The treatment did not increase the embryo euploidy rate but resulted in three natural conceptions and two conceptions with IVF [63].

26.5 Conclusion

In women with POI and profound DOR, ovarian cortical activation has been attempted via ovarian autotransplantation with or without conditioned culture systems or with an ovarian injection of platelet-rich plasma. In addition, several stem cell-based therapies were proposed for a similar population of those with poor ovarian response or poor embryo quality with ART. In that respect, OSC mitochondria have been injected into the retrieved oocytes with no proven improvement in pregnancy rates as of yet. Bone marrow MSCs have been used in a limited number of women with POI with some endocrinologic response. Bone marrow-derived CD-133+ stem cell infusion with ovarian artery catheterization has also been reported in women with a poor ovarian response with some encouraging results. All these interventions are still considered experimental but should be seen as milestones of progress in the management of women with POI, DOR, or POR.

References

1. Poirot C, Abirached F, Prades M, Coussieu C, Bernaudin F, Piver P. Induction of puberty by autograft of cryopreserved ovarian tissue. Lancet. 2012;379(9815):588.
2. Ernst E, Kjaersgaard M, Birkebaek NH, Clausen N, Andersen CY. Case report: stimulation of puberty in a girl with chemo- and radiation therapy-induced ovarian failure by transplantation of a small part of her frozen/thawed ovarian tissue. Eur J Cancer. 2013;49(4):911–4.

3. Donnez J, Dolmans MM, Pellicer A, Diaz-Garcia C, Sanchez Serrano M, Schmidt KT, et al. Restoration of ovarian activity and pregnancy after transplantation of cryopreserved ovarian tissue: a review of 60 cases of reimplantation. Fertil Steril. 2013;99(6):1503–13.
4. Demeestere I, Simon P, Dedeken L, Moffa F, Tsepelidis S, Brachet C, et al. Live birth after autograft of ovarian tissue cryopreserved during childhood. Hum Reprod. 2015;30(9):2107–9.
5. Marconi G, Quintana R, Rueda-Leverone NG, Vighi S. Accidental ovarian autograft after a laparoscopic surgery: case report. Fertil Steril. 1997;68(2):364–6.
6. Girard FR. Ovarian autotransplantation. Cal State J Med. 1922;20(1):21–6.
7. Pincus G, Enzmann EV. The comparative behavior of mammalian eggs in vivo and in vitro: I. The activation of ovarian eggs. J Exp Med. 1935;62(5):665–75.
8. Bastings L, Beerendonk CC, Westphal JR, Massuger LF, Kaal SE, van Leeuwen FE, et al. Autotransplantation of cryopreserved ovarian tissue in cancer survivors and the risk of reintroducing malignancy: a systematic review. Hum Reprod Update. 2013;19(5):483–506.
9. Donnez J, Dolmans MM. Ovarian cortex transplantation: 60 reported live births brings the success and worldwide expansion of the technique towards routine clinical practice. J Assist Reprod Genet. 2015;32(8):1167–70.
10. Silber S. Ovarian tissue cryopreservation and transplantation: scientific implications. J Assist Reprod Genet. 2016;33(12):1595–603.
11. Silber S. How ovarian transplantation works and how resting follicle recruitment occurs: a review of results reported from one center. Womens Health (Lond). 2016;12(2):217–27.
12. Menon V, Edwards RL, Lynch SS, Butt WR. Luteinizing hormone-releasing hormone analog in treatment of hypergonadotrophic amenorrhoea. Br J Obstet Gynecol. 1983;90(6):539–42.
13. Ishizuka B, Kudo Y, Amemiya A, Ogata T. Ovulation induction in a woman with premature ovarian failure resulting from a partial deletion of the X chromosome long arm, 46, X, del(X) (q22). Fertil Steril. 1997;68(5):931–4.
14. Suzuki N, Yoshioka N, Takae S, Sugishita Y, Tamura M, Hashimoto S, et al. Successful fertility preservation following ovarian tissue vitrification in patients with primary ovarian insufficiency. Hum Reprod. 2015;30(3):608–15.
15. Matt DW, Kauma SW, Pincus SM, Veldhuis JD, Evans WS. Characteristics of luteinizing hormone secretion in younger versus older premenopausal women. Am J Obstet Gynecol. 1998;178(3):504–10.
16. Schildkraut JM, Schwingl PJ, Bastos E, Evanoff A, Hughes C. Epithelial ovarian cancer risk among women with polycystic ovary syndrome. Obstet Gynecol. 1996;88(4 Pt 1):554–9.
17. Futterweit W, Deligdisch L. Effects of androgens on the ovary. Fertil Steril. 1986;46(2):343–5.
18. Futterweit W, Deligdisch L. Histopathological effects of exogenously administered testosterone in 19 female to male transsexuals. J Clin Endocrinol Metab. 1986;62(1):16–21.
19. Risma KA, Clay CM, Nett TM, Wagner T, Yun J, Nilson JH. Targeted overexpression of luteinizing hormone in transgenic mice leads to infertility, polycystic ovaries, and ovarian tumors. Proc Natl Acad Sci U S A. 1995;92(5):1322–6.
20. Umehara T, Kawai T, Kawashima I, Tanaka K, Okuda S, Kitasaka H, et al. The acceleration of reproductive aging in Nrg1(flox/flox);Cyp19-Cre female mice. Aging Cell. 2017;16(6):1288–99.
21. Wood CD, Vijayvergia M, Miller FH, Carroll T, Fasanati C, Shea LD, et al. Multi-modal magnetic resonance elastography for noninvasive assessment of ovarian tissue rigidity in vivo. Acta Biomater. 2015;13:295–300.
22. Kawamura K, Cheng Y, Suzuki N, Deguchi M, Sato Y, Takae S, et al. Hippo signaling disruption and Akt stimulation of ovarian follicles for infertility treatment. Proc Natl Acad Sci U S A. 2013;110(43):17474–9.
23. Pan D. Hippo signaling in organ size control. Genes Dev. 2007;21(8):886–97.
24. Zhao B, Tumaneng K, Guan KL. The Hippo pathway in organ size control, tissue regeneration, and stem cell self-renewal. Nat Cell Biol. 2011;13(8):877–83.
25. Hergovich A. Mammalian Hippo signaling: a kinase network regulated by protein-protein interactions. Biochem Soc Trans. 2012;40(1):124–8.
26. Holbourn KP, Acharya KR, Perbal B. The CCN family of proteins: structure-function relationships. Trends Biochem Sci. 2008;33(10):461–73.

O. Bukulmez

27. Stein IF, Cohen MR, Elson R. Results of bilateral ovarian wedge resection in 47 cases of sterility; 20-year-end results; 75 cases of bilateral polycystic ovaries. Am J Obstet Gynecol. 1949;58(2):267–74.
28. Costello MF, Ledger WL. Evidence-based management of infertility in women with polycystic ovary syndrome using surgery or assisted reproductive technology. Womens Health (Lond). 2012;8(3):291–300.
29. Kaipia A, Hsueh AJ. Regulation of ovarian follicle atresia. Annu Rev Physiol. 1997;59:349–63.
30. Welt CK. Primary ovarian insufficiency: a more accurate term for premature ovarian failure. Clin Endocrinol. 2008;68(4):499–509.
31. Bidet M, Bachelot A, Bissauge E, Golmard JL, Gricourt S, Dulon J, et al. Resumption of ovarian function and pregnancies in 358 patients with premature ovarian failure. J Clin Endocrinol Metab. 2011;96(12):3864–72.
32. Daan NM, Hoek A, Corpeleijn E, Eijkemans MJ, Broekmans FJ, Fauser BC, et al. Reproductive characteristics of women diagnosed with premature ovarian insufficiency. Reprod Biomed Online. 2016;32(2):225–32.
33. Reddy P, Liu L, Adhikari D, Jagarlamudi K, Rajareddy S, Shen Y, et al. Oocyte-specific deletion of Pten causes premature activation of the primordial follicle pool. Science. 2008;319(5863):611–3.
34. Fan HY, Liu Z, Cahill N, Richards JS. Targeted disruption of Pten in ovarian granulosa cells enhances ovulation and extends the life span of luteal cells. Mol Endocrinol. 2008;22(9):2128–40.
35. Adhikari D, Gorre N, Risal S, Zhao Z, Zhang H, Shen Y, et al. The safe use of a PTEN inhibitor for the activation of dormant mouse primordial follicles and generation of fertilizable eggs. PLoS One. 2012;7(6):e39034.
36. McGee EA, Hsueh AJ. Initial and cyclic recruitment of ovarian follicles. Endocr Rev. 2000;21(2):200–14.
37. Gavish Z, Peer G, Roness H, Cohen Y, Meirow D. Follicle activation and 'burn-out' contribute to post-transplantation follicle loss in ovarian tissue grafts: the effect of graft thickness. Hum Reprod. 2014;29(5):989–96.
38. Smitz J, Dolmans MM, Donnez J, Fortune JE, Hovatta O, Jewgenow K, et al. Current achievements and future research directions in ovarian tissue culture, in vitro follicle development and transplantation: implications for fertility preservation. Hum Reprod Update. 2010;16(4):395–414.
39. Meirow D, Roness H, Kristensen SG, Andersen CY. Optimizing outcomes from ovarian tissue cryopreservation and transplantation; activation versus preservation. Hum Reprod. 2015;30(11):2453–6.
40. Meirow D, Levron J, Eldar-Geva T, Hardan I, Fridman E, Zalel Y, et al. Pregnancy after transplantation of cryopreserved ovarian tissue in a patient with ovarian failure after chemotherapy. N Engl J Med. 2005;353(3):318–21.
41. Silber S, Kagawa N, Kuwayama M, Gosden R. Duration of fertility after fresh and frozen ovary transplantation. Fertil Steril. 2010;94(6):2191–6.
42. Kawamura K, Cheng Y, Sun YP, Zhai J, Diaz-Garcia C, Simon C, et al. Ovary transplantation: to activate or not to activate. Hum Reprod. 2015;30(11):2457–60.
43. Novella-Maestre E, Herraiz S, Rodriguez-Iglesias B, Diaz-Garcia C, Pellicer A. Short-term PTEN inhibition improves in vitro activation of primordial follicles, preserves follicular viability, and restores AMH levels in cryopreserved ovarian tissue from cancer patients. PLoS One. 2015;10(5):e0127786.
44. McLaughlin M, Kinnell HL, Anderson RA, Telfer EE. Inhibition of phosphatase and tensin homolog (PTEN) in human ovary in vitro results in increased activation of primordial follicles but compromises development of growing follicles. Mol Hum Reprod. 2014;20(8):736–44.
45. Gurtner GC, Werner S, Barrandon Y, Longaker MT. Wound repair and regeneration. Nature. 2008;453(7193):314–21.
46. Stellos K, Kopf S, Paul A, Marquardt JU, Gawaz M, Huard J, et al. Platelets in regeneration. Semin Thromb Hemost. 2010;36(2):175–84.

47. Gkini MA, Kouskoukis AE, Tripsianis G, Rigopoulos D, Kouskoukis K. Study of platelet-rich plasma injections in the treatment of androgenetic alopecia through a one-year period. J Cutan Aesthet Surg. 2014;7(4):213–9.
48. Sills ES, Rickers NS, Li X, Palermo GD. First data on in vitro fertilization and blastocyst formation after intraovarian injection of calcium gluconate-activated autologous platelet-rich plasma. Gynecol Endocrinol. 2018;34(9):756–60.
49. Johnson J, Canning J, Kaneko T, Pru JK, Tilly JL. Germline stem cells and follicular renewal in the postnatal mammalian ovary. Nature. 2004;428(6979):145–50.
50. Johnson J, Bagley J, Skaznik-Wikiel M, Lee HJ, Adams GB, Niikura Y, et al. Oocyte generation in adult mammalian ovaries by putative germ cells in bone marrow and peripheral blood. Cell. 2005;122(2):303–15.
51. White YA, Woods DC, Takai Y, Ishihara O, Seki H, Tilly JL. Oocyte formation by mitotically active germ cells purified from ovaries of reproductive-age women. Nat Med. 2012;18(3):413–21.
52. Zou K, Yuan Z, Yang Z, Luo H, Sun K, Zhou L, et al. Production of offspring from a germline stem cell line derived from neonatal ovaries. Nat Cell Biol. 2009;11(5):631–6.
53. Dunlop CE, Telfer EE, Anderson RA. Ovarian stem cells – potential roles in infertility treatment and fertility preservation. Maturitas. 2013;76(3):279–83.
54. Zhang H, Zheng W, Shen Y, Adhikari D, Ueno H, Liu K. Experimental evidence showing that no mitotically active female germline progenitors exist in postnatal mouse ovaries. Proc Natl Acad Sci U S A. 2012;109(31):12580–5.
55. Stimpfel M, Skutella T, Cvjeticanin B, Meznaric M, Dovc P, Novakovic S, et al. Isolation, characterization, and differentiation of cells expressing pluripotent/multipotent markers from adult human ovaries. Cell Tissue Res. 2013;354(2):593–607.
56. Virant-Klun I, Stimpfel M, Cvjeticanin B, Vrtacnik-Bokal E, Skutella T. Small SSEA-4-positive cells from human ovarian cell cultures: related to embryonic stem cells and germinal lineage? J Ovarian Res. 2013;6:24.
57. Zou K, Hou L, Sun K, Xie W, Wu J. Improved efficiency of female germline stem cell purification using fragilis-based magnetic bead sorting. Stem Cells Dev. 2011;20(12):2197–204.
58. Telfer EE, Anderson RA. The existence and potential of germline stem cells in the adult mammalian ovary. Climacteric. 2019;22(1):22–6.
59. Tilly JL, Sinclair DA. Germline energetics, aging, and female infertility. Cell Metab. 2013;17(6):838–50.
60. Oktay K, Baltaci V, Sonmezer M, Turan V, Unsal E, Baltaci A, et al. Oogonial precursor cell-derived autologous mitochondria injection to improve outcomes in women with multiple IVF failures due to low oocyte quality: a clinical translation. Reprod Sci. 2015;22(12):1612–7.
61. Labarta E, de Los Santos MJ, Herraiz S, Escriba MJ, Marzal A, Buigues A, et al. Autologous mitochondrial transfer as a complementary technique to intracytoplasmic sperm injection to improve embryo quality in patients undergoing in vitro fertilization-a randomized pilot study. Fertil Steril. 2019;111(1):86–96.
62. Gavrilova-Jordan LSB, Andaloussi EA, Sportes C, Pantin J, Al-Hendy A, editors. Bone marrow-derived human mesenchymal stem cells transplantation in the ovary restores steroidogenesis in women with premature ovarian insufficiency. 100th annual meeting of the Endocrine Society; 2018 March 17–March 20, 2018. Endocrine Reviews: Chicago; 2018.
63. Herraiz S, Romeu M, Buigues A, Martinez S, Diaz-Garcia C, Gomez-Segui I, et al. Autologous stem cell ovarian transplantation to increase reproductive potential in patients who are poor responders. Fertil Steril. 2018;110(3):496–505 e1.

Chapter 27
Oocyte Cryopreservation at an Earlier Age

Rachel M. Whynott and Hakan E. Duran

27.1 Brief History of Oocyte Cryopreservation

The idea to preserve items for future use dates back to the early humans, who learned to preserve food in order to travel larger distances and to help survive famine [1]. Over time, a variety of ways to preserve items of importance have been developed, such as the use of preservatives/desiccants, dehydration, and freezing [1]. The first reports of successfully preserving human gametes involved sperm, and in 1953, the first human was born from a frozen sperm sample [1, 2]. The first birth from a frozen oocyte did not occur until 1986, 33 years later [3]. This was two years after the first live birth from a cryopreserved embryo [2]. Furthermore, another live birth from a frozen oocyte was unable to be replicated for several more years [1]. The original patients possibly benefiting from oocyte cryopreservation were those diagnosed with cancer, who did not have a partner, or had ethical reasons for why they did not feel comfortable cryopreserving embryos [4].

Why was the cryopreservation and thaw of an oocyte more difficult than either for sperm or embryos? The meiotic spindles of oocytes are very sensitive to temperature changes, and oocytes have a large volume to surface ratio, significant water content, and a single membrane [5, 6]. Slow-freezing was the original method of oocyte cryopreservation, which involved placing embryos in the presence of low concentrations of cryoprotectant agents and slowly lowering the temperature until frozen [7]. The water content in the ooplasm forms ice crystals during this procedure, which may physically interrupt the meiotic spindle. Different recipes for various cryoprotectants and protocols for freezing and thawing did not help improve the overall efficiency of the slow-freeze method; there is only a 2% live birth rate per oocyte [8]. Vitrification was then discovered, which involves exposure of the oocyte

R. M. Whynott · H. E. Duran (✉)
Department of Obstetrics and Gynecology, Division of Reproductive Endocrinology and Infertility, University of Iowa, Iowa City, IA, USA
e-mail: hakan-duran@uiowa.edu

© Springer Nature Switzerland AG 2020
O. Bukulmez (ed.), *Diminished Ovarian Reserve and Assisted Reproductive Technologies*, https://doi.org/10.1007/978-3-030-23235-1_27

to higher concentrations of cryoprotectants in very small volumes followed by plunging in liquid nitrogen to maximize the rapidity of cooling [2, 7]. This freezes oocytes in a state that has been described as "glass-like," minimizes ice crystal formation, and improves oocyte survival and pregnancy rates [1, 2, 7, 9]. Due to the higher rates of success by vitrification, oocyte cryopreservation was no longer considered experimental, starting in 2012 [1, 2, 6, 7]. The number of cycles to cryopreserve oocytes has been on the rise ever since. Women may cryopreserve oocytes for several reasons, including in the setting of imminent gonadotoxic treatments such as chemotherapy or for banking in the setting of aging without a partner.

27.2   Rationale of Cryopreserving Oocytes in a Young Patient

27.2.1   "Need-Based"

Women of reproductive age may find themselves in a situation where a gonadotoxic agent (such as an alkylating agent-based chemotherapy or pelvic radiation) may be recommended for treatment of a number of disease states, including cancers. In the United States, approximately 70,000 men and women ages 15 to 39 are diagnosed with cancer every year [10]. Some of these individuals might not have children or may not have completed their families. This can increase the stress and devastation a new diagnosis such as cancer can have on a patient, even if the disease, with treatment, has an otherwise good prognosis [11]. The most commonly applied technique to safeguard a woman's reproductive potential after a course of gonadotoxic treatment is controlled ovarian stimulation with oocyte retrieval in order to cryopreserve oocytes or embryos for later use [12]. This is ideally done before any gonadotoxic treatment is administered and can be performed by any modern Assisted Reproductive Technology (ART) Center. Other methods, such as ovarian tissue cryopreservation and sole use of GnRH agonists before and during gonadotoxic treatment to protect oocytes in situ, are still considered experimental or controversial and are outside the scope of this chapter.

Since fertility preservation for women became available, both the occurrence of counseling and the numbers of patients undergoing these procedures have increased over time [13]. A study of over 5000 patients revealed that most women counseled for fertility preservation had been diagnosed with breast cancer (41%), followed by lymphoma (28%) [13]. Only 7% of the patients had a benign disease that required a gonadotoxic therapy [13]. Of the benign diseases, the most common one was systemic lupus erythematosus, at 24.8% [13].

A study published by Quinn et al. in 2017 found that baseline antral follicle counts and outcomes of ovarian stimulation in regard to mature oocyte numbers were similar between age-matched patients with breast cancer and healthy women who were undergoing planned oocyte cryopreservation [14]. Another, larger study evaluated a number of other malignancies, including sarcomas, Hodgkin's and non-Hodgkin's lymphomas, gastrointestinal, cerebral, gynecological cancers, and a group of remaining malignancies in comparison to breast cancer patients to determine if oocyte yield was decreased [13]. They discovered that oocyte yield was not affected by malignancy type (other than ovarian cancer) but by maternal age in their group of patients [13]. This has been shown in several other studies as well [15–17].

Treatments most associated with decreased fertility include alkylating agent-based chemotherapies such as cyclophosphamide, pelvic radiation therapy (mostly due to effects on the ovaries rather than the uterus), and high-dose cranial radiation therapy (impairs pituitary function) [10]. The effects are typically dependent on dose and also on the age of the female undergoing the therapy [18]. Higher dosing and older women tend to have worse outcomes. However, even if a woman maintains her fertility after her cancer treatment, her pregnancy and live birth rates are typically lower than that of an average woman of the same age [18]. When a woman presents for discussion of oocyte cryopreservation, it is important to have an open discussion with the medical team that includes the oncologist and reproductive endocrinologist, regarding the plan for cancer treatment, if the treatment can be reasonably delayed to allow for an ovarian stimulation cycle and oocyte retrieval, as well as the likelihood of effects on fertility at the end of treatment.

27.2.2 Planned Oocyte Cryopreservation ("Anticipated Gamete Exhaustion," "Elective," "Social")

Teenage pregnancies in the United States have decreased by 51% from 2007 to 2016 [19]. The birth rate for women in their 20s decreased by 4% in just 1 year (2015 to 2016) and has been declining steadily each year since 2006 [19]. The birth rates for these two age groups have been at record lows, while birth rates for women in their 30s and 40s are at their highest since the 1960s [19]. As a result, the general fertility rate has been declining from 2007 to 2013 and continuing in 2015 and 2016 [19]. The average age of a first-time mother in the United States is now 26.6, a record high for this country [19].

What is influencing the trend toward delaying childbirth? It is likely multifactorial. In part, it may be due to improved contraceptive methods and improved access to these methods [20]. It may also be affected by the decision to delay childbearing until after certain educational, financial, or career goals are met [20–23]. However, most women state that they are waiting for the right partner before pursuing pregnancy [22–24]. With the rate of marriage on the decline in the United States and the rate of births by unmarried women declining as well, this is not surprising [19, 25]. As women are often delaying childbirth for reasons outside of their control, there is a push to move away from terminology suggesting that planned oocyte cryopreservation is "elective," "social," or "non-medical," but rather as possible preventative medicine for anticipated gamete exhaustion [26]. It has been argued that women protecting their gametes by cryopreservation prior to gonadotoxic therapies are undergoing preventive medicine and those women protecting their gametes from the threat of time are doing the same thing- possibly preventing infertility in the future [26]. Fertility preservation without a "medical indication/necessity" has been available for men for several decades, and with the streamlining of oocyte cryopreservation, it appears to be the time for this to be an option available for women as well.

27.3 Are There Limitations for Offering Oocyte Cryopreservation?

27.3.1 Lower Age Limit?

A lower age limit for oocyte cryopreservation becomes important when a patient is planned to undergo a gonadotoxic therapy at a very young age. As discussed in a previous section, there are several treatments for fertility preservation that are under investigation, such as ovarian tissue cryopreservation and in vitro maturation of oocytes, which may be useful in the future for pre-pubertal females [27, 28]. As of the time of this writing, the accepted methods of controlled ovarian hyperstimulation, oocyte retrieval, and vitrification are used for females who have already undergone puberty. Treatments for females who have not yet gone through puberty are considered experimental [29]. If a young patient has recently gone through puberty and is interested in oocyte preservation, discussion with the patient and her parents is warranted to review what is involved in the process, including injections, blood tests, and ultrasounds. Depending on the patient's body habitus, it may be possible to perform follicular monitoring abdominally, but still perform transvaginal oocyte retrieval while the patient is sedated for decreased discomfort. For religious, cultural or other reasons, families may not be supportive of a vaginal ultrasound or pelvic examination at any point in the process, and it is best to discuss these issues ahead of the treatment so alternative options can be explored.

27.3.2 Upper Age Limit?

Is there an upper age threshold, where a practitioner should not recommend or allow a patient to undergo oocyte cryopreservation? The American Society for Reproductive Medicine (ASRM) prefers that those who wish to be oocyte donors donate between the ages of 21 and 34, to decrease the cytogenetic risks associated with oocyte age [30]. There are no recommendations from ASRM regarding an upper age limit for patients attempting to use or cryopreserve their own oocytes, although counseling regarding the risks of doing so should be provided [31]. Success rates have been shown to be higher when patients have cryopreserved oocytes at

≤35 years of age [4]. However, cryopreservation of oocytes at age 38 that are then used at age 40 may be more successful than attempts at natural pregnancy or with assisted reproduction at age 40 [4]. Providers in the United States are varied in their practice, and each clinic may have its own age threshold for women to proceed with their own eggs [31]. It may be reasonable to assess a patient's ovarian reserve and then counsel her accordingly, to see if the possible benefits would outweigh the risks and costs of undergoing stimulation, retrieval, and storage [9, 32].

If the opportunity arises, patients should be encouraged to proceed with oocyte cryopreservation at a younger age, to avoid the risks of genetic abnormalities in older oocytes, as well as the risk of diminished ovarian reserve with age and the lower likelihood of a live birth with fewer cryopreserved oocytes, probably also with lower quality [32]. Unfortunately, the average age of a female inquiring about planned oocyte preservation is between 36 and 38 years old [20, 24]. It is important to continue the education of females about the age-related decline in fertility while giving honest facts about the success rates of oocyte cryopreservation resulting in a live birth at a later time point in their lives. Any woman considering oocyte cryopreservation should also be informed about the timeline for embryo transfer and the maximum age that the individual reproductive center would offer an embryo transfer based on obstetric and other risks associated.

27.4 Ovarian Stimulation Protocol Considerations

When a woman is undergoing oocyte cryopreservation, providers do not have to be concerned about how the stimulation will affect the endometrial lining or pregnancy in a fresh cycle. In addition, women undergoing oocyte cryopreservation are more likely to be high responders, as they are not in the clinic for infertility and may be at higher risk of ovarian hyperstimulation syndrome (OHSS). Strategies such as the use of GnRH antagonist protocols with agonist-only triggers to reduce the risks of OHSS should be considered in individuals with good ovarian reserve.

In situations where time is of the essence, such as in oocyte cryopreservation cases for cancer, consideration can be given to some of the newer strategies for ovarian stimulation, such as random-start and double stimulation cycles. These strategies take advantage of the theory that follicular growth occurs in waves and that two or more cohorts of follicles can grow and provide oocytes without unnecessary delay [33].

In a random-start stimulation cycle, stimulation is started without regard given to where the patient is in her menstrual cycle. This reduces the possibility of potential delay for controlled ovarian stimulation and consequently the delay in gonadotoxic treatment. This may allow an additional number of patients that may be able to take advantage of oocyte cryopreservation as the delay to cancer treatment can be significantly shorter. One study comparing random-start cancer patients matched with women undergoing conventional ovarian stimulation due to male, tubal, or uterine factor infertility revealed that the duration of stimulation was one day longer in the random-start patients, but the total number of oocytes and total mature oocytes were higher [34]. In a study comparing cancer patients undergoing random-start versus early follicular phase start stimulations, oocyte and embryo numbers were similar between the groups [35]. A 2017 systematic review of 19 publications also suggested that random-start ovarian stimulation is an effective option for cancer patients given similar outcomes as traditional protocols but with a shorter duration [36].

In a double stimulation cycle, a patient undergoes two stimulations and two oocyte retrievals within one 28-day "cycle" or time frame. This could potentially increase the total number of oocytes or embryos obtained in the same time period as a conventional stimulation cycle. A 2018 study compared follicular phase stimulation with immediate subsequent luteal phase stimulation in women with diminished ovarian reserve to see if the oocyte and embryo quantity and quality were comparable between the phases and if it would increase the total number of oocytes and embryos obtained [37]. The oocyte and embryo quality was found to be similar between the phases and more oocytes and embryos were obtained in the time period than if only a single stimulation had occurred [37]. This result has been shown in previous smaller studies as well [38, 39]. This protocol was utilized in a small study of ten cancer patients undergoing oocyte cryopreservation, and there were no delays in treatment or diagnoses of OHSS [40]. The use of the double stimulation protocol has been mostly studied in poor responders. Additional studies reviewing the safety in cancer patients given their typically normal ovarian reserve are needed.

27.5 Reported Recovery Rates and Performance After Oocyte Warming

Oocyte recovery rates and performance after warming are impacted by the patient's age at cryopreservation, the method of cryopreservation (vitrification versus slow-freeze), as well as the individual ART center's success rates. Survival rates are approximately 85–95% for vitrified oocytes, with younger oocytes surviving more readily than those harvested at an older age [2, 4, 41, 42]. Each center's individual success rates may differ, but in general, there is an approximate 4–7% live birth rate per warmed vitrified oocyte and 2% per thawed slow-freeze oocyte [6, 8, 43]. Many recent studies have reported comparable outcomes from cryopreserved oocytes through the vitrification method versus using fresh oocytes [2, 42, 44, 45]. However, a recent retrospective analysis of data from 2013 to 2015 from the Society for Assisted Reproductive Technology (SART) revealed that the live birth rate from fresh donor oocytes was 11.4% higher than that from frozen donor oocytes [46]. This finding is unlikely to impact a patient's interest in oocyte cryopreservation, as she may have personal or medical reasons for delaying pregnancy, and using her own fresh oocytes may not be an option. Furthermore, patients may prefer to try ART with their own genetic material than using fresh donor oocytes, especially when choosing the former does not preclude the latter. Nevertheless, there are physical changes happening in oocyte by cryopreservation, some of which are irreversible (such as zona hardening) and may help explain some of the discrepancies in outcome.

There have been several tools designed to assist providers in counseling patients regarding an optimal number of oocytes to attain for cryopreservation [41, 44]. To use these tools, a discussion of the patient's goals is involved. This discussion should query a patient's acceptable percentage risk of not having a live birth at a later date and how many children they ultimately desire. In 2013, a Gallup poll revealed 47% of women aged 30–49 desired two children total and 25% desired three children [47]. This can help guide the patient and the practitioner to decide how many oocyte cryopreservation cycles will be necessary to obtain a reasonable number of oocytes to approach the patient's goals or to have a discussion regarding how realistic the patient's expectations are. These tools are also created based upon particular programs' success rates and vary in whether they account for embryo euploidy, etc. Providers need to take these factors into account when using these tools for assistance in counseling patients.

27.6   Discussion on Feasibility of Oocyte Cryopreservation in Young Patients and Future Prospects

As discussed previously, oocyte cryopreservation is becoming a widely available option for women desiring an attempt to achieve pregnancy at a later date, regardless of their reasoning. A criticism of oocyte cryopreservation is that the numbers of women returning to use their vitrified oocytes thus far are comparatively few, but as oocyte cryopreservation is a relatively new technology, these numbers may increase over time. A study of 1468 women who underwent oocyte cryopreservation for a reason other than cancer from 2007 to 2015 revealed that 9.3% of the patients had returned to use their oocytes, at an average of 2.1 years later [4]. Most of these women had vitrified oocytes due to age, whereas 12% had a medical condition other than cancer for which they cryopreserved oocytes in advance [4]. Most of the women were single at time of oocyte cryopreservation, and half returning to use their oocytes had since found a partner [4]. The other half of the women returning used donor sperm when using their oocytes [4]. Reasons for not returning might include natural pregnancy or the decision to not pursue pregnancy at all.

Despite the relatively low numbers of women returning to use their cryopreserved oocytes, a study of 201 women who underwent oocyte cryopreservation from 2012 to 2016 revealed that most of the women (89%) reported they were happy that they underwent fertility preservation, even if they were to never come back to use the oocytes [48]. Most of the women felt that oocyte cryopreservation provided them with increased control over their reproductive planning (88%) [48]. Regret was noted in 16% of the women who had undergone oocyte cryopreservation, and this feeling was linked to a perception of lower adequacy of information, less emotional support during the process, and if they had fewer than ten oocytes retrieved [48]. This highlights the need for robust pretreatment counseling, including realistic expectations for the treatment and for the possibility of the need for additional procedures in the future (needing additional cycles for a greater total number of oocytes, undergoing oocyte warming and embryo transfer in the future). Patients can also be referred to additional resources for emotional and mental support during the process.

After proper counseling, oocyte cryopreservation can be a useful treatment for women hoping to have a chance for a pregnancy at a later date. As oocyte cryopreservation becomes more prevalent, continued follow-up of patients and whether or not they eventually use their cryopreserved oocytes will be an area for research. Additional advocacy is warranted to help women with the financial aspect of the treatment, as cost is often a barrier to those who are interested and well-informed, regardless of their motive for oocyte cryopreservation. It is our hope that women who wish to become mothers who have not yet found the right partner or who have been diagnosed with a devastating illness will be able to have a practical chance to realize that dream.

References

1. Ali J, AlHarbi NH, Ali N. Chapter 1. Historical background on gamete and embryo cryopreservation. Methods Mol Biol. 2017;1568:3–20.
2. Mature oocyte cryopreservation: a guideline. Fertil Steril. 2013;99:37–43.
3. Chen C. Pregnancy after human oocyte cryopreservation. Lancet. 1986;327:884–6.
4. Cobo A, Garcia-Velasco JA, Coello A, Domingo J, Pellicer A, Remohi J. Oocyte vitrification as an efficient option for elective fertility preservation. Fertil Steril. 2016;105:755–64.e8.
5. Shaw JM, Oranratnachai A, Trounson AO. Fundamental cryobiology of mammalian, oocytes and ovarian tissue. Theriogenology. 2000;53:59–72.
6. Potdar N, Gelbaya TA, Nardo LG. Oocyte vitrification in the 21st century and post-warming fertility outcomes: a systematic review and meta-analysis. Reprod Biomed Online. 2014;29:159–76.
7. Levi Setti PE, Porcu E, Patrizio P, Vigiliano V, de Luca R, d'Aloja P, et al. Human oocyte cryopreservation with slow freezing versus vitrification. Results from the National Italian Registry data, 2007–2011. Fertil Steril. 2014;102:90–5.e2.
8. Essential elements of informed consent for elective oocyte cryopreservation: a Practice Committee opinion. Fertil Steril. 2008;90:S134–5.
9. Saumet J, Petropanagos A, Buzaglo K, McMahon E, Warraich G, Mahutte N. No. 356-egg freezing for age-related fertility decline. J Obstet Gynaecol Can. 2018;40:356–68.
10. Coccia PF, Pappo AS, Beaupin L, Borges VF, Borinstein SC, Chugh R, et al. Adolescent and young adult oncology, version 2.2018, NCCN Clinical Practice Guidelines in Oncology. J Natl Compr Canc Netw. 2018;16:66–97.
11. Assi J, Santos J, Bonetti T, Serafini PC, Motta ELA, Chehin MB. Psychosocial benefits of fertility preservation for young cancer patients. J Assist Reprod Genet. 2018;35:601–6.
12. von Wolff M, Dittrich R, Liebenthron J, Nawroth F, Schuring AN, Bruckner T, et al. Fertility-preservation counselling and treatment for medical reasons: data from a multinational network of over 5000 women. Reprod Biomed Online. 2015;31:605–12.

13. von Wolff M, Bruckner T, Strowitzki T, Germeyer A. Fertility preservation: ovarian response to freeze oocytes is not affected by different malignant diseases-an analysis of 992 stimulations. J Assist Reprod Genet. 2018;35:1713–9.
14. Quinn MM, Cakmak H, Letourneau JM, Cedars MI, Rosen MP. Response to ovarian stimulation is not impacted by a breast cancer diagnosis. Hum Reprod. 2017;32:568–74.
15. Lefebvre T, Mirallie S, Leperlier F, Reignier A, Barriere P, Freour T. Ovarian reserve and response to stimulation in women undergoing fertility preservation according to malignancy type. Reprod Biomed Online. 2018;37:201–7.
16. Garcia-Velasco JA, Domingo J, Cobo A, Martinez M, Carmona L, Pellicer A. Five years' experience using oocyte vitrification to preserve fertility for medical and nonmedical indications. Fertil Steril. 2013;99:1994–9.
17. Almog B, Azem F, Gordon D, Pauzner D, Amit A, Barkan G, et al. Effects of cancer on ovarian response in controlled ovarian stimulation for fertility preservation. Fertil Steril. 2012;98:957–60.
18. van Dorp W, Haupt R, Anderson RA, Mulder RL, van den Heuvel-Eibrink MM, van Dulmen-den Broeder E, et al. Reproductive function and outcomes in female survivors of childhood, adolescent, and young adult cancer: a review. J Clin Oncol. 2018;36:2169–80.
19. Martin J, Hamilton BE, Osterman MJK, Driscoll A, Drake P. Births: final data for 2016. National Vital Statistics Reports from the Centers for Disease Control and Prevention. 2018;67.
20. Fritz R, Jindal S. Reproductive aging and elective fertility preservation. J Ovarian Res. 2018;11:66.
21. Heck KE, Schoendorf KC, Ventura SJ, Kiely JL. Delayed childbearing by education level in the United States, 1969–1994. Matern Child Health J. 1997;1:81–8.
22. Hammarberg K, Kirkman M, Pritchard N, Hickey M, Peate M, McBain J, et al. Reproductive experiences of women who cryopreserved oocytes for non-medical reasons. Hum Reprod. 2017;32:575–81.
23. Cooke A, Mills TA, Lavender T. Advanced maternal age: delayed childbearing is rarely a conscious choice a qualitative study of women's views and experiences. Int J Nurs Stud. 2012;49:30–9.
24. Baldwin K, Culley L, Hudson N, Mitchell H, Lavery S. Oocyte cryopreservation for social reasons: demographic profile and disposal intentions of UK users. Reprod Biomed Online. 2015;31:239–45.
25. System CNNVS. Provisional number of marriages and marriage rate: United States, 2000–2016.
26. Stoop D, van der Veen F, Deneyer M, Nekkebroeck J, Tournaye H. Oocyte banking for anticipated gamete exhaustion (AGE) is a preventive intervention, neither social nor nonmedical. Reprod Biomed Online. 2014;28:548–51.
27. Abir R, Ben-Aharon I, Garor R, Yaniv I, Ash S, Stemmer SM, et al. Cryopreservation of in vitro matured oocytes in addition to ovarian tissue freezing for fertility preservation in paediatric female cancer patients before and after cancer therapy. Hum Reprod. 2016;31:750–62.
28. Revel A, Revel-Vilk S, Aizenman E, Porat-Katz A, Safran A, Ben-Meir A, et al. At what age can human oocytes be obtained? Fertil Steril. 2009;92:458–63.
29. Loren AW. Fertility issues in patients with hematologic malignancies. Hematology Am Soc Hematol Educ Program. 2015;2015:138–45.
30. Medicine ASfR. Recommendations for gamete and embryo donation: a committee opinion 2013.
31. Klitzman RL. How old is too old? Challenges faced by clinicians concerning age cutoffs for patients undergoing in vitro fertilization. Fertil Steril. 2016;106:216–24.
32. Dondorp W, de Wert G, Pennings G, Shenfield F, Devroey P, Tarlatzis B, et al. Oocyte cryopreservation for age-related fertility loss. Hum Reprod. 2012;27:1231–7.
33. Sighinolfi G, Sunkara SK, La Marca A. New strategies of ovarian stimulation based on the concept of ovarian follicular waves: from conventional to random and double stimulation. Reprod Biomed Online. 2018;37(4):489–97.

34. Kim JH, Kim SK, Lee HJ, Lee JR, Jee BC, Suh CS, et al. Efficacy of random-start controlled ovarian stimulation in cancer patients. J Korean Med Sci. 2015;30:290–5.
35. Muteshi C, Child T, Ohuma E, Fatum M. Ovarian response and follow-up outcomes in women diagnosed with cancer having fertility preservation: comparison of random start and early follicular phase stimulation – a cohort study. Eur J Obstet Gynecol Reprod Biol. 2018;230:10–4.
36. Danis RB, Pereira N, Elias RT. Random start ovarian stimulation for oocyte or embryo cryopreservation in women desiring fertility preservation prior to gonadotoxic cancer therapy. Curr Pharm Biotechnol. 2017;18:609–13.
37. Cimadomo DVaiarelli A, Colamaria S, Trabucco E, Alviggi C, Venturella R, et al. Luteal phase anovulatory follicles result in the production of competent oocytes: intra-patient paired case-control study comparing follicular versus luteal phase stimulations in the same ovarian cycle. Hum Reprod. 2018; https://doi.org/10.1093/humrep/dey217.
38. Ubaldi FM, Capalbo A, Vaiarelli A, Cimadomo D, Colamaria S, Alviggi C, et al. Follicular versus luteal phase ovarian stimulation during the same menstrual cycle (DuoStim) in a reduced ovarian reserve population results in a similar euploid blastocyst formation rate: new insight in ovarian reserve exploitation. Fertil Steril. 2016;105:1488–95.e1.
39. Cardoso MCA, Evangelista A, Sartorio C, Vaz G, Werneck CLV, Guimaraes FM, et al. Can ovarian double-stimulation in the same menstrual cycle improve IVF outcomes? JBRA Assist Reprod. 2017;21:217–21.
40. Tsampras N, Gould D, Fitzgerald CT. Double ovarian stimulation (DuoStim) protocol for fertility preservation in female oncology patients. Hum Fertil. 2017;20:248–53.
41. Goldman RH, Racowsky C, Farland LV, Munne S, Ribustello L, Fox JH. Predicting the likelihood of live birth for elective oocyte cryopreservation: a counseling tool for physicians and patients. Hum Reprod. 2017;32:853–9.
42. Almodin CG, Minguetti-Camara VC, Paixao CL, Pereira PC. Embryo development and gestation using fresh and vitrified oocytes. Hum Reprod. 2010;25:1192–8.
43. Cil AP, Turkgeldi L, Seli E. Oocyte cryopreservation as a preventive measure for age-related fertility loss. Semin Reprod Med. 2015;33:429–35.
44. Doyle JO, Richter KS, Lim J, Stillman RJ, Graham JR, Tucker MJ. Successful elective and medically indicated oocyte vitrification and warming for autologous in vitro fertilization, with predicted birth probabilities for fertility preservation according to number of cryopreserved oocytes and age at retrieval. Fertil Steril. 2016;105:459–66.e2.
45. Grifo JA, Noyes N. Delivery rate using cryopreserved oocytes is comparable to conventional in vitro fertilization using fresh oocytes: potential fertility preservation for female cancer patients. Fertil Steril. 2010;93:391–6.
46. Kushnir VA, Darmon SK, Barad DH, Gleicher N. New national outcome data on fresh versus cryopreserved donor oocytes. J Ovarian Res. 2018;11:2.
47. Newport F, Wilke J. Desire for children still norm in U.S. Gallup 2013.
48. Greenwood EA, Pasch LA, Hastie J, Cedars MI, Huddleston HG. To freeze or not to freeze: decision regret and satisfaction following elective oocyte cryopreservation. Fertil Steril. 2018;109:1097–104.e1.

Chapter 28
Ovarian Cortical Tissue Biopsy and Freezing for Autotransplantation

Trisha Shah and Erkan Buyuk

28.1 Introduction

Ovarian tissue cryopreservation and autotransplantation is an effective alternative method for fertility preservation. Human ovary autotransplantation involves ovarian tissue extraction, freezing and then thawing of the ovarian tissue with subsequent transplantation to the same patient once the patient is cured of her disease. Parkes et al. initially introduced the concept of ovarian tissue cryopreservation and auto-transplantation, performing ovarian tissue grafting in the rat model in 1953 [1]. Several decades later, there was subsequent success with restoration of fertility following ovarian autotransplantation using in vivo sheep models [2]. In humans, in vitro studies were first noted to be successful in 1996 [3]. The first report of restoration of human ovarian function in vivo following autotransplantation of frozen-thawed tissue was published in 2000 [4]. Shortly after in 2004, the first report of a live birth following ovarian tissue cryopreservation (OTC) and autotransplantation emerged [5]. While this fertility preservation method is still considered experimental given its nascent stages, it has nonetheless become a bourgeoning practice globally for the past 20 years. There have been hundreds of ovarian transplantation procedures spanning 21 countries, resulting in over 130 live births to date [6, 7]. The American Society of Clinical Oncology has updated its recommendations in 2018 to reflect inclusion of ovarian tissue cryopreservation and transplantation as part of fertility preservation strategies, indicating its importance when discussing fertility preservation in patients with cancer [8].

T. Shah · E. Buyuk (✉)
Montefiore's Institute for Reproductive Medicine and Health, Department of Obstetrics and Gynecology & Women's Health, Albert Einstein College of Medicine, Montefiore Medical Center, Bronx, NY, USA
e-mail: ebuyuk@montefiore.org

© Springer Nature Switzerland AG 2020
O. Bukulmez (ed.), *Diminished Ovarian Reserve and Assisted Reproductive Technologies*, https://doi.org/10.1007/978-3-030-23235-1_28

28.2   Indications for Ovarian Cortical Tissue Biopsy and Freezing

Ovarian cortical tissue biopsy and freezing for fertility preservation can be utilized in many circumstances. Its indication in the setting of malignant or nonmalignant systemic diseases requiring chemotherapy, radiotherapy or bone marrow transplant has materialized [9]. Approximately 17 per 100,000 females are diagnosed with cancer under age 20, and approximately 10% of women with cancer are diagnosed during their reproductive years. Given advances in cancer diagnosis and treatment, however, the 5-year childhood survival rate is greater than 80% [7, 10]. The malignancies that constitute the most frequent indications for fertility preservation include breast cancer, hematologic malignancies, and solid malignancies such as sarcoma. Among nonmalignant systemic diseases, women requiring hematopoietic stem cell transplantation for hematologic diseases such as sickle cell anemia or aplastic anemia or women who have autoimmune diseases refractory to immunosuppressive therapy are candidates for cryopreservation of their ovarian tissue [11]. Malignancies represent approximately 85% of those seeking ovarian tissue cryopreservation, while non-malignant diseases represent about 15% [6].

When there is ovarian exposure to cytotoxic chemotherapy or radiotherapy, there can be significant irreversible damage to ovarian primordial follicles, follicular recruitment, and growth or direct damage to the oocytes leading to loss of fertility. Alkylating chemotherapeutic agents, ionizing radiotherapy to the pelvis and abdomen, or cranial or total body irradiation bear the highest risk of cytotoxic insult to the ovaries and can lead to subsequent fertility loss [12]. The nonsurgical relative risk of premature ovarian failure (POI) is up to 13 times after exposure to chemotherapy and radiation [13]. The extent of loss of fertility varies by age at diagnosis and treatment, cancer type and stage, as well as varying cytotoxic drugs, doses, site, and fractionation of the chemotherapy or radiotherapy. These can also have profound effects on pregnancy, with data showing poorer pregnancy outcomes given increased rates of miscarriage, prematurity, and low birth weights [14]. Ovarian cortical tissue biopsy can offer unique advantages in oncofertility, given its application for prepubertal females, those with hormone-sensitive malignancy, or those who require immediate treatment with gonadotoxic therapy, as compared to embryo or oocyte cryopreservation.

Other indications for ovarian cortical tissue biopsy and freezing include ovarian diseases such as benign bilateral ovarian tumors, those at a high risk of ovarian torsion, or severe and recurrent ovarian endometriosis [15]. It may also be encouraged in cases with a high risk of POI with genetic or family history [7]. As elective methods of fertility preservation for personal reasons are becoming more prevalent, this technique of autotransplantation may also become utilized for that purpose.

28.3   Technique of Ovarian Tissue Biopsy and Freezing

Obtaining ovarian tissue is ideally performed prior to the initiation of gonadotoxic treatments. In the literature, it has been obtained via laparoscopy, robot-assisted laparoscopy, minilaparotomy, or laparotomy and can also be performed at the time of oophoropexy or surgical removal of pelvic or abdominal malignancy. A partial oophorectomy (>50% of the ovary) or total oophorectomy can be performed for ovarian tissue cryopreservation (OTC) [9]. A total oophorectomy would require extraction with a large vascular pedicle in cases where a future whole-ovary autotransplantation is contemplated, although no successful whole-ovary autotransplantation has been performed in humans. The majority of ovarian follicles are found in the ovarian cortex, thus obtaining even small amounts of cortical tissue can result in a large yield of oocytes. Prior to freezing, the ovarian cortex is separated from the medulla and can be cut into strips measuring 1mm x 5mm x 10mm using a tissue slicer to ensure perfusion of cryoprotectant and revascularization during autotransplantation. Ovarian cortex can be cryopreserved via the slow freeze method or vitrification [16, 17].

Slow freeze involves exposure of cortical ovarian tissue to cryoprotectants followed by cooling of the tissue slowly to approximately −140 °C at a programmable low rate (~1 °C/min), after which the tissue is stored in liquid nitrogen at −196 °C. Protocols have been well developed for freezing and thawing using this method, and the majority of live births documented thus far have utilized this technique. Vitrification involves exposure of cortical ovarian tissue to higher doses of cryoprotectants than those used in slow freezing, followed by ultra-rapid cooling to −196 °C at very fast rates (~20,000 °C/min) by direct immersion into liquid nitrogen. Vitrification offers several advantages in that it is a technically less difficult and shorter process that is more cost effective, while still carrying a low risk of intracellular crystallization. However, it requires the use of higher concentrations of cryoprotectants, which may increase the risk of cellular toxicity and osmotic trauma. As this is a newer method used for ovarian tissue cryopreservation, there have only been two live births utilizing this method to date [9, 18].

In a systematic in vitro comparison of oocyte viability using morphologic criteria after vitrification and slow freezing, Keros et al. demonstrated that both techniques had similar outcomes with preservation of oocytes, while preservation of supporting cells and matrix of the stroma were better after vitrification of human ovarian tissue [19]. This potentially suggests that vitrification may result in better outcomes than slow freeze. To date, there has been no prospective study comparing clinical outcomes of each cryopreservation technique with human ovarian tissue, as vitrification in this setting has not been utilized for a long enough period of time. Using either method of cryopreservation for the whole ovary would result in a higher risk of cryoinjury due to inadequate diffusion of cryoprotectants throughout the entire ovary.

Another critical aspect performed in an experienced laboratory aside from cryo-preservation is the evaluation of ovarian tissue prior to and after freezing. This should be performed in an attempt to prevent reintroduction of malignant cells or transplanting nonviable or poorly functioning ovarian tissue. Histological examination, transmission electron microscopy, immunohistochemistry, terminal deoxynucleotidyl transferase-mediated biotinylated deoxyuridine triphosphate nick end-labeling (TUNEL) assay, polymerase chain reaction (PCR), estradiol and progesterone production in vitro, and xenografting can be used for this purpose [9].

28.4 Technique of Autotransplantation

Autotransplantation of ovarian cortical tissue can be performed surgically as either orthotopic transplantation or heterotopic transplantation [5, 20, 21]. Orthotopic autotransplantation of ovarian tissue involves transplanting frozen-thawed cortical ovarian tissue back to the same patient into pelvic sites such as the remaining ovary, ovarian fossa, or broad ligament [22]. Heterotopic autotransplantation of ovarian tissue involves transplanting frozen-thawed cortical ovarian tissue back to the same patient into extrapelvic sites such as the forearm or abdomen. This technique was described by Oktay et al. by placing cortical strips of tissue between the fascia and subcutaneous tissue in the forearm [23]. They additionally described an abdominal approach using the same suture pull-through technique as employed in the forearm in a breast cancer patient [22, 24].

These methods of OTC are similar in that they both do not require prior ovarian stimulation as needed with oocyte or embryo cryopreservation, which can delay gonadotoxic treatment. It can additionally be used in prepubertal females or hormone-sensitive malignancies. While both techniques can restore endocrine function, heterotopic transplantation cannot result in a spontaneous pregnancy, and thus would require further ART. Heterotopic transplantation, however, may be preferred in cases of patients that are poor surgical candidates given severe pelvic adhesions or have insufficient pelvic vasculature to support transplantation after pelvic radiotherapy (Table 28.1). Tissue monitoring may also be easier in heterotopic transplantation [11, 25, 26].

Table 28.1 Comparison of orthotopic and heterotopic autotransplantation

	Orthotopic autotransplantation	Heterotopic autotransplantation
Site of transplantation	Pelvic	Extrapelvic
Prior stimulation of ovary required	No	No
Restoration of endocrine function	Yes	Yes
Ability for spontaneous pregnancy	Yes	No, requires IVF

Given that both of these techniques involve avascular grafting, there is a risk of post-grafting ischemia and follicular atresia. In fact, it has been shown that only 7% of the follicle loss is due to freezing/thawing process, while most of the follicles are lost due to ischemia/reperfusion injury [27]. One method to avoid the ischemia/reperfusion injury is autotransplantation of a frozen thawed whole ovary with its vascular pedicle back to the same patient [28]. It is a surgically challenging procedure, given difficult vascular and microvascular anastomoses, and has a higher risk of postoperative vascular complications that may compromise the entire ovary. Although live birth following autotransplantation of the whole ovary has been successfully shown in sheep, there are no human live births to date using autotransplantation of a whole ovary [29]. Although it remains a biologically plausible option, given clinical success rates of orthotopic and heterotopic autotransplantation, it may be reserved for rare circumstances [28].

28.5 Clinical Outcomes with Autotransplantation

The time to return of ovarian function following autotransplantation of frozen-thawed cortical ovarian tissue is varied in the literature but may resume 2–9 months postoperatively [9]. There is a varied rate of return of endocrine function, with two large meta-analyses reporting rates from 63.9% to 95%, respectively [6, 30]. The mean lifespan of the grafted tissue varies and can depend on the fraction of the ovary that was obtained, or the total surface area that was transplanted. The mean duration of the transplanted tissue is 4–5 years; however, there are reports lasting as long as 10 years to result in subsequent pregnancies [18].

In terms of its safety, there have been no reports in the literature of a recurrence of original cancer in correlation with orthotopic transplantation. Jadoul et al. were able to track surgical complications from 140 women who underwent OTC using responses of surveys and report four minor complications and one major complication resulting in reoperation for intra-abdominal hemorrhage. Patients reported a 96% satisfaction rate overall with the process. These data support the use of OTC, given its low complication and high satisfaction rates [31].

While there is no international registry established, it is estimated that the live birth rate per cortical ovarian tissue transplant is ~30%, which is widely supported in the literature [32–35]. The largest meta-analysis to date includes data from 545 cases at a single institution: 4% of these women had autotransplantation with a live birth rate of 33% [31]. Two other large global meta-analyses both reviewing over 300 cases found live birth rates of ~27% and 37%, respectively, which are also consistent with prior data [6, 30]. The number of live births worldwide has exceeded 130 pregnancies, with exponential rates noted since 2014 (Fig. 28.1). Studies report that up to half of these pregnancies were spontaneous [6]. One series even reports three live births from one single ovarian-tissue reimplantation procedure [18].

Neonatal outcome data of 40 of these live births have been reviewed and demonstrated that the mean gestational age at birth was 39 weeks and the mean weight at

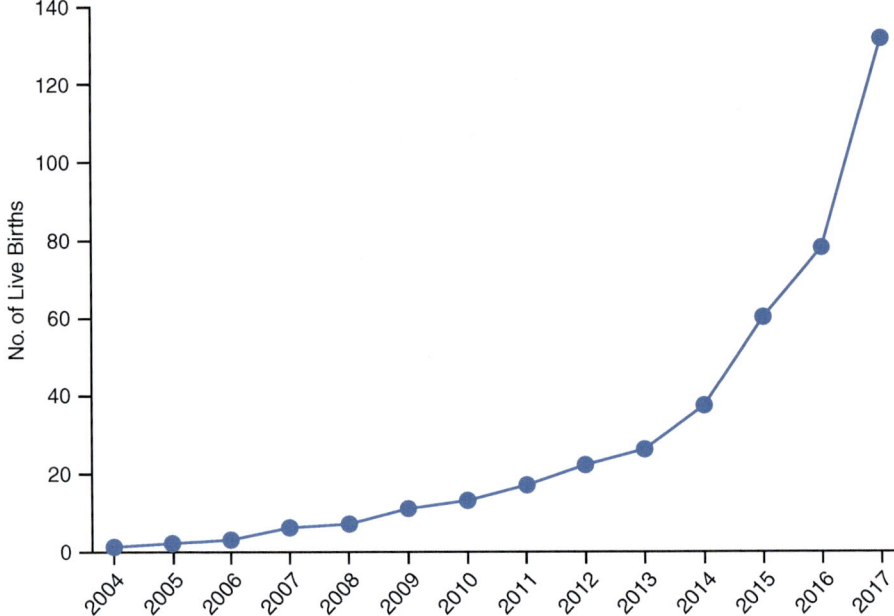

Fig. 28.1 Live births following orthotopic autotransplantation from 2004 to 2017. (Donnez and Dolmans [7])

birth was 3168 g, consistent with other singleton pregnancies at birth. There has been only 1 fetal anomaly documented in 93 live births, which is consistent with the 1–2% rate of congenital anomaly in the general population [6, 18].

28.6   Limitations of Autotransplantation

While the success of autotransplantation has been revolutionary, these aforementioned methods have the limitation of carrying an additional risk of reintroducing malignant cells, particularly in instances of ovarian malignancies or in malignancies that may metastasize to the ovaries. Dolmans et al. used PCR-based studies to show malignant cell contamination of cryopreserved ovarian tissue from leukemia patients [36]. Despite evidence that frozen-thawed ovarian tissue with malignant contamination did not result in transmission of the disease xenografted to mice or that improvement in isolation technique involving washing the follicles three times showed no evidence of malignant cells, these methods are currently contraindicated in humans [37, 38]. Thus, in cases of leukemia or other cancers with high likelihood of ovarian involvement, alternative methods such as in vitro maturation (IVM) or ovarian follicle transplantation (artificial ovary) are needed.

28.7   In Vitro Maturation

IVM is a technique by which preantral follicles are extracted and isolated, and the final stages of maturation are completed in vitro in culture media. Immature oocytes progress from germinal vesicles in prophase I through meiosis I to reach metaphase II (MII). This stage of nuclear maturation, and additionally cytoplasmic maturation, need to occur in order to undergo fertilization and are under the control of epigenetic factors [39]. The first human live birth with this technique was documented in 1991; however, given overall lower success rates and the improvements of oocyte and embryo cryopreservation, the use of IVM has declined in clinical practice [40]. This method of fertility preservation, however, is favorable because it eliminates or reduces gonadotropin stimulation in the patient. This is particularly critical for those in which elevations in estradiol with stimulation are contraindicated, such as thromboembolism or hormone-sensitive malignancies. It also serves as an alternative for those who cannot delay gonadotoxic treatment. It can additionally be used for those with PCOS or those that are at a high risk of ovarian hyperstimulation syndrome.

There are two sources to obtain immature oocytes to employ the principles of IVM: [1] The first scenario involves a minimal controlled ovarian hyperstimulation (COH) or no prior COH, followed by aspiration of the ovarian follicles to obtain oocytes, and [2] the second scenario involves ovarian tissue freezing, thawing, followed by in vitro culture of the tissue for IVM, which also may include the use of an artificial ovary [41].

28.7.1   Obtaining Follicles for IVM via Aspiration

The process of oocyte aspiration has been described in IVM. Factors such as type of needle, aspiration pressures, or use of a mesh cell strainer often differ from protocols associated with oocyte retrieval in IVF given follicular sizes less than 10 mm in IVM [41]. Clinical outcomes for IVM for fertility preservation are promising although large prospective studies are lacking. In a large retrospective study of 192 IVM cycles using oocyte aspiration with no COH in women with cancer who require urgent chemotherapy, 105 IVM cycles (54.7%) resulted in cryopreservation of oocytes, and 82 IVM cycles (42.7%) resulted in cryopreservation of embryos. The results were comparable irrespective of the phase of the cycle in which oocyte aspiration occurred: early follicular, late follicular, or luteal [42]. When directly comparing oocyte aspiration with IVM to conventional IVF for fertility preservation in over 600 combined cycles, IVF had a statistically higher median number of oocytes collected and high rates of resultant oocyte and embryo cryopreservation. Of 33 cycles in which pregnancy was attempted, LBR per cycle was 31% following IVF and 7% following IVM, although these differences did not reach statistical significance [43].

28.7.2   Obtaining Follicles for IVM via OTC

Obtaining immature oocytes isolated from ovarian tissue has been described in the literature and can be followed by in vitro maturation and subsequent cryopreservation. In a small retrospective case series of four patients, the women underwent retrieval of immature oocytes from the antral follicles of the excised ovarian tissue, with a success of a total of eight mature oocytes vitrified [44]. This method led to an ongoing clinical pregnancy by Segers et al. in 2015, thus illustrating its clinical promise [45]. Sermondade et al. examined 54 patients who underwent oocyte vitrification after IVM associated with oocyte aspiration and compared primordial follicle density in OTC subsequently obtained in the same patient. This was an attempt to use antimullerian hormone (AMH) levels and antral follicle count (AFC) as clinical predictors of the number of oocytes cryopreserved after IVM. They deduced that an AMH and AFC of >3.5 ng/mL and >19 follicles, respectively, are required for obtaining at least eight frozen mature oocytes after IVM. They additionally found significant correlation of serum AMH with primordial follicles in the OTC sample. The primordial follicle density also correlated with the number of mature oocytes cryopreserved [46]. These data support the potential use of OTC as a method to obtain oocytes and the combined technique of follicle aspiration, followed by OTC, to increase chances of pregnancy. These clinical parameters may influence counseling of appropriate options of fertility preservation, although more studies are needed [47].

28.7.3   Artificial Ovary

The artificial ovary is a 3-D biocompatible and biodegradable matrix in which isolated follicles and ovarian stromal cells can be encapsulated and transplanted to patients. It serves as an important conduit for ovarian material because ovarian follicles are surrounded by a basal membrane, excluding them from the stromal environment, capillaries, and nerves. Isolation would then eliminate the risk of transmission of malignant cells during autotransplantation. Several research groups have contributed to both in vitro and animal in vivo studies [48–52]. The technique for developing an artificial ovary was based on the preliminary studies using suspension in plasma clots [53]. Studies in other fields had developed fibrin scaffolding as a matrix because it can facilitate cell proliferation, transplantation, and delivery of growth factors [54, 55]. This was applied to the ovary, where a fibrinogen droplet and the isolated ovarian stromal cells suspended in media were combined together. Thrombin was subsequently added to create the fibrin clot. In vitro studies showed two fibrin clot formulations had reproducible degradation of the fibrin network, had survival and proliferation of stromal cells, and had increasing stromal cell density [56]. This was then applied to a murine animal model with autotransplantation in a fibrin scaffold. Luyckx et al. showed that isolated murine preantral follicles survived and developed, supporting ovarian cells proliferated, and grafted endothelial cells proliferated with the formation of capillaries, all after 1 week of autotransplantation of fibrin matrices. Because of the successful fibrin matrix formulations, they recovered a greater number of follicles after autografting (32%), compared to 20.3% using human follicles grafted in a plasma clot in a prior study [53, 57]. Further murine studies showed secondary follicles were more likely to survive and develop than primordial primary follicles in a fibrin matrix after 1 week of grafting, which may imply that the composition of the fibrin matrix supports already existing larger follicles [58]. In 2016, Paulini et al. showed that isolated human follicles were able to survive after encapsulation in fibrin clots when xenografted in murine models [59]. Future studies are needed in this field using human follicles and transplantation, as this may be a favorable technique for fertility preservation.

Once the follicles are aspirated or isolated with either aforementioned method, they undergo maturation in vitro. There are several protocols describing maturation media; however, the addition of hormonal additives to the culture media seems to increase implantation rates [60]. FSH aids with expansion of the cumulus-oocyte complex (COC) and contributes to subsequent oocyte maturation, while LH and hCG facilitate resumption of meiosis and the final stages of maturation following what would be an LH surge and ovulation in vivo. Proteins are found in maturation media, although sources can vary from maternal serum and human follicular fluid to human serum albumin (HSA). Serum containing complex components including growth factors and amino acids may also be added [41].

To date, there have only been four live births as a result of IVM for fertility preservation in cancer patients; however, there are >1400 births as a result of IVM, with estimates >5000 births worldwide [43, 61]. Neonatal outcomes of children conceived using IVM has been described in the literature as being similar to conventional IVF [62–64]. A 2017 prospective single-blinded study compared outcomes at first trimester screening, 21 weeks of gestation, birth, and at 2 years of age and found no increased risks of offspring as a result of IVM compared to both IVF and ICSI controls [65]. IVM is still considered an experimental technique of fertility preservation, and more studies are needed to better elucidate the safety and efficacy as it is applied in clinical settings [66].

28.8   Future

Ovarian cortical tissue biopsy and freezing for autotransplantation has proven to be a valid method for fertility preservation, although it is still considered experimental. Future steps in this field should be taken to allow for broader clinical implementation. An international registry would support improved collection of data and tracking of clinical outcomes, with the eventual goal of allowing this technique to be no longer considered experimental. The need for developing selection criteria to guide clinical decision making has not been standardized, and a consensus on important factors may guide our ability to counsel patients on fertility preservation options. This technique boasts several advantages over currently used methods of oocyte and embryo cryopreservation, thus having the potential to provide a patient with more choices. Its shortcomings are attempted to be overcome using methods like IVM and the creation of an artificial ovary, although more research is needed to incorporate these techniques in routine clinical setting.

References

1. Parkes AS, Smith AU. Regeneration of rat ovarian tissue grafted after exposure to low temperatures. Proc R Soc Lond B Biol Sci. 1953;140(901):455–70.
2. Gosden RG, Baird DT, Wade JC, Webb R. Restoration of fertility to oophorectomized sheep by ovarian autographs at e196 degrees C. Hum Reprod. 1994;9:597–603.
3. Newton H, Aubard Y, Rutherford A, Sharma V, Gosden R. Low temperature storage and grafting of human ovarian tissue. Hum Reprod. 1996;11(7):1487–91.
4. Oktay K, Karlikaya G. Ovarian function after transplantation of frozen, banked autologous ovarian tissue. N Engl J Med. 2000;342(25):1919.
5. Donnez J, Dolmans MM, Demylle D, Jadoul P, Pirard C, Squifflet J, et al. Livebirth after orthotopic transplantation of cryopreserved ovarian tissue. Lancet (London, England). 2004;364(9443):1405–10.
6. Gellert SE, Pors SE, Kristensen SG, Bay-Bjorn AM, Ernst E, Yding Andersen C. Transplantation of frozen-thawed ovarian tissue: an update on worldwide activity published in peer-reviewed papers and on the Danish cohort. J Assist Reprod Genet. 2018;35(4):561–70.
7. Donnez JA, Dolmans M. Fertility preservation in women. N Engl J Med. 2017;377(17):1657–65.
8. Kutluk Oktay BEH, Partridge AH, Quinn GP, Reinecke J, Taylor HS, Hamish Wallace W, Wang ET, Loren AW. Fertility preservation in patients with cancer: ASCO clinical practice guideline update. J Clin Oncol. 2018;38(19):1994–2001.
9. Salama M, Woodruff TK. New advances in ovarian autotransplantation to restore fertility in cancer patients. Cancer Metastasis Rev. 2015;34(4):807–22.
10. Siegel R, Ma J, Zou Z, Jemal A. Cancer statistics, 2014. CA Cancer J Clin. 2014;64:9–29.
11. Demeestere I, et al. Orthotopic and heterotopic ovarian tissue transplantation. Hum Reprod Update. 2009;15(6):649–65.
12. Marci R, et al. Radiations and female fertility. Reprod Biol Endocrinol. 2018;16(1):112.
13. Andersen AN. Chemotherapy risks to fertility of childhood cancer survivors. Lancet (London, England). 2016;17(5):540–1.
14. Bea G. Reproductive outcomes after a childhood and adolescent young adult cancer diagnosis in female cancer survivors: a systematic review and meta-analysis. J Adolesc Young Adult Oncol. 2018;7:627–42.
15. Kitajima M, Dolmans M, Donnez O, Masuzaki H, Soares M, Donnez J. Enhanced follicular recruitment and atresia in cortex derived from ovaries with endometriomas. Fertil Steril. 2014;101:1031–7.
16. Nagy ZP, Varghese AC, Agarwal A, editors. Cryopreservation of mammalian gametes and embryos: methods and protocols. New York: The Humana Press; 2017.
17. Practice Committee of American Society for Reproductive Medicine. Ovarian tissue cryopreservation: a committee opinion. Fertil Steril. 2014;101(5):1237–43.
18. Jensen AK, Macklon KT, Fedder J, Ernst E, Humaidan P, Andersen CY. 86 successful births and 9 ongoing pregnancies worldwide in women transplanted with frozen-thawed ovarian tissue: focus on birth and perinatal outcome in 40 of these children. J Assist Reprod Genet. 2017;34(3):325–36.
19. Keros V, Xella S, Hultenby K, Pettersson K, Sheikhi M, Volpe A, et al. Vitrification versus controlled-rate freezing in cryopreservation of human ovarian tissue. Hum Reprod. 2009;24:1670–83.

20. Oktay K, Tilly J. Livebirth after cryopreserved ovarian tissue autotransplantation. Lancet (London, England). 2004;364(9451):2091–2; author reply 2–3
21. Kim SS, Hwang IT, Lee HC. Heterotopic autotransplantation of cryobanked human ovarian tissue as a strategy to restore ovarian function. Fertil Steril. 2004;82(4):930–2.
22. Oktay K, Buyuk E. Ovarian transplantation in humans: indications, techniques and the risk of reseeding cancer. Eur J Obstet Gynecology Reprod Biol. 2004;113(Suppl 1):S45–7.
23. Oktay KBE, Rosenwaks Z, Rucinski J. A technique for transplantation of ovarian cortical strips to the forearm. Fertil Steril. 2003;80:193–8.
24. Oktay K, Buyuk E, Veeck L, Zaninovic N, Xu K, Takeuchi T, Opsahl M, Rosenwaks Z. Embryo development after heterotopic transplantation of cryopreserved ovarian tissue. Lancet (London, England). 2004;363(9412):837–40.
25. Sonmezer M, Oktay K. Orthotopic and heterotopic ovarian tissue transplantation. Best Pract Res Clin Obstet Gynaecol. 2010;24(1):113–26.
26. Donnez J, Dolmans M. Transplantation of ovarian tissue. Best Pract Res Clin Obstet Gynaecol. 2014;28(8):1188–97.
27. Baird DT, Webb R, Campbell BK, Harkness LM, Gosden RG. Long-term ovarian function in sheep after ovariectomy and transplantation of autografts stored at −196 C. Endocrinology. 1999;140:462–71.
28. Martinez-Madrid B, Dolmans M, Van Langendonckt A, Defrere S, Donnez J. Freeze-thawing intact human ovary with its vascular pedicle with a passive cooling device. Fertil Steril. 2004;82:1390–4.
29. Arav A, Revel A, et al. Oocyte recovery, embryo development and ovarian function after cryopreservation and transplantation of whole sheep ovary. Hum Reprod. 2005;20(12):3554–9.
30. Pacheco F, Oktay K. Current success and efficiency of autology ovarian transplantation: a meta-analysis. Reprod Sci. 2017;24(8):1111–20.
31. Jadoul P, Guilmain A, Squifflet J, Luyckx M, Votino R, Wyns C, et al. Efficacy of ovarian tissue cryopreservation for fertility preservation: lessons learned from 545 cases. Hum Reprod. 2017;32(5):1046–54.
32. Dittrich R, Hackl J, Lotz L, Hoffmann I, Beckmann MW. Pregnancies and live births after 20 transplantations of cryopreserved ovarian tissue in a single center. Fertil Steril. 2015;103(2):462–8.
33. Stoop D, et al. Fertility preservation for age-related fertility decline. Lancet (London, England). 2014;384:1311–9.
34. Van der Ven H, Liebenthron J, Beckmann M, Toth B, Korell M, Krüssel J, Frambach T, Kupka M, Hohl MK, Winkler-Crepaz K, et al. Ninety-five orthotopic transplantations in 74 women of ovarian tissue after cytotoxic treatment in a fertility preservation network: tissue activity, pregnancy and delivery rates. Hum Reprod. 2016;31:2031–41.
35. Donnez J, Dolmans M. Ovarian cortex transplantation: 60 reported live births brings the success and worldwide expansion of the technique towards routine clinical practice. J Assist Reprod Genet. 2015;32:1167–70.
36. Dolmans MM, Marinescu C, Saussoy P, Van Langendonckt A, Amorim C, Donnez J. Reimplantation of cryopreserved ovarian tissue from patients with acute lymphoblastic leukemia is potentially unsafe. Blood. 2010;116:2908–14.
37. Dolmans MM, Luyckx V, Donnez J, Andersen CY, Greve T. Risk of transferring malignant cells with transplanted frozen-thawed ovarian tissue. Fertil Steril. 2013;99:1514–22.
38. Tea G. Cryopreserved ovarian cortex from patients with leukemia in complete remission contains no apparent viable malignant cells. Blood. 2012;120(22):4311–6.
39. Practice Committees of the American Society for Reproductive Medicine and the Society for Assisted Reproductive Technology. In vitro maturation: a committee opinion. Fertil Steril. 2013;99(3):663–6.
40. Cha KY, Koo JJ, Ko JJ, Choi DH, Han SY, Yoon TK. Pregnancy after in vitro fertilization of human follicular oocytes collected from nonstimulated cycles, their culture in vitro and their transfer in a donor oocyte program. Fertil Steril. 1991;55(1):109.

41. Walls ML, Hart RJ. In vitro maturation. Best Pract Res Clin Obstet Gynaecol. 2018;53:60–72.
42. Creux H, et al. Immature oocyte retrieval and in vitro oocyte maturation at different phases of the menstrual cycle in women with cancer who require urgent gonadotoxic treatment. Fertil Steril. 2017;107:198–204.
43. Creux H, et al. Thirteen years' experience in fertility preservation for cancer patients after in vitro fertilization and in vitro maturation treatments. J Assist Reprod Genet. 2018;35(4):583–92.
44. Huang JY, et al. Combining ovarian tissue cryobanking with retrieval of immature oocytes followed by in vitro maturation and vitrification: an additional strategy of fertility preservation. Fertil Steril. 2008;89:567–72.
45. Segers I, et al. In vitro maturation (IVM) of oocytes recovered from ovariectomy specimens in the laboratory: a promising "ex vivo" method of oocyte cryopreservation resulting in the first report of an ongoing pregnancy in Europe. J Assist Reprod Genet. 2015;32(8):1221–31.
46. Sermondade N, et al. Serum antimüllerian hormone is associated with the number of oocytes matured in vitro and with primordial follicle density in candidates for fertility preservation. Fertil Steril. 2019;111(2):357–62.
47. Hart R. Optimizing the opportunity for female fertility preservation in a limited time-frame for patients with cancer using in vitro maturation and ovarian tissue cryopreservation. Fertil Steril. 2019;111(2):258–9.
48. Amorim CA, Van Langendonckt A, David A, Dolmans MM, Donnez J. Survival of human preantral follicles after cryopreservation of ovarian tissue, follicular isolation and in vitro culture in a calcium alginate matrix. Hum Reprod. 2009;24:92–9.
49. Shikanov S, Xu M, Woodruff TK, Shea LD. Interpenetrating fibrin-alginate matrices for in vitro ovarian follicle development. Biomaterials. 2009;30:5476–85.
50. Hornick JE, Duncan FE, Shea LD, Woodruff TK. Isolated primate primordial follicles require a rigid physical environment to survive and grow in vitro. Hum Reprod. 2012;27:1801–10.
51. Smith RM, Shikanov A, Kniazeva E, Ramadurai D, Woodruff TK, Shea LD. Fibrin-mediated delivery of an ovarian follicle pool in a mouse model of infertility. Tissue Eng Part A. 2014;20:3021–30.
52. Rajabzadeh AR, Eimani H, Mohseni Koochesfahani H, Shahvardi AH, Fathi R. Morphological study of isolated ovarian preantral follicles using fibrin gel plus platelet lysate after subcutaneous transplantation. Cell J. 2015;17:145–52.
53. Dolmans MM, Martinez-Madrid B, Gadisseux E, Guiot Y, Yuan WY, Torre A, Camboni A, Van Langendonckt A, Donnez J. Short-term transplantation of isolated human ovarian follicles and cortical tissue into nude mice. Reproduction. 2007;134:253–62.
54. Boehler RM, Graham JG, Shea LD. Tissue engineering tools for modulation of the immune response. BioTechniques. 2011;51:239–40.
55. Chiu CL, Hecht V, Duong H, Wu B, Tawil B. Permeability of three-dimensional fibrin constructs corresponds to fibrinogen and thrombin concentrations. Biores Open Access. 2012;1(97):134–40.
56. Luyckx V, et al. First step in developing a 3D biodegradable fibrin scaffold for an artificial ovary. J Ovarian Res. 2013;6:83.
57. Luyckx V, et al. A new step toward the artificial ovary: survival and proliferation of isolated murine follicles after autologous transplantation in a fibrin scaffold. Fertil Steril. 2014;101(4):1149–56.
58. Chiti MC, et al. Influence of follicle stage on artificial ovary outcome using fibrin as a matrix. Hum Reprod. 2016;31(2):427–35.
59. Paulini F, et al. Survival and growth of human preantral follicles after cryopreservation of ovarian tissue, follicle isolation and short-term xenografting. Reprod Biomed Online. 2016;33:425–32.
60. Yang ZY, Chian RC. Development of in vitro maturation techniques for clinical applications. Fertil Steril. 2017;108(4):577–84.
61. Chian RC, Xu CL, Huang JY, Ata B. Obstetric outcomes and congenital abnormalities in infants conceived with oocytes matured in vitro. Facts Views Vis Obgyn. 2014;6:15–8.

62. Soderstrom-Antilla V, Salokorpi T, Pihlaja M, Serenius-Sirve S, Suikkari AM. Obstetric and perinatal outcome and preliminary results of development of children born after in vitro maturation of oocytes. Hum Reprod. 2006;21:1508–13.
63. Buckett WM, Chian RC, Holzer H, Dean N, Usher R, Tan SL. Obstetric outcomes and congenital abnormalities after in vitro maturation, in vitro fertilization, and intracytoplasmic sperm injection. Obstet Gynecol. 2007;110:885–91.
64. Fadini R, Mignini Renzini M, Guarnieri T, Dal Canto M, de Ponti E, Sutcliffe A, et al. Comparison of the obstetric and perinatal outcomes of children conceived from in vitro or in vivo matured oocytes in in vitro maturation treatments with births from conventional ICSI cycles. Hum Reprod. 2012;27:3601–8.
65. Roesner S, von Wolff M, Elsaesser M, Roesner K, Reuner G, Pietz J, et al. Two-year development of children conceived by IVM: a prospective controlled single-blinded study. Hum Reprod. 2017;32:1341–50.
66. Practice Committee of American Society for Reproductive Medicine. Fertility preservation in patients undergoing gonadotoxic therapy or gonadectomy: a committee opinion. Fertil Steril. 2013;100(5):1214–23.

Index

Printed by Printforce, the Netherlands